Handbook of Pediatric Epilepsy

NEUROLOGICAL DISEASE AND THERAPY

Series Editor

WILLIAM C. KOLLER

Department of Neurology
University of Kansas Medical Center
Kansas City, Missouri

1. Handbook of Parkinson's Disease, *edited by William C. Koller*
2. Medical Therapy of Acute Stroke, *edited by Mark Fisher*
3. Familial Alzheimer's Disease: Molecular Genetics and Clinical Perspectives, *edited by Gary D. Miner, Ralph W. Richter, John P. Blass, Jimmie L. Valentine, and Linda A. Winters-Miner*
4. Alzheimer's Disease: Treatment and Long-Term Management, *edited by Jeffrey L. Cummings and Bruce L. Miller*
5. Therapy of Parkinson's Disease, *edited by William C. Koller and George Paulson*
6. Handbook of Sleep Disorders, *edited by Michael J. Thorpy*
7. Epilepsy and Sudden Death, *edited by Claire M. Lathers and Paul L. Schraeder*
8. Handbook of Multiple Sclerosis, *edited by Stuart D. Cook*
9. Memory Disorders: Research and Clinical Practice, *edited by Takehiko Yanagihara and Ronald C. Petersen*
10. The Medical Treatment of Epilepsy, *edited by Stanley R. Resor, Jr., and Henn Kutt*
11. Cognitive Disorders: Pathophysiology and Treatment, *edited by Leon J. Thal, Walter H. Moos, and Elkan R. Gamzu*
12. Handbook of Amyotrophic Lateral Sclerosis, *edited by Richard Alan Smith*
13. Handbook of Parkinson's Disease: Second Edition, Revised and Expanded, *edited by William C. Koller*
14. Handbook of Pediatric Epilepsy, *edited by Jerome V. Murphy and Fereydoun Dehkharghani*

Additional Volumes in Preparation

Handbook of Tourette's Syndrome and Related Tic and Behavioral Disorders, *edited by Roger Kurlan*

Handbook of Cerebellar Disease, *edited by Richard Lechtenberg*

Handbook of Cebrovascular Diseases, *edited by Harold P. Adams, Jr.*

Parkinsonian Syndromes: Diagnosis and Treatment, *edited by Matthew Stern and William C. Koller*

Handbook of Pediatric Epilepsy

edited by

Jerome V. Murphy
Fereydoun Dehkharghani

University of Missouri
and Children's Mercy Hospital
Kansas City, Missouri

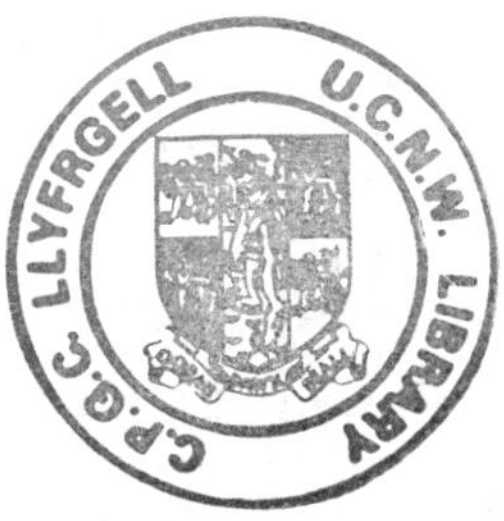

Marcel Dekker, Inc. **New York • Basel • Hong Kong**

UWB Heulog Library
WL 385 H236 1992
30110004583200

Library of Congress Cataloging-in-Publication Data

Handbook of pediatric epilepsy / edited by Jerome V. Murphy, Fereydoun Dehkharghani.
p. cm. -- (Neurological disease and therapy ; v. 14)
Includes bibliographical references and index.
ISBN 0-8247-8725-0 (alk. paper)
1. Epilepsy in children. I. Murphy, Jerome V. II. Dehkharghani, Fereydoun. III. Series.
[DNLM: 1. Epilepsy--diagnosis. 2. Epilepsy--in infancy & childhood. 3. Epilepsy--therapy. W1 NE33LD v. 14]
RJ496.E6H36 1992
618.9'2853--dc20
DNLM/DLC
for Library of Congress 92-49814
CIP

This book is printed on acid-free paper.

Copyright © 1993 by Marcel Dekker, Inc. All Rights Reserved.

Neither this book nor any part may be reproduced or transmitted in any form or by any means, electronic or mechanical, including photocopying, microfilming, and recording, or by any information storage and retrieval system, without permission in writing from the publisher.

Marcel Dekker, Inc.
270 Madison Avenue, New York, New York, 10016

Current printing (last digit):
10 9 8 7 6 5 4 3 2 1

PRINTED IN THE UNITED STATES OF AMERICA

To all those who provide medical and emotional support to children with seizures and to their families

Preface

Of all severe neurologic diseases seen by physicians the most common is undoubtedly epilepsy, or recurrent seizures. The incidence of epilepsy is about 49 cases per 100,000 population. Considering that 75% of epilepsies begin before age 20, and about a third before the age of five, epilepsy is definitely a pediatric illness.

Not only is epilepsy more common in children than in adults, but the types of seizures and classes of epilepsy seen in children are different. Almost all epilepsies observed in adults are also seen in children. And children exhibit unique forms of epilepsy not seen in their older counterparts. Examples of unique pediatric epilepsies are neonatal seizures, with their subtle symptomatology; metabolic and neurocutaneous disorders with seizures as part of their initial clinical presentation; the myoclonic epilepsies of infants and children; febrile convulsions; the Landau–Kleffner syndrome of acquired aphasia; childhood absence seizures; and the Lennox–Gastaut syndrome. Not only are these seizure disorders unique in childhood, but their treatment involves the use of drugs uncommon to adults (e.g., steroids, special diets, or pyridoxine).

It is very important that primary caretakers of children be knowledgeable in the diagnosis and treatment of pediatric epilepsies, as the number of pediatric neurologists available to care for children with epilepsy is small. If one compares the large number of children with recurrent seizures with the number of child neurologists in this country and realizes that most of the child neurologists are located in large medical centers, it is obvious that most children with epilepsy cannot be followed consistently by a pediatric neurologist. Therefore, these children must receive neurologic care from their primary medical caretaker with some assistance by physicians trained in adult neurologic diseases. We hope this book facilitates the delivery of pediatric neurologic care by educating the primary care physician on the treatment of seizures and epilepsies.

In the past 10 years there have been many advances and innumerable publications related to the cause, classification, effect, natural history, and treatment of pediatric epilepsy. In this book the authors distill this knowledge to provide a source where the primary caretakers of children may easily find the information necessary to provide optimal care to most children with epilepsy. Our goal is to provide knowledge not only on the specific epilepsies seen in children and their treatment, but also on more practical matters, such as events that may mimic epilepsy, practices applying to driver's licenses, activities of a child with epilepsy, when to start treatment with antiepileptic drugs, how to follow a patient being so treated, when that treatment can be withdrawn, and community services available for the families of children with epilepsy.

To this end the book is organized in the following fashion. The first three chapters address issues that need to be discussed with the families of children with epilepsy, the definition of epilepsy, principles of using antiepileptic drugs, and the classification of epilepsies and seizures. The next six chapters cover the specific treatment of pediatric seizures according to their classification. In chapters 10 through 16 other medical aspects of epilepsy are described: the medical and cognitive effects of epilepsy and its treatment on the individual, the risk of epilepsy in other family members, diagnostic procedures helpful in patients with epilepsy, available surgeries in patients with intractable epilepsy, and the interaction of pregnancy and epilepsy. The remaining two chapters are devoted to nonmedical issues faced by the patient and his or her family, issues that come up following the diagnosis and during treatment: available community support services for epilepsy and legal difficulties encountered by the person with epilepsy.

We believe this book will serve as a valuable reference for those responsible for the primary medical care of pediatric patients who have epileptic seizures.

JEROME V. MURPHY
FEREYDOUN DEHKHARGHANI

Contents

Contributors

V. Elving Anderson, Ph.D. Professor of Genetics and Cell Biology, Department of Genetics and Cell Biology, University of Minnesota, Minneapolis, Minnesota

Stanley Berent, Ph.D. Professor of Psychology and Director of Neuropsychology, Departments of Psychiatry, Neurology, and Psychology, University of Michigan, Ann Arbor, Michigan

Valerie Lynn Curtis, M.D. Assistant Professor of Neurology, Department of Neurology, University of Texas Health Science Center at Houston, Houston, Texas

Fereydoun Dehkharghani, M.D. Associate Professor of Pediatrics (Neurology), University of Missouri, and Director of the Neurophysiology Laboratory, Children's Mercy Hospital, Kansas City, Missouri

Kevin Farrell, M.B.ChB, FRCPE, FRCPC Associate Professor, Department of Pediatrics, University of British Columbia, Vancouver, British Columbia, Canada

Bruno Giordani, Ph.D. Assistant Professor of Psychology, Department of Psychiatry, University of Michigan, Ann Arbor, Michigan

W. Allen Hauser, M.D. Professor of Neurology and Public Health, G.H. Sergievsky Center, College of Physicians and Surgeons, Columbia University, New York, New York

Nyrma Hernandez, ACSW Deputy Executive Vice President, Epilepsy Foundation of America, Landover, Maryland

Jerome V. Murphy, M.D. Professor, University of Missouri, and Chief of Neurology, Children's Mercy Hospital, Kansas City, Missouri

David Field Oliver, Esq. Trial Department, Smith, Gill, Fisher & Butts, Kansas City, Missouri

R. Eugene Ramsay, M.D. Professor of Neurology, Director of Comprehensive Epilepsy Center, Department of Neurology, University of Miami School of Medicine, Miami, Florida

Nancy Santilli, RN, PNP, MN Associate Director, Comprehensive Epilepsy Program, Department of Neurology, University of Virginia Health Sciences Center, Charlottesville, Virginia

Robert C. Vannucci, M.D. Professor of Pediatrics and Neuroscience, Department of Pediatrics, Division of Pediatric Neurology, Pennsylvania State University School of Medicine, The Milton S. Hershey Medical Center, Hershey, Pennsylvania

Jerome Y. Yager, M.D. Assistant Professor, Department of Pediatrics, Division of Pediatric Neurology, Royal University Hospital, Saskatoon, Saskatchewan, Canada

Handbook of Pediatric Epilepsy

1

Approach to the Patient Who May Have Epilepsy

JEROME V. MURPHY
University of Missouri
and Children's Mercy Hospital
Kansas City, Missouri

I. DEFINITIONS

(See Table 1.) The word *epilepsy* is derived from the Greek verb *epilambanein* which meant to seize or to attack [1, pp. 21–23]. Therefore, during a seizure the person was seized or attacked by an external force or spirit. The body was invaded and the spirit that took residence caused the patient to convulse and foam. Based on this theory, patients relied on certain spiritual remedies (e.g., lichen of horses, genitals of seals, testicles of the hippopotamus, and human blood) to effect a release from the invading spirit [1, pp. 28–80]. Even Galen claimed that some people with epilepsy or arthritis were cured by drinking a solution of burned human bones [1, pp. 28–80]. Although the word *epilepsy* persists, the spiritual connotation of the word has been replaced.

It is difficult to define a *seizure* definitively just as it is difficult verbally to describe accurately any complex activity. The founding father of modern neurology, John Hughlings Jackson, defined a seizure as the name for an *occasional, sudden, excessive, rapid, and local discharge of gray matter* [1, pp. 328–346]. This definition, which was proven after the invention of the electroencephalogram (EEG), was novel and is useful. The concept of a local discharge of gray matter is not always true. Many pediatric seizures apparently involve an electric change in a large area of cortex, or all cerebral cortex, at the onset of the seizure.

Table 1 Definitions

Seizure	Generally involuntary event accompanied by a sudden, rapid, and abnormal discharge of cortical neurones
Epilepsy	Recurrent unprovoked seizures
Aura	Change in the patient preceding and forewarning a seizure
Ictus	Event, usually a seizure
Postictal	Pertaining to the patient's state after the seizure

The important part of this definition of a seizure is that the clinical event has to be accompanied by an electrical change or discharge in neurones, or a paroxysmal change in the recorded electroencephalogram concurrent with the event. That is how the word *seizure* will be used in this book. (The phrase *epileptic seizure* has been used elsewhere to differentiate these events from nonepileptic seizures. To facilitate reading, the word *seizure* as used herein refers to epileptic seizures.) This electrical change may be evident on a standard EEG. Very rarely, if the electrical activity is restricted to a small area of brain, and if the area is distant from the recording scalp electrodes (e.g., in the mesial temporal cortex), the standard EEG may show little change during the event. This can make a correct diagnosis difficult.

It is important to remember that a seizure is a clinical event, generally without known provocation, which is caused by a paroxysmal change in the electrical activity of neurones recognizable on EEG. There are other paroxysmal changes which are normal findings (e.g., sleep spindles, rhythmic midtemporal discharges, and positive spike rates of 14 and 6 per second) on EEG. These changes are not accompanied by an involuntary clinical event, and therefore are not seizures. These electrical phenomena do not indicate a predisposition to seizures.

The EEG may also display spike and slow-wave abnormalities without recognized changes in the patient, and the electroencephalographer may refer to such changes as subclinical seizures. We have seen patients whose EEG demonstrates numerous bursts of generalized spike and wave discharges, at times continuous, who do not have clinical symptoms (see Fig. 1). Such EEG abnormalities are only consistent with, or suggestive of, a seizure disorder; they are not diagnostic without a concurrent clinical event. The only exception would be a patient paralyzed with neuromuscular blocking agents, or someone in deep coma. Terms such as *subclinical seizure* should be avoided, as a seizure is an observed clinical event which is known to be accompanied by an electrical change in cerebral neurones.

Fortunately, most seizures can be recognized as such from a precise description of the event, including the aura and any postictal change. An abnormal EEG is not essential to a correct diagnosis. Just as an abnormal EEG is not always diagnostic of a seizure disorder, a normal EEG does not rule out epilepsy. Many

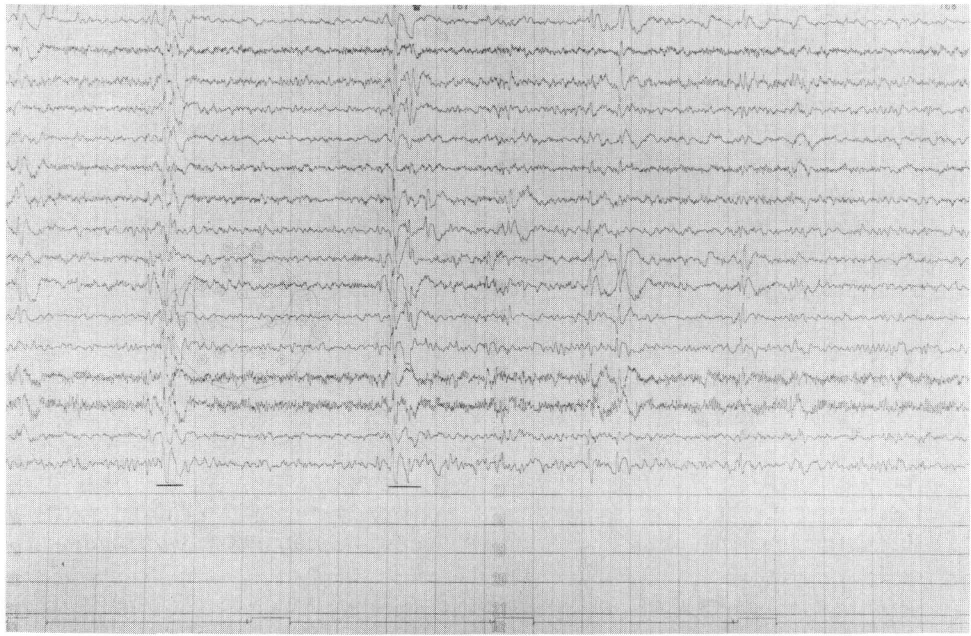

Figure 1 EEG of a patient treated for 2 years with AEDs for suspected seizures. During the generalized bursts of intermixed spikes and slow waves (underlined), the patient had no change in awareness or performance. The EEG was normal during the events thought to be seizures. Lacking clinical changes corresponding to a change in the EEG, it was concluded that the patient did not have epilepsy, despite the clearly abnormal EEG.

children with epilepsy will have a normal EEG in between seizures, or interictally [6,7]. The EEG is helpful but not always diagnostic (see Chapter 12).

Initially, the word *epilepsy* denoted either a single convulsion or the condition characterized by recurrent convulsions [1, pp. 21–23]. Now we call a single convulsion, or other event, as defined above, a seizure, and *epilepsy* refers to *unprovoked recurring seizures* [2,3]. Most experts interested in epilepsy would not include febrile convulsions or hypoglycemic seizures (reactive seizures) in this definition, as they are provoked seizures. Similarly, numerous seizures occurring only in a brief interval (e.g., 1 day) would not generally be considered by itself as epilepsy.

It becomes obvious that the definition of epilepsy given above can be difficult to apply. Since the seizures of epilepsy are random events, more common at some times than others, they must have some precipitants, or provocations, only some of which are known (e.g., sleep deprivation, hyperventilation, stress). Febrile seizures, as an example, share many features with epilepsy: (1) one-third of patients with a single convulsion will have a recurrence, (2) the natural history is one of spontaneous resolution, and (3) the convulsion itself is indistinguishable from the convulsion of a patient with epilepsy. Nevertheless, recurrent febrile seizures are not considered an epilepsy (see Chapter 8).

The diagnosis of epilepsy does not depend on routine EEG findings, or on any other study, unless the event being evaluated occurs during the EEG. Epilepsy is a clinical diagnosis made by a physician on the basis of (1) a description of a typical event, (2) knowledge that the described event is characteristic of a seizure, and (3) a history that the event is recurrent.

Many patients have a warning that a seizure is about to recur, and this is referred to as an *aura*. The expression of an aura is very variable and frequently vague. For Dostovyesky, as described in *The Idiot*, the aura was an "inner light" [4]. Auras, if present, are not always followed by a seizure. Parents may be able to recognize the warning or aura and predict that their child will have a seizure that day based on (1) a change in behavior, and (2) past observations of such an association. Older patients may describe certain feelings or odors that warn them of an approaching seizure. Similarly, they may learn that an intervention, such as intense thought, can abort the seizure.

Postictal changes refer only to the patient's generally depressed neurologic state after the seizure. The patient may not have a postictal state (i.e., he or she may be fully alert immediately after the seizure stops). More commonly, the postictal state consists of slowly ($\leq$24 h) resolving lethargy. Other postictal symptoms can be hemiparesis, vomiting, or headache. Todd's postictal weakness refers to a focal weakness (e.g., a hemiparesis) following a seizure and should not last more than 24 h. This probably relates to postictal inhibition of involved neurones, or focal cerebral edema [5].

Another helpful observation in the diagnosis of a seizure is the patient's state of alertness or awareness during the seizure. It is important to assess whether consciousness is intact, impaired, or lost. If both hemispheres are diffusely involved in epileptic activity (i.e., the seizure is generalized), the patient is unable to interact with, or record, his or her environment. If only one hemisphere, or a limited area of brain, is involved in the seizure, the patient may be aware of what is happening and may be able to do something to avoid injury or to draw attention to himself. By definition, consciousness is impaired in partial complex seizures (see Chapter 3).

An accurate description of the clinical and electrical events that comprise the seizure will permit the proper *classification of the seizure* [10]. This is helpful in the selection of optimal therapy. Following classification of the seizure the next important step is the *classification of the epilepsy* or the epileptic syndrome that the recurrent seizures represent [10]. This classification allows one to make an accurate determination of cause and prognosis. To classify the epilepsy the physician must determine if the disorder is due to a previous event (e.g., encephalitis or trauma) or if it is idiopathic. If this is an idiopathic event, one must determine the type of seizure, the age of the child at the onset of seizures, and the presence of other clinical features for the accurate classification of the epilepsy. Both the classification of the seizure and the classification of the epilepsy are described in Chapter 3.

II. RECURRENT EVENTS THAT CAN MIMIC EPILEPSY

There are numerous paroxysmal events that occur in childhood which can simulate seizures. Some events may actually be accompanied by a convulsion (e.g., breath holding), but they should not be categorized as epilepsy, and treatment with antiepileptic drugs (AEDs) is not beneficial. Recurrent events occurring in childhood that simulate epilepsy include *paroxysmal vertigo*, *breath-holding spells*, *cardiogenic syncope*, *periodic behaviors in a child with an abnormal EEG*, *paroxysmal kinesigenic choreoathetosis*, *shuddering attacks*, *night terrors*, *Tourette syndrome*, *pseudoseizures*, *migraine*, and *rages*. Generally, an accurate clinical description of the event and an awareness of the disorder is sufficient to differentiate it from epilepsy. (See Table 2 for a summary.) At times a video-EEG, with simultaneous recording of the event and the cerebral electrical accompaniment, is necessary to make this distinction.

1. Paroxysmal vertigo. This may be a disorder of the labyrinthine system of the inner ear [11]. The patient suddenly experiences vertigo and clutches tightly onto a stable object until the symptom passes. Pallor, nystagmus, vomiting, and diaphoresis accompany the attack. Recovery is immediate. Attacks diminish in intensity over a period of months. The follow-up of children with paroxysmal vertigo indicates that many of them subsequently develop migraine headaches [12]. Therefore, prophylactic treatment of the vertigo with antimigrainous agents may provide relief if treatment is necessary. Observations that help differentiate this from a seizure are the continued alertness of the frightened and crying child during the event, the absence of typical tonic or clonic movements, and the absence of a period of postictal lethargy.

2. Breath-holding spells. Breath-holding spells occur in children in the first 2 years of life and generally resolve by school age [13,14]. They are of two varieties, pallid and cyanotic, and both can terminate in a tonic attack accompanied by clonic activity. In the pallid breath-holding spell the child will just start a vigorous cry in response to distress, rapidly lose consciousness, and appear pale. These breath-holding spells are thought to be secondary to vagally mediated asystole.

In the cyanotic variety the cry is prolonged and the loss of consciousness is accompanied by cyanosis, secondary to apnea. The specific feature of breath-holding that distinguishes it from epilepsy is that all events are precipitated by

Table 2 Recurrent Events That Mimic Epilepsy

Event	Differentiation from epilepsy
Paroxysmal vertigo	Patient is frightened and crying; no loss of awareness
Breath-holding spells	Loss of consciousness and accompanying convulsion is always provoked by an event that makes the child cry
Cardiogenic syncope	Abnormal EKG; patient has episodic loss of consciousness without consistent convulsive movement
Periodic behaviors	Event is without a sudden onset and the EEG is normal during the event; the behavior is specific to a certain environment
Paroxysmal kinesigenic choreoathetosis	Event generally occurs on arising, and movements are not typical of seizures or accompanied by change in alertness
Shuddering attacks	Brief shivering spells with continued awareness
Night terrors	Brief nocturnal episodes of terror without typical convulsive movements
Tourette syndrome	Repetitive movements of parts of upper body without loss of awareness or impairment of performance
Pseudoseizures	No EEG changes, save movement artifact during event; thrashing movements are observed rather than tonic or clonic movements
Migraine	Severe headache followed by sleep from which the patient can be roused; headaches usually accompanied by photophobia, sonophobia, nausea, and pallor
Rages	Provoked and goal-directed; see ''Periodic behaviors''

emotional or physical trauma. The convulsion is never a spontaneous event interfering suddenly with an activity.

Breath-holding spells can be aborted by startling the child, as with a squirt from a water gun, during the vigorous cry [15; E. Christopherson, personal communication]. If that does not work, a studious lack of attention to the event is recommended. Regardless of how these episodes are managed, the outcome is excellent. There is no increased risk of subsequent epilepsy and AEDs drugs are never indicated.

3. Cardiogenic syncope. When severe enough to cause cerebral hypoperfusion and hypoxia, some cardiac arrhythmias can be difficult to distinguish from seizures. The patient usually has a warning of a faint feeling and then loses consciousness [16]. A convulsion can occur due to the cerebral ischemia. The arrhythmias are distinguished from seizures by (1) the aura of a faint feeling, (2) the presence of episodic loss of consciousness without convulsive movements, and (3) an abnormal electrocardiogram. Many EEG laboratories routinely record the EKG on one of the EEG channels, permitting documentation of an abnormal cardiac rhythm. As an example, see Fig. 1 in Chapter 4.

4. Daydreaming. Daydreaming, as well as other episodic symptoms, may be mistakenly interpreted as seizures [17] in the following scenario. A child has scholastic difficulties and the physician is asked by the child's teacher to eliminate medical causes of this problem, involving staring and other repetitive behaviors. An EEG demonstrates nonrelevant spikes or paroxysms of spike-and-wave activities and a mistaken diagnosis of epilepsy is made (see Fig. 1). AED therapy may be pursued for years.

With the aid of a video-EEG a second physician will demonstrate that the events in question represent a behavior and will conclude that the child has pseudoseizures. In reality the original physician made an erroneous diagnosis. This erroneous sequence of events may be avoided by remembering three principles: (1) an abnormal EEG does *not* diagnose epilepsy unless the electrical abnormality accompanies an event called a seizure [6,18]; (2) generalized seizures, especially absence seizures, have a sudden and dramatic onset; and (3) a behavior is frequently situation specific (e.g., in school but not at home). The child with daydreaming, as well as other behaviors, drifts into the state; seizures are generally random events that have an abrupt onset with interruption of a normal activity.

5. Paroxysmal kinesigenic choreoathetosis. In 1940, Mount and Reback described a fascinating nonepileptic movement disorder of childhood [19,20]. Movement after prolonged rest (e.g., getting up from a chair at the end of a class) provokes a less-than-5-min episode of uncontrolled awkward movements (choreoathetosis) without falling and without alteration of consciousness. One mother described her son as acting "as if he had a poker up his rectum." Although this is not an epilepsy, it frequently can be controlled by carbamazepine [21], valproic acid [22], phenytoin [23], or clonazepam [24,25]. In some patients these movements are spontaneous, (i.e., nonkinesigenic).

6. Shuddering attacks. These are brief (<20 s) attacks of shivering motion without loss of consciousness which are increased during periods of excitement [26]. They do not occur in sleep and do not respond to AEDs. In one report shuddering attacks was associated with the presence of familial essential tremor [27].

7. Night terrors. Night terrors or pavor nocturnus is a sleep disorder with episodes of extreme distress with the child appearing terrified. The episode lasts less than 1 min and the child has no recall for the event. According to one report, this behavior can be eliminated in a week by awakening the child 10 min before the suspected episode if they occur at a consistent time, or by arousing the child right at the first sign of a spell (i.e., sweating, tachycardia, or movement) [28]. Treatment with AEDs is ineffective.

8. Tourette syndrome. This syndrome is defined as the presence of motor and vocal tics for at least a year. Common tics are eye blinking, nose movements, tossing of the head, throat clearing, sniffing, and high-pitched squeaks [29]. Only a minority of patients have coprolalia or copropraxia. Distinction

from a seizure disorder is fairly easy. The movements are not those associated with seizures. The patient is aware of the movements, and can mimic them, but he or she is unable to suppress them for prolonged periods. These tics do not interfere directly with activities. When they do cause disruptions, treatment with haloperidol, pimozide, or clonidine may provide relief [30].

9. Pseudoseizures. These can be extremely difficult to distinguish from a true epileptic attack, although this problem has been greatly facilitated by the use of video-EEGs [31]. In most pseudoseizures the patient has nonsynchronous flailing of the extremities and side-to-side head movements [32,33]. In generalized clonic seizures the limbs are synchronously jerking, with brief episodes of stillness, and the head flexes forward, or moves up and to one side, or extends backward. However, the distinction between pseudoseizures and seizures can be hard [34].

When pseudoseizures occur in patients who are known to have epilepsy, the distinction is not easily made. The situation is abetted when every unexplained event, following the diagnosis of epilepsy, is considered a seizure. Unfortunately, whereas most epilepsies can be controlled with appropriate medications, pseudoseizures have a variable response to AED therapy. A placebo effect can occur when pseudoseizures are treated as an epilepsy. A correct diagnosis is essential prior to initiating therapy to avoid this pitfall. Psychiatric intervention may be helpful in relieving the symptoms [35,36].

10. Migraine headaches. Typical migraine headaches are easily distinguishable from epilepsy. The pains of migraine has a slow onset, and the patient never loses alertness. Confusion between the two specific diagnoses may arise (1) when the aura of a migraine is not consistently followed by its intense throbbing headache, (2) from the EEG abnormalities frequent in migraineurs [37, pp. 66–75], (3) from the more-than-expected association of the two illnesses in the same person [37, pp. 126–137], and (4) when a headache follows an unrecognized seizure [38].

In children the aura of a migraine is frequently accompanied by visual symptoms (i.e., loss of vision, hemianopsia, scotomota, flashing lights, or visual distortions). These prodromal symptoms are followed by an increasingly severe headache without disturbance of consciousness. Studies have documented (1) the frequency of EEG abnormalities in patients with migraine [37, pp. 126–137]. The EEG changes in patients with migraine are generalized slowing seen after the headache, a nonspecific finding, or more focal changes. The latter probably relates to the recurrent ischemia of a migraine attack. The conclusion that epilepsy and migraine coexist in the same person more than one would expect is derived from hospital-based studies.

There are three specific situations in which migraine and epilepsy are difficult to distinguish: basilar artery migraine, occipital epilepsy, and migraine after minor head trauma. In basilar artery migraine, brain stem ischemia can produce loss of consciousness and dysfunction of brain stem. Symptoms of the latter include diminished awareness, ataxia, weakness, and visual loss [37, pp. 103–109].

The second situation, occipital epilepsy, is more frequently confused with basilar migraine. These children have episodic spells preceded by visual changes similar to those seen in migraine. This visual aura is followed by more typical epileptic activity, such as fluttering of the eyelids and hemiconvulsions. The EEG commonly demonstrates occipital spike and wave discharges, suppressed by eye opening (see Chapter 5).

In the third situation, migraine after minor head trauma, vomiting, headache, and loss of consciousness recurrently follow minor head trauma. A positive family history of migraine headaches and the minor nature of the preceding head trauma distinguish this from posttraumatic seizures [40].

11. Rages. Rages are generally distinguishable from seizures by a careful description of the event itself and by the observation that the behavior or rage is provoked even though the reaction is very inappropriate. The rage itself is generally goal directed, with the child destroying a toy or attempting to injure someone [41]. On the contrary, a seizure consists of nonpurposeful activities. Injuries that occur during a seizure are nonintentional and nonrewarding. Although a video-EEG will differentiate between a rage and a seizure, we have found it difficult to provoke a rage in the video-EEG unit.

III. NONMEDICINAL CONSIDERATIONS IN CHILDREN WITH EPILEPSY

A. Activities

Chilren with controlled seizures should be able to enjoy the same activities as those enjoyed by similarly skilled children without seizures. Traumatic sports such as football carry no increased risk for children with epilepsy. Obviously, a child whose seizures are not completely controlled should avoid activities that put him or her in a position that were a seizure to occur, life or limb would be endangered. These decisions need to be made on a case-by-case basis [42].

Like anyone else, children with epilepsy can participate in water sports as long as a lifeguard is present. Available studies indicate that under these conditions children with epilepsy carry no increased risk of drowning than that of children without epilepsy [43–45] save under very specific circumstances [46]. The increased risk of drowning in epilepsy comes from children in unsupervised water, as in the bathtub. As school-age children prefer not to be watched when they bathe, we recommend that children with epilepsy take showers, not baths. Showers are not without hazard, but drowning is not one of them.

Exercise itself is not thought to aggravate a seizure disorder. In the only available study of its kind, young persons with epilepsy had EEGs recorded in three situations: resting, during 3 min of hyperventilation, and during 15 min on an ergometer. During exercise the number of epileptogenic discharges decreased, and during hyperventilation, the number increased. Therefore, exercise itself may even be beneficial [47].

B. Who Needs to Know That the Child Has Epilepsy?

This seemingly innocuous question can be difficult to answer. As long as members in the community harbor erroneous concepts as to the cause of epilepsy (e.g., it is due to brain damage), families should be reluctant to establish general public awareness of their child's diagnosis. On the other hand, transient caretakers, such as baby-sitters, should know what to do during a seizure, avoiding the knee-jerk reaction of mouth-to-mouth resuscitation, dialing the proverbial 911, and/or inserting something into the mouth.

As to whether or not the diagnosis of epilepsy needs to be on a child's school health record depends on the availability of such records to potential employers and the attitude and knowledge of teachers about epilepsy. If the teacher attributes a learning difficulty to epilepsy, or if the child is put on one side of a classroom to facilitate observation of, and care for, a seizure, the teacher's knowledge of that child's diagnosis has done that child a disservice. If, on the other hand, appropriate information on epilepsy is a part of all educational services, such inappropriate attitudes would not be present and the diagnosis of epilepsy would not be an embarrassment.

C. Driving Licenses

This topic is discussed further in Chapter 16. It is a difficult problem, with each state having antithetical driving laws that govern the rights of individuals, all with a similar condition (recurrent seizures), to drive [49].

As an example, a person with epilepsy in Missouri only needs a letter from a physician supporting the person's claim to be competent to drive safely. The bordering state, Kansas, requires that the person be seizure-free one year before he or she may drive. Wisconsin requires only three seizure-free months, but then driving is frequently limited to a certain radius of home (e.g., 100 miles). In some states (e.g., California) a physician is obliged to report seizures to the state licensing bureau, violating confidentiality, and encouraging the underreporting of seizures by the patient.

Whether or not a person with epilepsy should drive depends on numerous factors: (1) the time of the seizures (if they occur only during sleep, daytime driving might not carry a risk), (2) the presence of a distinct aura (if this precedes a seizure by a sufficient time interval, the patient may be able to stop driv ing despite being in a congested area), (3) the presence of alternative transportation (public transportation would be preferred in many large cities even by those without epilepsy), and (4) the necessity to drive (i.e., business or pleasure?) [49].

The actual risk of an automobile accident in someone with epilepsy is extremely small relative to other causes of accidents. As a cause of accidents it equals the frequency of sudden and unexpected death while driving as a contributing cause to such accidents [49]. Nevertheless, the accidents that do occur when a person with epilepsy has a seizure while driving can be disastrous, with severe mortality and morbidity to driver, passengers, and bystanders [50]. As with alcoholic inebriation, alternative forms of transportation have to be made available to a patient with poorly controlled epilepsy.

On the other hand, the urge to drive a car can exert a positive influence in an adolescent. If the teenager with epilepsy realizes that obtaining a driver's license may be a necessary rite of passage, they should be more compliant, and even compulsive, about adhering to AED regimens.

D. Frequency of Administering Medications

If possible, and depending on the pharmacokinetics of the particular AED, it should be administered twice a day or less. If multiple doses are required, it may be easier to administer AEDs before and after school rather than during school hours. If school is involved in the administration of medications, (1) more people have to be notified of changes in medicinal regimens, and (2) the student can be perceived as different by his peers, as he has to go to the nurse every day to receive medication. The less frequently that drugs are given during the day, the less frequently the parent or child has to remember the time of the dose, and therefore the higher the likelihood is that there will be good compliance with medical regimens.

E. Alcohol Consumption

This topic obviously has little concern for the child with epilepsy. Occasionally, an older child may participate in a ritual glass of wine at a family repast, or the young college student may consider it appropriate to learn his or her tolerance of alcohol. There is no question that repeated consumption of large amounts of alcohol is associated with seizures, but the exact etiology is unclear [51]. There is no evidence that the consumption of moderate amounts of alcohol adversely effects the control of seizures [52]. In one study of patients with epilepsy, they consumed one to three glasses of an alcoholic beverage twice a week for 16 weeks. No change in the frequency of seizures or in AED concentrations in serum were observed during this period [53]. Based on this, the young adult with epilepsy should avoid excessive consumption of ethanol but may participate in the largely ceremonial tasting of wine at meals.

IV. REFERRAL TO A NEUROLOGIST

In patient's with epilepsy there are occasions when referral to someone with additional experience in epilepsy is desirable. The utilization of such services frequently depends on the availability of such talent in the extended community. The most experienced person in such a situation is a pediatric neurologist. If none is available, others who can help are a general neurologist, the staff of an epilepsy center, or a neurosurgeon. Frequently, the local affiliate of the Epilepsy Foundation of America will be able to educate the family in epilepsy and thereby reduce their concerns. If there is no local affiliate, the family can call the national office at 1-800-EFA-1000 for further assistance.

Reasons to consider referral for additional help include the following: (1) seizures that are intractable to the initial AED(s), (2) unusual seizure disorders with which the primary practitioner is not familiar, (3) apparent intolerance of recommended AEDs, (4) continuing anxiety or concerns of the family, and (5) obtaining information on current recommendations for the duration of therapy.

1. Intractable seizures. When seizures are intractable to the initial AED(s), the logical referral is to a neurologist for additional suggestions. Nevertheless, if seizures persist, the next logical step is referral to a center for the treatment for epilepsy to consider the use of other therapeutic interventions (e.g., investigational drugs or neurosurgery). These avenues should be pursued within several years of onset of the disorder because seizures that are not controlled within 5 years of onset generally become intractable to all therapies (i.e., the earlier the seizures are controlled, the better, in the long run, for the patient).

2. Unusual seizure disorders with which the primary practitioner is not familiar. Unusual epilepsies that need the attention of an experienced person, such as a pediatric neurologist, include infantile spasms and the Lennox–Gastaut syndrome. These epilepsies have distinct etiologies that may or may not be evident at their onset, and their treatment may require unique therapies (e.g., ACTH or steroids).

3. Apparent intolerance of recommended AEDs. Drug intolerance can pose a severe dilemma. As an example, a young mentally retarded child with epilepsy may develop gum hypertrophy while receiving phenytoin, hyperactivity on phenobarbital, and a falling white blood cell concentration when given carbamazepine. Each drug is effective in controlling seizures, but none appear to be well tolerated. A physician with more experience in treating pediatric epilepsies may be able to suggest other AEDs, recognize interactions between AEDs, determine that the side effect of one of the drugs is transient and not dangerous, or decide that treatment with AEDs is not beneficial to the patient.

4. Continuing anxiety or concerns of the family. Parental concerns about their child's epilepsy, even when it is medically managed in appropriate fashion, can be generated by (1) the frequently expressed fear that the child would die

during a convulsion, (2) a feeling of guilt that a parental action (e.g., punishing or immunizing the child) might have provoked the event, (3) nagging questions that because the seizure comes from the brain, their child has an abnormal brain, and (4) a not uncommon belief that such unnatural agents as AEDs, being given daily, are unnatural toxins. These concerns may be resolved by discussions with other families having a child with epilepsy, contact with the local epilepsy chapter (see above), or by referral to a qualified psychologist. These actions will facilitate appropriate medical management.

Although specialty referrals are necessary at times, most children with epilepsy can be medically managed by their primary medical caretaker and do not need to be referred to a neurologic specialist.

REFERENCES

1. Temkin O. The falling sickness. Baltimore: The Johns Hopkins University Press, 1971.
2. Ferry PC, Banner W Jr, Wolf RA. Seizure disorders in children. Philadelphia: JB Lippincott Company, 1986:31.
3. Holmes GL. Diagnosis and management of seizures in children. Philadelphia: WB Saunders Company, 1987:1.
4. Dostovyesky F. The idiot. New York: Modern Library, 1983:221–223.
5. Aicardi J. Epilepsy in children. New York: Raven Press, 1986:114.
6. Lewis DV, Freeman JM. The electroencephalogram in pediatric practice: its use and abuse. Pediatrics 1977; 60:324–30.
7. Klass DM, Westmoreland BF. Nonepileptogenic epileptiform electroencephalographic activity. Ann Neurol 1985; 18:627–35.
8. Mizrahi EM. Electroencephalogric/polygraphic/video monitoring in childhood epilepsy. J Pediatr 1984; 105:1–9.
9. Holmes GL. Prolonged electroencephalographic videotape monitoring in children. Am J Dis Child 1982; 136:608–11.
10. Dreifuss F. Classification of epileptic seizures and the epilepsies. Pediatr Clin NA 1989; 36:265–79.
11. Koenigsberger M, Chutorian AM, Gold AP, Schvey MS. Benign paroxysmal vertigo of childhood. Neurology. 1970; 20:1108–13.
12. Curatolo P, Sciaretto A. Benign paroxysmal vertigo and migraine. Dev Med Child Neurol 1987; 29:405–6.
13. Lombroso C, Lerman P. Breatholding spells (cyanotic and pallid infantile syncope). Pediatrics 1967; 39:563–81.
14. Gordon N. Breatholding spells. Dev Med Child Neurol 1987; 29:811–14.
15. Singh NN, Watson JE, Winton ASW. Treating self-injury: water mist spray versus facial screening or forced arm exercise. J Appl Behav Anal 1986; 19:403–10.
16. Rutter N, Southall DP. Cardiac arrhythmias misdiagnosed as epilepsy. Arch Dis Child 1985; 60:54–70.
17. Donat JF, Wright FS. Episodic symptoms mistaken for seizures in the neurologically impaired child. Neurology 1990; 40:156–57.

18. Dehkharghani D, Ahmed I, Murphy JV. The inappropriate management of children who have nonepileptic events and generalized EEG discharges. Ann Nuerol 1989; 26:472.
19. Mount LA, Reback S. Familial paroxysmal choreoathetosis; preliminary report on a hitherto undescribed clinical syndrome. Arch Neurol Psychiatr 1940; 44:841–47.
20. Kertesz A. Paroxysmal kinesigenic choreoathetosis: an entity within the paroxysmal choreoathetosis syndrome. Description of 10 cases, including 1 autopsied. Neurology 1967; 17:680–90.
21. Kato M, Shukuro A. Paroxysmal kinesigenic choreoathetosis: report of a case relieved by carbamazepine. Arch Neurol 1969; 20:508–13.
22. Suber DA, Riley TL. Valproic acid and normal computerized tomograhic scan in kinesiogenic familial choreoathetosis. Arch Neurol 1980; 37:327.
23. Homan RW, Vasko MR, Blaw M. Phenytoin plasma concentrations in paroxysmal kinesigenic choreoathetosis. Neurology 1980; 30:673–76.
24. Lance JW. Familial paroxysmal dystonic choreoathetosis and its differentiation from related syndromes. Ann Neurol 1977; 2:285–93.
25. Tibbles JAR, Barnes SE. Paroxysmal dystonic choreoathetosis of Mount and Reback. Pediatrics 1980; 65:149–51.
26. Holmes GL, Russman BS. Shuddering attacks evaluation using electroencephalographic frequency modulation radiotelemetry and videotape monitoring. Am J Dis Child 1986; 40:72–73.
27. Vanasse M, Bedard P, Andermann F. Shuddering attacks in children: an early clinical manifestation of essential tremor. Neurology 1976; 26:1027–30.
28. Lask B. Novel and nontoxic treatment for night terrors. Br Med J 1988; 297:592.
29. American Psychiatric Association, Committee on Nomenclature and Statistics. Diagnostic and statistical manual of mental disorders, 3d ed. Washington, DC: American Psychiatric Association, 1980.
30. Bruun RD. (1984) Gille de la Tourette's syndrome. An overview of clinical experience. J Am Acad Child Psychiatr 1984; 23:126–33.
31. Luther JS, McNamara JO, Carwile S, Miller P, Hope V. Pseudoepileptic seizures: methods and video analysis to aid diagnosis. Ann Neurol 1982; 12:458–62.
32. Gates JR, Ramani V, Whalen S, Loewson R. Ictal characteristics of pseudoseizures. Arch Neurol 1985; 42:1183–87.
33. Gulick TA, Spinks IP, Kind DW. Pseudoseizures: ictal phenomena. Neurology 1982; 32:24–30.
34. King DW, Gallagher BB, Murvin AJ, Smith DB, Marcus DJ, Hartlage LC. Pseudo seizures: diagnostic evaluation. Neurology 1982; 32:18–23.
35. Aylward GP. Description of a therapeutic approach to pseudoseizures in adolescents. Community Ment Health J 1984; 20:155–58.38.
36. Wyllie E, Friedman D, Rorhner AD, Luders H, Dinner D, Morris H III, Cruse R, Erenberg G, Kotagal P. Psychogenic seizures in children and adolescents: outcome after diagnosis by ictal video and electroencephalographic recording. Pediatrics 1990; 85:480–84.
37. Barlow CF. Headaches and migraine in children. Philadelphia: Spastics International Medical Publications, 1984.

38. Schon F, Blau JN. Post-epileptic headache and migraine. J Neurol Neurosurg Psychiatr 1987; 50:1148–52.
39. Panayiotopoulos CP. Benign childhood epilepsy with occipital paroxysms: a 15 year prospective study. Ann Neurol 1989; 26:51–56.
40. Haas DC, Lourie H. Trauma-triggered migraine: an explanation for the common neurological attacks after mild head injury. Review of the literature. J Neurosurg 1988; 68:181–88.
41. Elliott FA. The episodic dyscontrol syndrome and aggression. Neurol Clin 1984; 2:113–25.
42. O'Donohue NV. What should the child with epilepsy be allowed to do? Arch Dis Child 1983; 58:934–37.
43. Bachman DS. Physician's responsibilities for patients with epilepsy. Ann Neurol 1979; 6:279.
44. Pern JH. Epilepsy and drowning in childhood. Br Med J 1977; 1:1510–11.
45. Freeman JM. Epilepsy and swimming. Pediatrics 1985; 76:139.
46. Dreifuss FE. Epileptics and scuba diving. JAMA 1985; 253:1877–78.
47. Horyd W, Gryziak J, Niedzielska K. Effect of physical exertion on seizure discharges in the EEG of epilepsy patients. Neurol Neurochir Pol 1981; 15:545–52.
48. Spudis EV, Penry JK, Gibson P. Driving impairment caused by episodic brain dysfunction. Restrictions for epilepsy and syncope. Arch Neurol 1986; 43:558–64.
49. Fountain AJ, Lewis JA, Heck AF. Driving with epilepsy: a contemporary prospective. South Med J 1983; 76:481–84.
50. Gastaut H, Zifkin BG. The risk of automobile accidents with seizures occurring while driving: relation to seizure type. Neurology 1987; 37:1613–16.
51. Lechtenberg R, Worner TM. Seizure risk with recurrent alcohol detoxification. Arch Neurol 1990; 47:535–38.
52. Hauser WA, Ng SKC, Brust JCM. Alcohol, seizures, and epilepsy. Epilepsia 1988; 29 Suppl 2:S66–S88.
53. Hoppener RJ. Epilepsy and alcohol: the influence of social alcohol intake on seizures and treatment in epilepsy. Epilepsia 1983; 24:459–71.

2

Considerations in the Use of Antiepileptic Drugs

JEROME V. MURPHY
University of Missouri
and Children's Mercy Hospital
Kansas City, Missouri

I. INTRODUCTION

The focus of this chapter is on a discussion of general and practical issues pertinent to the use of antiepileptic drugs (AEDs). Some of these issues are discussed in more detail in other chapters. In this chapter we draw this information together in one place for the convenience of the reader.

It is frequently helpful to discuss some of these topics with the patient's family before initiating chronic drug therapy. If the parents or guardians have been well informed on the nature of epilepsy and its treatment, their input may be helpful in reaching decisions concerning the daily use of AEDs, which drug to use if several are equally effective, and so on. There are times when AED therapy is mandatory, but there are situations when the benefits of such chronic therapy are debatable (e.g., febrile seizures and benign rolandic epilepsy). A well-informed family will be able to participate in the periodic decision making that is necessary.

II. INDICATIONS FOR STARTING ANTIEPILEPTIC DRUGS

In general, intervention with medications should be undertaken when that intervention can alter the course of an illness for the betterment of the patient. The intervention has to be a reasonable compromise between the illness and the possible complications of therapy. If the intervention presents the risk of adversity equivalent to the disease being treated, the intervention is probably not indicated.

As an example, we would disagree with the statement by Aicardi that an imperative indication for the initiation of therapy is two or more seizures whatever the type of seizure [1]. If seizures are infrequent and brief, or if they are manifestations of a benign pediatric epilepsy (see Chapter 5), intervention with daily medications may not be warranted [2]. Such decisions must be made individually, and depend on the reaction of the family and the patient to the seizure.

The goal of therapy is to improve the quality of the child's life in the broadest sense and not just to reduce the number of seizures. Despite the relatively small risk of a recurrence after a first seizure, some would recommend AED therapy to prevent the injury that could accompany a second seizure [3]. Considering the unpredictable side effects and intolerances of AEDs, and the unproven efficacy of AEDs after a single first seizure (see below), chronic AED therapy should not be started after a single seizure [4]. Exceptions to this rule will be mentioned.

An algorithm is presented in Table 1 indicating steps to be taken and stepwise decisions to make in the initiation of AED therapy in a patient with epilepsy. The issues addressed in this chapter will help in following the steps of the algorithm.

A. Type of Epilepsy

Before initiating therapy, the basic determinations necessary to evaluate a pediatric seizure disorder are the type of seizure and the underlying etiology. (Information contained in the following chapters will aid in these determinations.) Knowledge of the type of seizure helps in AED selection, and knowledge of the epilepsy that is causing these seizures helps predict the effect of the epilepsy on the child's well-being and the prognosis for the illness. The effect of the epilepsy on the patient's general well-being can then be weighed against the detriments and possible side effects of chronic AED therapy to decide whether or not to initiate a program of daily medications.

B. Risk of Recurrence

Two important factors that help in the determination of whether or not to initiate chronic AED therapy are the risk of recurrent seizures and the attendant risk for injury or functional disability from each seizure. If the risk of recurrence is small but a recurrence would have significant sequelae (e.g., change of employment or loss of a driver's license), treatment with an AED in indicated.

Regarding the risk of a recurrent seizure, 36% of children with a first unprovoked convulsion, regardless of the specific epilepsy, have a recurrence in the first 12 months after the initial event [5]. This is true whether the first seizure is brief, prolonged (e.g., status epilepticus), or several seizures in one 24-h period.

Table 1 Algorithm for Treatment of Seizures

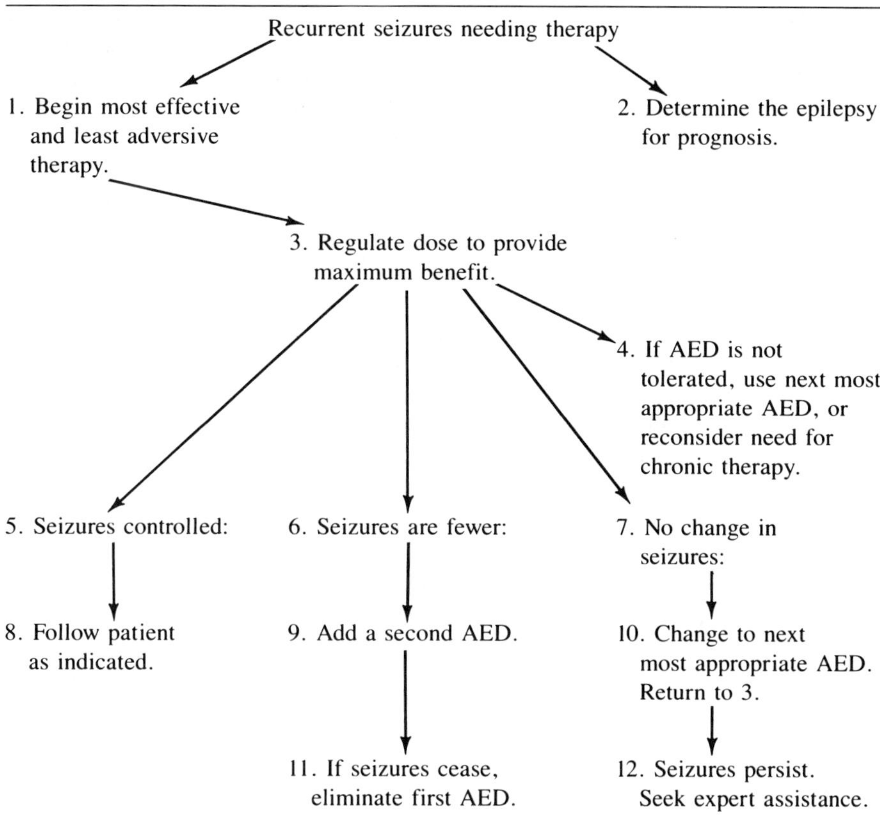

The results of an EEG and the presence of neurologic abnormalities can alter this recurrence risk. If the child with a single unprovoked seizure has an EEG with changes indicative of a seizure disorder, the likelihood of a recurrence increases from 36% to 52%. On the other hand, a normal EEG after a first seizure reduces the predictive risk of recurrence from 36% to 23%. If the first seizure occurs in a child with a neurologic handicap, (e.g., mental retardation, post-head trauma, post-meningitis), the risk of recurrence is higher and that risk depends on the nature of the original event [5].

It is generally desirable to learn seizure frequency before initiating chronic AED therapy. As stated earlier, if seizures are nocturnal, infrequent, or very mild events, not interfering with the child's well-being, the family may prefer not to use daily medications.

Besides the relatively low risk of a recurrence after a single unprovoked seizure, there are additional reasons not to recommend chronic AED therapy after a single event. First there is evidence that the recommendation to initiate chronic antiepileptic therapy after a single seizure may not alter the risk of a recurrence [5–8]. In the available studies of the risk of a second seizure after a first unprovoked seizure, the recurrence rate was the same whether or not chronic AED therapy was recommended after the first seizure. This reported lack of efficacy may relate to the failure of patient compliance to a medical regimen as the memory of the single frightening event fades.

Another reason not to recommend chronic AED therapy after a single event is that if one does start daily therapy after a single event, it may be difficult to differentiate the natural course of the epilepsy from the benefit or side effects of the drug. In one study where children were randomized to treatment or no treatment after a single seizure, the risk of recurrence equaled the complications of the therapy [9]. If there is concern that the next event would be prolonged, then rather than initiating chronic AED therapy, the family could be instructed on the treatment of prolonged seizures at home by the rectal instillation of the intravenous formulation of diazepam (see Chapter 7).

Despite these arguments against the use of chronic AED therapy after only one convulsion, there are some circumstances wherein chronic AED therapy may be indicated after only one seizure. These circumstances include (1) the effects of a recurrence on a patient's employment, (2) the potential and prolonged loss of a driver's license after another seizure, which depends on state regulations, and (3) an overwhelming familial anxiety about the effects of a recurrent seizure. The first two concerns would apply only to the older adolescent or adult with seizures. Obviously, the concerns of the patient's family are important and must be considered.

III. SELECTION OF AED

Once the decision has been reached to initiate AED therapy (i.e., the risk of further seizures is sufficient and they would impair the child's well-being), several factors help to determine which drug is best for that specific patient. These include type of seizure, potential adversities of each AED, cost, and the ability of the patient and the family to comply to a medical regimen. These considerations are sequentially listed in Table 2. Age is another factor, and this will be considered under specific complications and pharmacologic properties that relate to age.

A. Seizure Type

Most patients with *generalized clonic*, *tonic*, *tonic–clonic*, or *tonic–clonic–tonic seizures* will achieve seizure control using any of five available AEDs: carbamazepine, phenobarbital, phenytoin, primidone, and valproic acid [10–15] (see Chapter 4). The same five AEDs are also equally effective in the control of *par-*

Table 2 Sequential Considerations in the Selection of the Most Appropriate Antiepileptic Drug

1. AED is theoretically appropriate for the seizures.
2. It has the least risk of significant adversity.
3. The family is able to comply with program of administration and necessary follow-up studies.
4. The cost to the family is not prohibitive.
5. It works.

tial seizures and *partial seizures with secondary generalization* [11–19] (see Chapter 5). Therefore, in these specific generalized seizures and in all partial seizures, the specific type of seizure helps little in selecting the optimal antiepileptic drug. Other factors (e.g., cost, potential complications) should be used in selecting the most appropriate drug therapy.

In generalized *absence*, *febrile*, and *generalized myoclonic seizures*, the efficacious AEDs are somewhat more specific. Typical absence seizures can be controlled equally well with either ethosuximide or valproic acid [20]. Febrile seizures respond poorly to the chronic administration of AEDs and respond best to the periodic administration of liquid diazepam during fevers [21]. Valproic acid, clonazepam, and ACTH are commonly used in myoclonic seizures, and the reader is referred to Chapter 9 for further information.

B. Potential Adversities of AEDs

The risk and severity of possible side effects of AEDs must be considered in each individual case before initiating therapy. Most AEDs can affect performance and well-being on an individual basis [22,23]. With the exception of phenobarbital [24,25], this effect on performance is an unpredictable response. When such occurs, an appropriate change in AEDs is warranted. Examples of specific side effects that might influence the selection of an appropriate AED follow (see Chapter 10 for additional information).

1. Phenobarbital

As mentioned above, phenobarbital use has been related to a decline in intellectual test scores [24,25] and disturbances of behavior [23]. Therefore, its use in children is indicated only when therapy with other AEDs has failed. *Primidone*, which is metabolized to phenobarbital, has similar disadvantages [12]. The use of these two AEDs should be limited in children, and their effect on behavior and intellect needs to be monitored carefully when either is used.

2. Phenytoin

Five side effects commonly associated with phenytoin are gum hypertrophy, hypertrichosis, coarsening of facial features, the fetal hydantoin syndrome, and cognitive impairment. As demonstrated in a primate model and in the human, the gum hypertrophy associated with phenytoin usage relates to dental hygiene and the dose of phenytoin [26–29]. Therefore, a neurologically handicapped patient, in whom twice-daily brushing of teeth is performed inadequately, may not be an optimal candidate for therapy with phenytoin.

Hypertrichosis is reversible if phenytoin is withdrawn when the increase in body hair is first evident [30]. Coarsening of facial features has been associated with the use of phenytoin, but this has been reported only in ataxic patients receiving polypharmacy and with chronic phenytoin toxicity. It is not observed in patients on monotherapy whose phenytoin dose produces therapeutic concentrations in plasma [31,32].

One report has described cognitive impairment in volunteers given phenytoin [33]. This may represent an artifact of the test system used, in that phenytoin delays reaction time in persons receiving it. Serum concentrations of phenytoin were not measured in these volunteers.

The fetal hydantoin syndrome is another complication of phenytoin therapy and probably occurs in 5 to 10% of fetuses exposed to phenytoin in pregnancy [35]. It is also seen in fetuses exposed to carbamazepine [36]. (See Chapter 15 for further discussion of this topic.)

3. Clonazepam

The major side effects limiting usage of clonazepam are lethargy and drooling. Its use should be limited in patients sedated by other AEDs or in children in whom drooling is a problem. This adversity may be reduced by starting with low doses and gradually increasing it [37,38].

4. Carbamazepine

Carbamazepine has been very rarely associated with bone marrow suppression [39]. The value of routine hematologic monitoring is debatable considering this very low risk in children. Hyponatremia is a more frequent finding [40]. Therefore, carbamazepine may not be an optimal AED for children who have either renal disease or hematological difficulties.

At the initiation of its use carbamazepine has a long half-life, and therefore one should start it at a dose of 2.5 to 5 mg/kg body weight. Every several days the dose is increased until a dose of about 15 mg/kg is achieved. Due to its acquired short half-life, multiple (i.e., three or four) daily doses are required. These pharmacokinetic properties require the ability of the patient and his or her family to a complex regimen.

5. Valproic Acid/Divalproex Sodium

Minor complications of valproate therapy include excessive weight gain [41] and alopecia [42]. Its use compounds the problem in an already overweight child. Alopecia is rarely an indication for great concern, unless the family has not been forewarned of the transient nature of this complication.

Thrombocytopenia and pancreatitis are more serious problems [43,44]. Knowledge of the risk of these rare problems does not help in initiating valproate in a healthy patient, but it would not be indicated as the first AED in a patient with the potential for a bleeding diathesis.

Pregnant women who are receiving valproic acid or divalproex sodium have a 1% risk of delivering a child with spina bifida [45]. Obviously, this potential complication of valproate must be explained to young women whose seizures are controlled with valproic acid and who desire to start their family. Supplemental folic acid early in pregnancy may reduce the risk of spina bifida in the fetus [46,47].

The potential for a fatal hepatotoxicity has to be considered when using valproate. Therapy with valproate carries an overall risk of 1 in 49,000 for fatal hepatotoxicity. This complication occurs in the first 6 months of therapy with the drug [48]. Two factors increase this risk for this complication: (1) the use of polypharmacy, and (2) the use of valproate in the first 2 years of life. Using monotherapy these fatalities have occurred only in children below 10 years of age. When VPA is part of a polypharmacy program, the risk increases in children below 10 and the risk extends to all ages.

Using monotherapy, the risk of a fatal hepatotoxicity below the age of 2 appears higher than in older children, and if valproate is used with other AEDs in infants, the risk increases to 1 in 800 [48]. In consideration of this rare and potentially fatal complication, extra attention needs to be paid to infants receiving valproate. If possible, it should not be used in infants already receiving other AEDs (i.e., do not use valproate as part of a polypharmacy program unless the other AEDs will be rapidly withdrawn). As the fatal hepatotoxicity occurs in the first 6 months of valproate therapy, other AEDs can be added after this period.

C. Cost of Medication

The cost of individual AEDs varies considerably. The cost of a month's supply of frequently used AEDs for a hypothetical 32-kg 10-year-old, using brand-name drugs and manufacturers' recommended daily doses [49] is given in Table 3. (These are the charges used at the Children's Mercy Hospital Pharmacy in Kansas City, Missouri in July 1990.) If laboratory tests are required for monitoring patients on a specific AED, their cost should also be considered [50].

For purposes of cost containment some institutions have recommended using generic equivalents when available. One should take care in using generic AEDs and avoid them in patients whose epilepsy is difficult to control. Many AEDs have narrow therapeutic levels for efficacy, and substitutions might not be equivalent for that person. Reports of failure or adversities of such compounds are available [51–54]. Although some comparative studies involving series of patients indicate that differences between generic products and the brand-name

Table 3 Comparative Costs of Antiepileptic Drugs[a]

AED	Brand name	Daily dose	cost for 1 month[b]
Phenobarbital	N.A. (30-mg tablet)	90 mg	$ 7.50
Phenytoin	Dilantin (50-mg tablet)	175 mg	11.85
Carbamazepine	Tegretal (200-mg tablet)	600 mg	23.70
Valproic acid	Depakote (250-mg tablet)	750 mg	24.60
Ethosuximide	Zarontin (250-mg capsule)	500 mg	19.20

[a]Children's Mercy Hospital, Kansas City, Missouri, outpatient pharmacy charges.
[b]Using recommended doses for a 32-kg 10-year-old patient.

products are not therapeutically significant [55,56], the Food and Drug Administration has had to recall generic AEDs [57,58].

Both the American Academy of Neurology and the Epilepsy Foundation of America have published statements recommending more careful control of the generic AEDs. The physician should be notified if generic drugs are required for a patient and when the AED is being changed from one brand to another [59,60]. If the brand name of the generic AED is changed, more frequent determinations of blood levels of the AED may be necessary and could eliminate the cost savings of a generic AED.

D. Compliance

The ability of the patient and the patient's family to comply with complex drug regimens may influence selection of an appropriate AED. If prior experience indicates that there would be difficulty complying with an AED regimen requiring multiple daily doses and periodic dose changes, that patient may achieve better compliance by taking a long-acting AED, such as phenobarbital, phenytoin, or ethosuximide, all of which may be given once daily, if tolerated.

Similarly, a patient with a record of poor compliance may do better taking a drug that has the same starting and maintenance doses, avoiding the gradual incremental dosing needed when starting an AED such as carbamazepine or primidone. If it is perceived that frequent hematologic studies might be necessary for one drug and not another of equal efficacy, a family with a record of noncompliance would do better if their child received the latter AED. All these considerations imply that the AEDs under consideration would have equal theoretic efficacy and equal potential for adversity. These properties of individual AEDs will be described below.

IV. PHARMACOLOGICAL PROPERTIES OF INDIVIDUAL AEDS

Numerous pharmacokinetics properties of AEDs determine how they are used practically to minimize apparent intolerance of a potentially beneficial AED.

Table 4 Pharmacologic Properties of Common Antiepileptic Drugs

Drug	Dose (mg/kg/day) Starting	Maintenance	Number of daily doses	Therapeutic range (μg/mL plasma)
Phenobarbital	3–5[a]	Same	≥1	15–40 (r)[b]
Phenytoin	3–10[a]	Same	≥2[c]	10–20 (r)
Primidone	5	10–20	≥2	4–10 (t)[d]
Carbamazepine	5	15–30	≥3	5–12 (t)
Valproic acid	15–30	15–30	≥2	50–100 (t)
Ethosuximide	20	20	≥1	>40

[a]Lower doses are used in older children.
[b]r, random time of drawing blood.
[c]30 or 100 mg of Dilantin have a long half-life and can be given once daily.
[d]t, trough levels.

Age of patient, AED half-life, effect of incremental doses, and so on, must all be considered when such drugs are administered. See Table 4 for a summary of these properties.

A. Phenobarbital

Phenobarbital is a long-acting AED which can therefore be administered either several times a day or once daily, depending on patient tolerance. The maintenance dose is 3 to 6 mg/kg per day, with higher doses needed in younger children to achieve therapeutic concentrations in plasma. Infants may need a loading dose, and higher maintenance (see Chapter 5).

If a child is started on a maintenance dose, it will require 2 to 3 weeks to achieve a steady state and therefore a meaningful plasma concentration. If an earlier benefit is desirable, the child should receive a loading dose, either 20 mg/kg in 1 day, or 10 mg/kg per day for 2 to 3 days. The plasma concentration (i.e., level) of phenobarbital can be determined, and the maintenance dose adjusted, after the loading dose.

Phenobarbital is available in a syrup with a concentration of 4 mg/mL and in 15-, 30-, 60-, and 100-mg tablets. A parenteral form of the drug is available for intramuscular or intravenous use, and this can replace the oral preparations on a milligram-for-milligram basis when the patient is NPO.

B. Phenytoin

For the long-term treatment of epilepsy, a maintenance dose of 3 to 10 mg/kg per day of phenytoin is necessary. Younger children need higher doses, and adolescents need the adult maintenance of about 5 to 6 mg/kg per day. It is very difficult to achieve therapeutic plasma concentrations of phenytoin in the first year of life using oral preparations [61,62].

Generally, 10 days is needed to achieve a steady-state plasma concentration of phenytoin if starting with a maintenance dose. As with phenobarbital, this can be achieved earlier by using oral loading doses of about 10 mg/kg per day for the first 2 to 3 days of therapy.

When using phenytoin it must be remembered that its metabolism follows zero-order kinetics. It is metabolized by arene oxidase. When arene oxidase becomes saturated, small increases in the dose of phenytoin are accompanied by large increases in plasma concentrations [63]. For example, if the concentration of phenytoin is 7 μg/mL plasma and the dose is doubled, the new concentration could be toxic (i.e., >20 μg/mL plasma).

If one uses the brand-name drug Dilantin (Parke-Davis) in the 30- or 100-mg capsules, the prolonged half-life permits once-a-day dosing. The liquid suspensions (6 and 25 mg/mL) and the chewable tablet (50 mg) require multiple daily doses. As the suspension is available in two concentrations, caution must be used to avoid confusion when prescribing the liquid form of this AED. Fears that the suspension would settle, thereby producing inaccurate doses, have proven to be unfounded [64].

Phenytoin is available in a parenteral form for intravenous use. Intramuscular administration is not recommended due to its delayed absorption—as long as 5 days—from such sites [65]. It can be directly administered intravenously, or diluted in saline. Phenytoin is not soluble in dextrose solutions [66]. Slow administration has been recommended due to its cardiac toxicity. Cardiac complications have been recorded in adults but have not been noted in children [67]. Sloughing of overlying skin will occur if phenytoin extravasates at the intravenous site.

C. Primidone

Primidone has had diminishing use in this country and probably worldwide. It is metabolized to phenobarbital and phenylethylmalonamide (PEMA). All three compounds—PEMA, phenobarbital and primidone—have antiepileptic activity, but the antiepileptic effect of the drug seems derived primarily from the phenobarbital metabolite [68]. It is reasonable, then, not to use phenobarbital and primidone in combination.

The maintenance dose is about 10 to 20 mg/kg per day, but this should be achieved gradually to avoid sedation. Patients not previously exposed to phenobarbital need to be started on about one-third of maintenance for one week, two-thirds of maintenance the second week, and so on. If primidone is to replace phenobarbital, a full maintenance dose can be started, with immediate cessation of phenobarbital therapy.

Primidone is available in 50- and 250-mg tablets and in a 50-mg/mL solution. Parenteral formulations are not available. If it cannot be given by mouth for a transient period, parenteral phenobarbital may briefly replace primidone.

D. Carbamazepine

Initially, carbamazepine has a long half-life, and therefore the patient who is naive to this drug needs to start on low doses (e.g., 5 mg/kg per day) and increase every 3 to 7 days until one achieves a dose of about 15 mg/kg per day. Generally, patients need thrice-daily dosing to avoid the lethargy induced by high levels if twice-daily dosing is used. Carbamazepine is available in a 20-mg/mL solution, a chewable 100-mg tablet, and a 200-mg tablet. Parenteral forms are not available and the only route of administration is by mouth.

E. Clonazepam

Clonazepam is the only benzodiazepine available in this country for the chronic treatment of epilepsy. The benzodiazepines diazepam and lorazepam are useful in the treatment of status epilepticus, and clorazepate, another benzodiazepine, is generally used only as a secondary, add-on, AED.

The seizure control that accompanies the use of clonazepam can be transient, with the recurrence of seizures in several months [37,38]. In one series of 40 children on AED polypharmacy, withdrawal of clonazepam resulted only rarely in deterioration of seizure control [69].

Nevertheless, it is an effective drug for the control of partial complex, and myoclonic, seizures. Cases have been described in which absence status occurred when clonazepam was added to valproate monotherapy [70]. In the author's experience, this is a very infrequent occurrence when the two AEDs are used in combination.

Side effects may be avoided by starting the dose at 0.01 to 0.03 mg/kg per day and using weekly increments until one achieves a dose of 0.1 to 0.2 mg/kg per day in divided doses. Toxicity is encountered when the starting dose, or an increase in dose, is excessive [38]. Clonazepam is unique in that neither efficacy nor toxicity correlate with blood levels [71] (i.e., blood levels are probably not worth pursuing when using clonazepam). It is packaged in 0.5-, 1.0-, and 2.0-mg tablets, and parenteral forms are not available.

F. Valproic Acid

Valproic acid is the last major antiepileptic drug to be approved for marketing by the U.S. Food and Drug Administration (FDA), and this occurred in 1978. (No new major AEDs have been approved for use in the United States between 1978 and 1991, whereas at least three other major antiepileptic drugs became available in Europe in that interval.) Valproate has the broadest range of efficacy for the treatment of pediatric seizure disorders. It is effective in generalized tonic–clonic, absence, myoclonic, and partial seizures [70], but it has the major and rare side effect of a potentially fatal hepatotoxicity [48].

The manufacturer recommends starting this drug at half-maintenance doses (i.e., 15 mg/kg per day) and increasing it subsequently to 20 to 30 mg/kg per day. Utilizing divalproex sodium, we have been able to start the AED at maintenance without recognized untoward effect, and would recommend this. (As mentioned earlier, divalproex sodium and valproic acid are used herein interchangeably save where specifically stated.)

If given in combination with phenobarbital, valproic acid characteristically elevates the level of phenobarbital about 30% [72]. When given in combination with other AEDs, plasma levels of both AEDs may be reduced, and it may be difficult to achieve therapeutic levels, despite large increases in drug dose [72–76].

Valproic acid is available in a 50-mg/mL syrup and a 250-mg capsule. Divalproex sodium, whose formulation reduces gastrointestinal adversity, is available in 125-mg sprinkles, which can be mixed with food, and 125-, 250-, and 500-mg tablets. Parenteral preparations are not available, but the liquid formulation can be administered rectally [77,78]. We have diluted it with water to avoid mucosal irritation.

V. DETERMINATION OF DRUG LEVELS

Tables of ''therapeutic'' plasma concentrations of antiepileptic drugs are generally available in most laboratories that perform this determination, but these tables must be considered only as guidelines (see Table 2). These ranges are statistical derivations that may not apply to every patient. Many patients achieve control of their seizures at subtherapeutic concentrations or levels, and there is no reason to increase the dose to achieve a therapeutic level. Conversely, if the level is high and the patient is well, there is no obligation to lower the dose in most situations. If a patient has a therapeutic concentration of an AED in plasma, and there is no benefit, changing to another AED may be indicated. Indications for obtaining blood levels of AEDs are given elsewhere [79]. In general, a patient whose seizures are well controlled will not benefit from periodic determinations of plasma levels of the AED. If a patient is ill, blood levels of AEDs may help differentiate symptoms of toxicity from those of intercurrent illness.

When drawing blood for the determination of AED concentration, it is essential either to know if the drug has a short or a long half-life, or to draw all levels before a scheduled dose (i.e., at the trough level). AEDs with a short half-life (e.g., carbamazepine or valproate) have variable plasma concentrations through the day. Randomly drawn blood for levels of these drugs will vary considerably, and such randomly drawn levels are generally a useless guide for altering dose. Blood drawn at the time of a trough concentration is more reliable and consistent. Therefore, levels should be drawn at the trough state, or before a dose is taken, when the concentration is at its theoretic nadir, for the sake of consistency and for comparisons with stated therapeutic levels. Rather than recalling the pharmacokinetics of every AED, it is easiest to draw blood routinely for all levels before the morning dose of medication, delaying the dose until this is done.

VI. PROVING DRUG EFFICACY

To prove that an AED is effective, one must be able to prove that the seizures are reduced in number and/or severity concurrent with the use of an AED. More important, the patient's quality of life has to have improved similarly. If the patient is having generalized tonic–clonic seizures every several weeks, drug efficacy may be easy to determine. If seizures occur every several months, it may take 6 months to determine efficacy. In every patient it is wise to maintain a seizure calender, indicating when seizures occur and when AED changes are made to assess the benefits of each AED objectively.

VII. MONOTHERAPY VERSUS POLYPHARMACY

There seems to be little question that patients function better on monotherapy (one AED) than when they are receiving several AEDs [80,81]. In one study of the efficacy of an on-site seizure clinic at an institution for neurologically handicapped persons, the most commonly observed association with improved function was a reduction in the number of the patient's AEDs [82,83]. It is easier to avoid this kind of polypharmacy when each AED is introduced, as opposed to tackling the problem when the patient has been receiving antiepileptic polypharmacy for several years. After the patient has been receiving several AEDs for several years, the benefit of each AED is difficult to substantiate retrospectively.

A. Avoiding Polypharmacy at the Beginning

If one adheres to the algorithm in Table 1, this should not be a problem. When one initiates an AED, three things can occur: seizures cease, seizure frequency is reduced, or the selected AED is not tolerated. In the first case, therapy is continued until the patient is no longer at risk for having seizures. In the second case, a second drug is added. If complete control is achieved, the first AED is eliminated. If the second AED is not tolerated or ineffective, a third is tried and the second stopped. In the third case the initial AED is stopped and another tried. If an added-on AED controls seizures, it is essential to try to remove the prior AED(s) to achieve monotherapy.

B. Approach to the Patient Already Receiving AEDs

The task of proving drug efficacy and minimizing the number of AEDs becomes more difficult when the patient is already receiving several AEDs at the first evaluation (i.e., the prior physician considered polypharmacy essential for optimal seizure control). (In one study, similar control of seizures and improved function were achieved in 71% of such patients by substituting monotherapy with divalproex sodium for polypharmacy [84]. If a careful history indicates which drugs have been effective in seizure control, and which have impaired function, a rational plan for AED elimination and monotherapy can be formulated. If the history is not clear on this point, one should start by eliminating AEDs with sedative side effects (i.e., primidone or phenobarbital).

If all components of the polypharmacy regimen have been in place for years, the reduction and elimination of each AED should be done with weekly reductions over a 4- to 8-week period to achieve monotherapy. AEDs may be eliminated more rapidly if (1) the drug to be eliminated has been used by the patient for less than months or (2) the patient is hospitalized and close observation is possible should unmasked seizures be severe.

If a seizure occurs during such AED reduction, do not restart the AED unless it is clear that the seizure is caused by the AED reduction, and that increasing or resuming the AED will not impair the child's well-being. At times the child will be able to perform better on fewer AEDs, despite an increase in seizure frequency. Initially, families may be reluctant to pursue a course of AED reduction, but in the author's experience they are subsequently rewarded by the improved alertness of the patient when the number of AEDs is diminished.

VIII. INTERACTIONS OF AEDS WITH COMMONLY USED NONEPILEPTIC MEDICATIONS

There are certain interactions of AEDs with drugs that patients may take briefly or chronically. Erythromycin frequently elevates the plasma concentration of carbamazepine, producing carbamazepine toxicity [85]. AEDs also reduce the efficacy of birth control pills, and other forms of contraception may be indicated in sexually active girls receiving AEDs [86]. Antineoplastic agents will also reduce levels of AEDs [87].

IX. TERMINATING AED THERAPY

At the initiation of therapy with AEDs the patient and his or her family should realize that the taking of AEDs is not a lifelong commitment. If seizures can be eliminated for several years with medications, the AED(s) can usually be withdrawn successfully. It is not known if this resolution reflects the natural course of an epilepsy (i.e., to resolve spontaneously) or if the resolution is secondary to the chronic suppression of clinical seizures with AEDs.

Available studies have some differences concerning the utility of the EEG in predicting which patients will have a recurrence, but there is general agreement that up to 80% of patients who are seizure-free for 2 years may eliminate AED therapy without recurrence of their epilepsy [88–91].

In one study of 88 children seizure-free for at least 2 years, the presence of slowing or spikes on the EEG before AED withdrawal was a very powerful predictor of recurrence of the epilepsy when AEDs were withdrawn [88]. Almost every patient with abnormal slowing and spikes on their EEG before AED withdrawal had recurrent seizures within 12 months of drug withdrawal. In another study the age of the patient at the onset of the epilepsy was a factor of prognostic significance [89]. Children below 3 at the onset of their epilepsy carried a more favorable prognosis for eventually successful AED withdrawal.

It must be remembered that all these studies on AED withdrawal in children looked at pediatric epilepsies in general. Undoubtedly, in the future we will be able to make more accurate prognoses regarding the success of AED withdrawal by correctly diagnosing the underlying epilepsy and by knowing the natural history of that specific epilepsy [92].

Two issues that are faced when a child is 2 years without seizures are the rapidity of AED withdrawal and management of the patient with persistent EEG abnormalities. Observations on drug withdrawal indicate that withdrawal over 6 weeks is safe [88]. Briefer periods of withdrawal have not been studied. Therefore, our approach is to withdraw AED(s) at weekly or 2-weekly decrements one AED at a time over a period of more than 1 month. If seizures recur during withdrawal, that AED is increased to a former dose if that is to the child's benefit. If withdrawal is accompanied by improvement in alertness and performance when seizures recur, replacement with another AED may be desirable to avoid a return of the diminished alertness.

There are no studies of patients whose EEGs remain epileptiform after 2 years of successful medical control of seizures. Options to consider in this situation are (1) continued treatment for another year and a repeat EEG then, and (2) cautious AED withdrawal in the face of an epileptiform EEG and prolonged control of seizures. If one knows the specific epilepsy being treated, knowledge of the natural course of that epilepsy will help in the decision making. At least one study claims to demonstrate that EEG abnormalities are not predictive of seizure recurrence following the withdrawal of AEDs [91].

The selection of any of these three options has to be individualized for each patient, considering the patient's age and future plans, the nature of the prior seizures, possible drug adversity, and the desires of the patient and his or her family. There are patients who, due to the social, medical, or occupational ef fects of another convulsion, would prefer not to try to eliminate AEDs, and for these patients the issues of drug withdrawal are moot.

REFERENCES

1. Aicardi J. Epilepsy in children. New York: Raven Press, 1986: 335.
2. Freeman JM, Tibbles J, Camfield C, Camfield P. Benign epilepsy of childhood: a speculation and its ramifications. Pediatrics 1987; 79:864–68.
3. Haruda F. Status epilepticus: risks and treatment (letter). Pediatrics 1989; 84:1121.
4. Freeman JM. Status epilepticus: risks and treatment (letter). Pediatrics 1989; 84:1121–22.
5. Shinnar S, Berg AT, Moshé SL, Petix M, Maytal J, Kang H, Goldensohn ES, Hauser WA. Risk of seizure recurrence following a first unprovoked seizure in childhood: a prospective study. Pediatrics 1990; 85:1076–85.
6. Hauser VA, Anderson VE, Lowenson RB, McRoberts SM. Seizure recurrence after a first unprovoked seizure. N Engl J Med 1982:522–28.
7. Hirtz DG, Ellenberg JH, Nelson KB. The risk of recurrence of nonfebrile seizures in children. Neurology 1984; 34:637–41.
8. Camfield PR, Camfield CS, Dooley JM, Tibbles JAR, Fung T, Garner B. Epilepsy after a first unprovoked seizure in childhood. Neurology 1985; 35:1657–60.
9. Camfield P, Camfield C, Dooley J, Smith E, Garner B. A randomized study of carbamazepine versus no medication after a first unprovoked seizure in childhood. Neurology 1989; 39:851–52.
10. Wilder BJ, Ramsay RE, Murphy JV, Karas BJ, Marquardt K, Hammond EJ. Comparison of valproic acid and phenytoin in newly diagnosed tonic–clonic seizures. Neurology 1983; 33:1474–76.
11. Feely M, O'Callaghan M, Duggan G, Callaghan N. Phenobarbitone in previously untreated epilepsy. J Neurol Neurosurg Psychiatr 1980; 43:365–68.
12. White PT, Plott D, Norton J. Relative anticonvulsant potency of primidone. A double blind comparison. Arch Neurol 1966; 14:31–35.
13. Ramsay RE, Wilder BJ, Berger JR, Bruni J. A double blind study comparing carbamazepine with phenytoin as initial seizure therapy in adults. Neurology 1983; 33:904–10.
14. Huf R, Schain RJ. Long-term experiences with carbamazepine (Tegretol) in children with seizures. J Pediatr 1980; 97:310–12.
15. Callaghan N, Kenny RA, O'Neill B, Crowley M, Goggin T. A prospective study between carbamazepine, phenytoin and sodium valproate as monotherapy in previously untreated and recently diagnosed patients with epilepsy. J Neurol Neurosurg Psychiatr 1985; 48:639–44.
16. de Silva M, McArdle B, McGowan M, Neville BGR, Johnson AL, Reynolds EH. Monotherapy for newly diagnosed epilepsy: comparative trials and prognostic evaluation (abstract). Epilepsia 1989; 30:662.
17. Mattson RH, Cramer JA, Collins JF, Smith DB, Delgado-Escueto AV, Browne TR, Williamson PD, Treiman DM, McNamara JO, McCutchen CB, Homan RW, Crill

WE, Lubozynski, Rosenthal NP, Mayersdorf A. Comparison of carbamazepine, phenobarbital, phenytoin, and primidone in partial and secondarily generalized tonic–clonic seizures. N Engl J Med 1985; 313:145–51.

18. Bruni J., Albright P. Valproic acid therapy for complex partial seizures. Its efficacy and toxic effects. Arch Neurol 1983; 40:135–37.
19. Loiseau P, Cohadon S, Jogeix M, Legroux M, Dartigues JF. Efficacité du valproate de sodium dans les épilepsies partielles. Etude croisée valproate–carbamazepine. Rev Neurol 1984; 140:434–37.
20. Callaghan N, O'Hare J, O'Driscoll D, O'Neill B, Daly M. Comparative study of ethosuximide and sodium valproate in the treatment of typical absence seizures (petit mal). Child Neurol 1982; 24:830–36.
21. Knudsen FU. Effective short-term prophylaxis in febrile convulsions. J Pediatr 1985; 106:487–90.
22. Vining EPG, Shinnar SS, Mellits ED, Silverton S, Brandt J. Discontinuing antiepileptic drugs improves intellectual function (abstract). Ann Neurol 1986; 20:389.
23. Meador KJ, Loring DW, Huh K, Gallagher BB, King DW. Comparative cognitive effects of anticonvulsants. Neurology 1990; 40:391–94.
24. Farwell JR, Lee YJ, Hirtz DG, Sulzbacher SI, Ellenberg JH, Nelson B. Phenobarbital for febrile seizures: effects on intelligence and on seizures recurrence. N Engl J Med 1990; 322:364–69.
25. Vining EP, Mellits EP, Dorsen MM, Cataldo MF, Quaskey SA, Spielberg SP, Freeman JM. Psychologic and behavioural effects of antiepileptic drugs in children: a double-blind comparison between phenobarbital and valproic acid. Pediatrics 1987; 80:165–74.
26. Staple PH, Reed MJ, Mashimo PA. Diphenylhydantoin gingival hyperplasia in *Macaca arctoides*: a new human model. J Periodontol 1977; 48:325–36.
27. Staple PH, Reed MJ, Mashimo PA, Sedransk N, Umemoto T. Diphenylhydantoin gingival hyperplasia in *Macaca arctoides*: prevention by inhibition of dental plaque deposition. J Periodontol 1978; 49:310–25.
28. Pihlstrom BL, Carlson JF, Smith QT, Bastien SA, Keenan KM. (1980). Prevention of phenytoin associated gingival enlargement: a 15-month longitudinal study. J Peridontol 1980; 51:311–17.
29. Kapur RN, Girgis S, Little TM, Masotti RE. Phenytoin-induced gingival hyperplasia: its relationship to dose and serum level. Dev Med Child Neurol 1973; 15:483–87.
30. DeLorenzo RJ. Phenytoin. Mechanisms of action. In: Levy RH, Dreifuss FE, Meldrum BS, Mattson RH, Kiffin Penry J. eds. Antiepileptic drugs. New York: Raven Press, 1989:143–58.
31. Lefebvre EB, Haining RG, Labbe RF. Coarse facies, calvarial thickening, and hyperphostasia associated with long-term anticonvulsant therapy. N Engl J Med 1972; 286:1301–2.
32. Falconer MA, Davidson S. Coarse features in epilepsy as a consequence of anticonvulsant therapy. Lancet 1973; II:1112–14.
33. Thompson PJ, Huppert F, Trimble MR. Phenytoin and cognitive functions: effects on normal volunteers and implications for epilepsy. Br J Clin Psychol 1981; 20:155–62.

34. Dodrill CB, Temkin NR. Motor speed is a contaminating factor in evaluation of the "cognitive" effects of phenytoin. Epilepsia 1989; 30:453–57.
35. Buehler BA, Delimont D, van Waes M, Finnell RH. Prenatal prediction of risk of the fetal hydantoin syndrome. N Engl J Med 1990; 322:1567–72.
36. Jones KL, Lacro RV, Johnson KA, Adams J. Pattern of malformations in the children of women treated with carbamazepine during pregnancy. N Engl J Med 1989; 320:1661–66.
37. Mikkelsen B, Birket-Smith E, Brandt S, Holm P, Lund M, Thorn I, Vestermark S, Zander-Olsen P. Clonazepam in the treatment of epilepsy. A controlled clinical trial in simple absences, bilateral massive epileptic myoclonus, and atonic seizures. Arch Neurol 1976; 33:322–25.
38. Browne TR. Clonazepam. A review of a new anticonvulsant drug. Arch Neurol 1976; 33:326–32.
39. Hart RG, Easton JD. Carbamazepine and hematological monitoring. Ann Neurol 1982; 11:309–12.
40. Lahr MB. Hyponatremia during carbamazepine therapy. Clin Pharmacol Ther 1985; 37:693–96.
41. Egger J, Brett EM. Effects of sodium valproate in 100 children with special reference to weight. Br Med J 1981; 283:577–81.
42. Sherard ES, Steiman GS, Couri D. Treatment of childhood epilepsy with valproic acid: results of the first 100 patients in a 6 month trial. Neurology 1980; 30:31–35.
43. Loiseau P. Sodium valproate, platelet dysfunction and bleeding. Epilepsia 1981; 22:141–46.
44. Wylie E, Cruse RP, Erenberg G, Rothner AD. Pancreatitis associated with valproic acid therapy. Am J Dis Child 1984; 138:912–14.
45. Guibaud S, Simplot A, Boisson C, Pison H. Dépistage prenatal de 4 cas de spina bifida chez de mères traitees par le valproate. J Genet Hum 1987; 35:231–35.
46. Milunsky A, Jick H, Jick SS, Bruell CL, MacLaughlin DS, Rothman KJ, Willett W. Multivitamin/folic acid supplementation in early pregnancy reduces the prevalence of neural tube defects. JAMA 1989; 262:2847–52.
47. Dansky LV, Andermann E, Rosenblatt D, Sherwin AL, Andermann F. Anticonvulsants, folate levels, and pregnancy outcome: a prospective study. Ann Neurol 19 ; 21:176–82.
48. Dreifuss FE, Langer DH, Moline KA, Maxwell JE. Valproic hepatic fatalities. II. US experience since 1984. Neurology 1989; 39:201–7.
49. ER Barnhart, publisher Physicians' desk reference, 43d ed. Oradell, NJ: Medical Economics Company Inc., 1989.
50. Goldberg MA. Costs of anticonvulsant therapy. Ann Neurol 1981; 9:95.
51. MacDonald JT. Breakthrough seizures following substitution of Depakene capsules (Abbott) with a generic product. Neurology 1987; 37:1885.
52. Wyllie E, Pippenger CE, Rothner AD. Increased seizure frequency with generic primidone. JAMA 1987; 258:1216–17.
53. Hartley R, Aleksandrowicz J, Ng PC, McLain B, Bowmer CJ, Forsythe WI. Breakthrough seizures with generic carbamazepine? Dev Med Child Neurol 1990; 32:460–62.
54. Busch RL. Generic carbamazepine and erythema multiforme: generic-drug nonequivalency. N Engl J Med 1989; 321: 692–93.

55. Chen SS, Allen J, Oxley J, Richens A. (1982). Comparative bioavailability of phenytoin from generic formulation in the United Kingdom. Epilepsia 1982; 23:149–52.
56. Jumao-as A, Bella I, Craig B, Lowe J, Dasheid RM. (1989). Comparison of steady-state blood levels of two carbamazepine formulations. Epilepsia 1989; 30:67–70.
57. FDA recalls and court actions, extended sodium phenytoin capsules, USP, 100 mg, Sidmak. FDC Reports, Jan 18, 1988:T, G-8.
58. FDA recalls and court actions, carbamazepine tablets, USP, 200 mg, Pharmaceutical Basics, Inc. FDC Reports, Sept 5, 1988:T, G-9.
59. Report of the Therapeutics and Technology Assessment Subcommittee the American Academy of Neurology. Assessment: generic substitution for antiepileptic medication. Neurology 1989; 40:1641–43.
60. EFA Commentary. J Epilepsy 1990; 3:55–59.
61. Whelan HT, Handeles L, Haberkern CM, Neima AH. High intravenous dosage requirement in a newborn infant. Neurology 1983; 33:106–8.
62. Bourgeois BFD, Dodson WE. Phenytoin elimination in newborns. Neurology 1983; 33:173–78.
63. Browne TR, Chang T. Phenytoin transformation. In: eds. Antiepileptic drugs. 3d ed. Levy RH, Dreifuss FE, Mattson RH, Meldrum BS, Penry JK, New York: Raven Press, 1989: 197–213.
64. Sarkar MA, Garnett WR, Karnes HT. (1989). The effects of storage and shaking on the settling properties of phenytoin suspension. Neurology 1989; 39:207–9.
65. Kostenauder HB, Rapp RP, McGovren JP, Foster TS, Perrier DG, Blacker HM, Hulon WC, Kinkel AW. Bioavailability and single dose pharmacokinetics of intramuscular phenytoin. Clin Pharmacol Ther 1975; 18:449–56.
66. Cloyd JC, Gumnit RJ, McLain W Jr. Status epilepticus. The role of intravenous phenytoin. JAMA 1980; 244:1479–81.
67. Earnest MP, Marx JA, Drury LR. Complications of intravenous phenytoin for acute treatment of seizures. JAMA 1983; 249:762–65.
68. Oxley J, Hebdige S, Richens A. (1979). A comparison of phenobarbitone and primidone in the control of epilepsy in chronic epilepsy. Br J Clin Pharmacol 1979; 7:414P.
69. Specht U, Boenigk HE, Wolf P. Discontinuation of clonazepam after long-term treatment. Epilepsia 1990; 30:458–63.
70. Jeavons PM, Clark JE, Maheshwari MC. Treatment of generalized epilepsies of childhood and adolescence with sodium valproate ('Epilim'). Dev Med Child Neurol 1977; 19:9–25.
71. Naito H, Wachi M, Nishida M. Clinical effects and plasma concentrations of long-term clonazepam monotherapy in previously untreated epilepticus. Acta Neurol Scand 1987; 76:58–63.
72. Patel IH, Levy RH, Cutler RE. Phenobarbital–valproic acid interaction. Clin Pharmacol Ther 1980; 27:515–21.
73. Wilder BJ, Willmore LJ, Bruni J, Villareal HJ. Valproic acid: interaction with other anticonvulsant drugs. Neurology 1978; 28:892–96.
74. Sackellares JC, Sato S, Dreifuss FE, Penry JK. Reduction of steady-state valproate levels by other antiepileptic drugs. Epilepsia 1981; 22:437–41.

75. Henriksen O, Johannessen SJ. Clinical pharmacokinetic observations on sodium valproate: a 5-year follow-up study in 100 children with epilepsy. Acta Neurol Scand 1982; 65:504–23.
76. Cloyd JC, Kriel RL, Fischer HJ. Valproic acid pharmacokinetics in children II. Discontinuation of concomitant drug therapy. Neurology 1985; 35:1623–27.
77. Thorpy MJ. Rectal valproate syrup and status epilepticus. Neurology 1980; 30:1113–14.
78. Vajda FJE, Mihaly GW, Miles JL, Donnan GA, Bladin PF. Rectal administration of sodium valproate in status epilepticus. Neurology 1978; 28:897–99.
79. Dodson WE. Level off. Neurology 1989; 39:1009–10.
80. Mattson RH, Cramer JA. Crossover from polytherapy to monotherapy in primary generalized epilepsy. Am J Med 1988; 84 Suppl 1A:23–28.
81. Bennett HS. Reduction of polypharmacy for epilepsy in an institution for the retarded. Dev Med Child Neurol 1983; 25:735–37.
82. Wilkinson IA, Murphy JV, Georgeson R. Impact of an on-site seizure clinic on the welfare of mentally retarded, institutionalized patients. Arch Neurol 1982; 39:41–44.
83. Schmidt D, Richter K. Alternative single anticonvulsant drug therapy for refractory epilepsy. Ann Neurol 1986; 19:85–87.
84. Ramsay RE, Wilder BJ, Pellock JM, Dreifuss FE, Mattson RH, Smith DB, Penry JK, Sunder TR, Ahmann P, Spitz MC, Murphy JV, Leroy RF, Morris DD, Hansen RG, Pierce MW. Successful conversion from polytherapy to Depakote monotherapy in patients with primary generalized tonic–clonic seizures (abstract). Epilepsia 1989; 30:662–63.
85. Goulden KJ, Camfield P, Dooley JM, Fraser A, Meek DC, Renton KW, Tibbles JAR. Severe carbamazepine intoxication after coadministration of erythromycin. J Pediatr 1986; 109:135–38.
86. Mattson RH et al. Use of oral contraceptives by women with epilepsy. JAMA 1986; 256:238–40.
87. Nahum MP, Arush MWBA, Robinson E. Reduced carbamazepine level during chemotherapy in a child with malignant lymphoma. Acta Paediatr Scand 1990; 79:873–75.
88. Shinnar S, Vining EPG, Mellits ED, D'Souza BJ, Holden K, Baumgardner RA, Freeman JM. Discontinuing antiepileptic medication in children with epilepsy after two years without seizures. A prospective study. N Engl J Med 1985; 313:976–80.
89. Bouma PAD, Peters ACB, Arts RJHM, Stijnen T, Van Rossum J. Discontinuation of entiepileptic therapy. J Neurol Neurosurg Psychiatr 1987; 50:1579–83.
90. Callaghan N, Garrett A, Goggin T. Withdrawal of anticonvulsant drugs in patients free of seizures for two years. A prospective study. N Engl J Med 1988; 318:942–46.
91. Holowach J, Thurston DL, O'Leary J. Prognosis in childhood epilepsy: followup study of 148 cases in which therapy has been suspended after prolonged anticonvulsant control. N Engl J Med 1972; 286:169–74.
92. Ambrosetto G, Tassinari CA. (1990. Antiepileptic drug treatment of benign childhood epilepsy with rolandic spikes. Is it necessary? Epilepsia 1990; 31:802–5.

3

Classification of Epileptic Seizures and Epilepsies

FEREYDOUN DEHKHARGHANI
University of Missouri
and Children's Mercy Hospital
Kansas City, Missouri

The epilepsy is either hereditary, or acquired. It may further be distinguished into primary and symptomatic: The first is when the brain is immediately affected; and the other is when it is drawn into sympathy with some other part of the body, such as the stomach, spleen, uterus, intestines, etc.

Another distinction is taken from the age of the patient: whether its first attack appeared before, at, or after the time of puberty. Also, whether the disease be violent, or only gentle. Willis, 1742 [1]

Convulsions are of two kinds: the symptomatic, depending upon another disease, and the idiopathic, said to be an original complaint, and arising from a morbid affection of the brain, though the distinction, be not, perhaps, perfectly philosophical, or accurate. Underwood, 1743 [2]

I. BACKGROUND

A. Historical Perspective

Efforts to classify epileptic seizures have been recorded since the writings of Hippocrates (460–377 B.C.) [3]. He established the belief that epilepsy is a disease of the brain, not corporeal or supernatural [4]. Classification of epilepsy into two types of central or idiopathic and sympathetic or centripetal spans from the time of Galen (A.D. 130–200) to that of Esquirol (1838) [5]. This classification was based on involvement of the cerebrum and accumulation of ventricles with circulation of natural or diseased humor arising in other organs, acting in sympathy with the brain. The digestive system was considered the most important causative source of extracerebral epilepsy. Classification of epilepsies into two major groups—cerebral and extracerebral—remained unchanged until the mid-nineteenth century when all epilepsies were believed to caused by direct cerebral involvement. Cerebral mechanisms were divided into two categories: (1) independent of any cerebral lesion, known as functional, idiopathic, essential, or centrencephalic, and (2) secondary to brain lesions, known as lesional, organic, structural, or symptomatic. It was believed that symptomatic seizures were always partial or focal and idiopathic (functional) seizures were exclusively generalized. This concept was changed in the early 1940s when the EEG began playing its important role in recognition and classification of epilepsies.

By the mid-1950s, symptomatic generalized epilepsies were discovered and it was noted that diffuse or multifocal cortical lesions could give rise to generalized epilepsies [5]. This view is reflected in the proposed international classification of epilepsy by Gastaut in 1969 [6], which was presented in 1970 by Merlis [7]. Later, clinical observations revealed the existence of idiopathic partial epilepsies. Like the generalized idiopathic epilepsies, this type of epilepsy was assumed to be based on constitutional predisposition.

The idea of epileptic predisposition goes back to the end of the eighteenth century. The recognition of reflex epilepsies and the genetic predisposition for 3-Hz generalized spike/slow-wave complexes gave further support to the concept of the constitutional predisposition for epilepsy. The 3-Hz generalized spike/slow-wave complex is inherited as an autosomal dominant trait [8–10].

B. Purpose of Classification

The framework for this chapter is based on a proposal for the revised classification of (1) the epilepsies and epileptic syndromes published in 1989 [11] and (2) a proposal for revised clinical and electroencephalographic classifications of epileptic seizures published in 1981 [12] (refer to Tables 1, 2, and 3). A distinction between the two classifications should be appreciated.

The terms *idiopathic, primary, essential, cryptogenic*, and *secondary* will be defined and common epileptic syndromes discussed. The purpose of classification is to facilitate communication. Accurate classification of a patient's seizure should assist in the selection of an antiepileptic drug (AED) because most anticonvulsants have a different spectrum of efficacy. Some antiepileptic drugs are predominantly effective for absences, others for myoclonic or convulsive seizures. When the patient's epilepsy is classified under a known syndrome, the

Table 1 International Classification of Epileptic Seizures

I. Partial (focal, local) seizures
   A. Simple partial seizures (consciousness not impaired)
      1. With motor symptoms
      2. With somatosensory or special sensory symptoms
      3. With autonomic symptoms
      4. With psychic symptoms
   B. Complex partial seizures (with impairment of consciousness)
      1. Beginning as simple partial seizures and progressing to impairment of consciousness
         a. With no other features
         b. With automatisms
      2. With impairment of consciousness at onset
         a. With no other features
         b. With automatism
   C. Partial seizures evolving to secondarily generalized seizures
II. Generalized seizures (convulsive or nonconvulsive)
   A. Absence seizures
      1. Absence seizures
      2. Atypical absence seizures
   B. Myoclonic seizures
   C. Clonic seizures
   D. Tonic seizures
   E. Tonic–clonic seizures
   F. Atonic seizures (astatic seizures)
III. Unclassified epileptic seizures

Source: Adapted and modified from "Proposal for revised clinical and electroencephalographic classification of epileptic seizures," The Commission on Classification and Terminology of the International League Against Epilepsy, Epilepsia 1981; 22:489–501.

prognosis and clinical course can be better predicted. Some forms of epilepsy may not need aggressive treatment (e.g., benign rolandic seizures), and some are age limited with spontaneous resolution. In drug-resistant cases, selection of appropriate candidates for surgery, and decision on the type of surgery, mandate awareness of the natural history of that epilepsy in each case. Classification of epileptic disorders is a dynamic process and will undergo periodic updating as more is learned about seizure disorders.

C. Basis of Classification

Despite an enormous effort and numerous international conferences, there is no really satisfactory classification for epileptic disorders. The dichotomy between

Table 2 International Classification of Epilepsies and Epileptic Syndromes (Major Categories)

1. Localization related (partial epilepsy and syndromes)
   1.1 Idiopathic
   1.2 Symptomatic
   1.3 Cryptogenic
2. Generalized epilepsies and syndromes
   2.1 Idiopathic
   2.2 Idiopathic or symptomatic
   2.3 Symptomatic
      2.3.1 Nonspecific etiology
      2.3.2 Specific syndromes
3. Epilepsies and syndromes undetermined whether focal or generalized
   3.1 With both generalized and focal seizures
   3.2 Without unequivocal generalized or focal features
4. Special syndromes
   4.1 Situation-related seizures

Source: Adapted and modified from "Proposal for revised classification of epilepsies and epileptic syndromes," Epilepsia 1989; 30(4):389–99.

generalized and focal (localization-related) epilepsy remains the basis for the two main categories of the present classification. Each of these two major categories is further divided into idiopathic when there is no underlying cause other than when a possible hereditary predisposition is found, and symptomatic epilepsies. In a recent classification proposed by the International League Against Epilepsy (ILAE), in addition to the major headings of idiopathic, symptomatic, localization-related, and generalized, there are certain groups of epilepsies that fit neither the categories of generalized or localization-related groups nor idiopathic or symptomatic disorders. They are grouped under specific syndromes, an example being febrile seizures. The syndromic approach in classification of epilepsies attempts to subdivide the epileptic patients into relatively homogeneous groups on the basis of clinical and EEG criteria. The main disadvantage of this approach is that not all epilepsies are classifiable. For some epileptic syndromes genetic predisposition is well documented, and for others, the interaction of genetic and acquired factors is evident. Some authors believe that even in acquired epilepsies, genetic predisposition plays an important role. In this view there is no clear distinction between primary and secondary epilepsies [13].

Another approach is to view different epileptic syndromes from the vantage point of a neurobiological continuum. This approach may offer a unifying trend but does not have precision in diagnosis and accuracy in prognosis compared to the syndromic approach. This approach leads to several subclassifications of epilepsy which are important and needed to encompass so many varied clinical presentations. Both approaches can be used at the clinical level [14].

Present international classification assumes that some seizures have a focal origin while others involve both hemispheres simultaneously from the start. As discussed by Rodin [14], it could be argued, however, that all seizures have to begin somewhere in the brain and the difference between focal and generalized may reside merely in different sites of origin and the speeds with which pathological cerebral electrical activity spreads to distant parts of the brain and the periphery. In a series of more than 200 photographed seizures induced by bemegride (Megimide), a convulsant drug, Rodin found only two patients who showed complete symmetry in the initial aspect of the clinical attack [15]. The dichotomy of generalized/partial, and acquired/genetic should not prevent the search for the biological continuum as a unifying theory. Evolution of seizure patterns from the neonatal period to infancy, and disappearance of infantile spasm and changing pattern of Lennox–Gastaut to multifocal seizures and other age-related epilepsies, have given support to the neurobiological continuum in different epilepsies.

D. Justification for Classifications

1. Seizures

The 1981 international classification of epileptic seizures (ICES) has been widely used in clinical drug trials and in epidemiological studies. In the Graniere [18] study, 94% of patients were classifiable. In a recent study of 1,220 cases, 82.5% of the seizures were classifiable. In this study, 56% of the patients had partial seizures and 26.5% had generalized seizures. Other investigators have found that 90 to 97% of the cases are classifiable [19,20]. Gastaut records 81.6% as classifiable. In Keranen's study [20], patients with partial seizures accounted for 56% and patients with generalized seizures for 26.5% of all cases. Granieri found 33% partial and 60% generalized seizures. Other investigators have reported predominance of partial seizures, which may represent underrepresentation of patients with generalized seizures in populations derived from epilepsy clinics. Partial seizures with complex symptomatology have been the most common type of epilepsy in most clinical studies (35 to 56% of classifiable cases) [16,17,21]. Previous studies have shown that the frequency of generalized seizures is higher in children than in adults [19].

2. Epilepsy

The international classification of epilepsy has been used in several major clinical studies and epidemiological surveys [16,17] and has been found relevant and useful; based on several reports, 76 to 98% of cases are classifiable. Many of these studies have used international classification of epileptic seizures as a basis for the recognition and presentation of the clinical seizures.

Table 3 Classification of Epilepsies and Epileptic Syndromes

1. Localization related (focal, local, partial) epilepsies and syndromes
    1.1 Idiopathic with age-related onset
        Benign childhood epilepsy with centrotemporal spikes
        Childhood epilepsy with occipital paroxysms
        Primary reading epilepsy
    1.2 Symptomatic (this category comprises syndromes of great individual variability based on seizure types, clinical features, anatomical localization, and etiology
        Chronic progressive epilepsia partialis continua of childhood (Rasmussen syndrome)
        Frontal lobe epilepsies
            Supplementary motor seizures
            Cingulate seizures
            Anteriofrontopolar seizures
            Orbitofrontal seizures
            Dorsolateral seizures
            Opercular seizures
            Epilepsies of the motor cortex
            Kojewnikow syndrome
        Temporal lobe epilepsies
            Amygdalohippocampal (mesiobasal limbic or primary rhinencephalic) seizures
            Lateral temporal seizures
        Parietal lobe epilepsies
        Occipital lobe epilepsies
        Syndromes characterized by seizures with specific mode of precipitation
            Reflex epilepsies
            Startle epilepsy
            Memory or pattern-stimulated epilepsy
    1.3 Cryptogenic (presumed to be symptomatic but etiology unknown)
2. Generalized epilepsies and syndromes
    2.1 Idiopathic (with age-related onset, listed in order of age of appearance)
        Benign neonatal familial convulsions
        Benign neonatal convulsions
        Benign myoclonic epilepsy in infancy
        Childhood absence epilepsy (pyknolepsy, petit mal)
        Juvenile absence epilepsy
        Juvenile myoclonic epilepsy (impulsive petit mal)
        Epilepsy with grand mal seizures (GTCS) on awakening
        Other generalized ideopathic epilepsies not defined above
        Epilepsies with seizures precipitated by specific modes of activation
    2.2 Cryptogenic or symptomatic epilepsies (in order of age of appearance)
        West syndrome (infantile spasms)
        Lennox–Gastaut syndrome

Epilepsy with myoclonic–astatis seizures
Epilepsy with myoclonic absences

2.3 Symptomatic

2.3.1 Nonspecific etiology
- Early myoclonic encephalopathy
- Early infantile epileptic encephalopathy with EEG suppression-burst pattern
- Other symptomatic generalized epilepsies not defined above

2.3.2 Specific syndromes (many disease states complicated by seizures as presenting or predominate features)
- Malformations
  - Aicardi syndrome
  - Lissencephaly–pachygyria
  - Phacomatoses
  - Hypothalamic hamartoma
- Proven or suspected inborn errors of metabolism
  - Neonate
    - Hyperglycinemia (early myoclonic encephalopathy with erratic myoclonus partial seizures and suppression burst on EEG)
    - Glycericacidemia
  - Infant
    - Phenylketonuria
    - Biopterine deficiency
    - Tay–Sacks
    - Sandhoff
    - early infantile type of ceroid-lipofuscinosis
    - Pyridoxine dependency
  - Child
    - Late infantile ceroid-lipofuscinosis with
    - myoclonic, atonic, astatic seizures
    - Infantile type of Huntington disease with dystonia, atypical myoclonus, GTC
  - Child and adolescent
    - Juvenile form of Gaucher
    - Juvenile form of ceroid-lipofuscinosis (Spielmeyer–Vogt disease)
    - Lafora disease
    - Degenerative progressive myoclonic epilepsy
    - Dyssynergia cerebellaris myoclonia with epilepsy (Ramsey–Hunt syndrome)
    - Cherry red spot myoclonus syndrome
    - Ramsey–Hunt-like syndrome with mitochondrial myopathy and abnormalities of lactate and pyruvate metabolism
  - Adult
    - Kuf disease

(**Table 3** cont.)

3. Epilepsies and syndromes undetermined as to whether they are focal or generalized
    3.1 With both generalized and focal seizures
        Neonatal seizures
        Severe myoclonic epilepsy in infancy
        Epilepsy with continuous spikes waves during slow-wave sleep
        Acquired epileptic aphasia (Landau–Kleffner syndrome)
        Other indetermined epilepsies not defined above
    3.2 Without unequivocal generalized or focal features (sleep grand mal)
4. Special syndromes
    4.1 Situation-related seizures
        Febrile convulsions
        Isolated seizures or isolated status epilepticus
        Seizures occurring only when there is an acute metabolic or toxic event

Source: Adapted and modified from "Proposal for revised classification of epilepsies and epileptic syndromes," Epilepsia 1989; 30(4):389–99.

II. DEFINITIONS

A. Seizures

More than a century ago, Hughlings Jackson defined an *epileptic seizure* as an occasional, sudden, extensive, and rapid discharge of some part of the cerebral hemisphere, clearly an electroclinical phenomenon. Later, Jackson suggested an anatomical physiological classification and promoted the concept of generalized and focal on clinical presentations of seizures [22].

Presently, epileptic seizures are defined as a brief, intermittent, involuntary, time-limited, sudden disturbance of brain function. Clinical manifestations of this disturbance depend on the site of the neurobiological changes in the brain. The clinical expression of a seizure represents dysfunction of a part of the cortex, and therefore this is determined by the function of that area of the brain.

From an electrophysiological point of view, epileptic seizures are the clinical manifestations of sudden excessive hypersynchronous, self-limiting abnormal cortical neuronal activity. These electrophysiological changes usually, but not always, can be recorded by EEG [6;23, pp. 3–21].

B. Epilepsy

The word *epilepsy*, in the general sense, is used to refer to the disorder associated with recurrent epileptic seizures. In a proposal for revised classification of epilepsies and epileptic syndromes published in 1989, an *epileptic syndrome* is defined as an epileptic disorder characterized by a cluster of signs and symptoms customarily occurring together. This includes such items as the type of seizure, etiology, anatomy, precipitating factors, age of onset, severity, chronicity, diurnal and circadian cycling, and sometimes prognosis. There is a great deal of semantic inconsistancy and confusion in classification and terminology of epileptic conditions. Misleading and outdated terminology continues to reappear in lectures and publications.

Epileptic syndromes are recognized by their characteristic electrophysiological manifestation, their clinical seizure type, and constellation of other recognizable signs and symptoms. Many of them have identifiable ages of onset, family histories, and clinical courses. Of all signs and symptoms, recurrent seizures remain the primary manifestation of a syndrome and helps to separate epileptic syndromes from another heredodegenerative or progressive metabolic illness whose course may become complicated by recurrent seizures. For example, phenylketonuria is a metabolic disorder whose course is complicated by seizures. Benign rolandic epilepsy is a seizure disorder without other signs.

C. Reactive Epileptic Seizures

Differentiation of reactive epileptic seizures from reflex epilepsies can be difficult. *Reactive epileptic seizures*, single or repeated, are a type of seizure that occur only when provoked by transient noxious events. They do not occur spontaneously and their interictal EEG is normal. Reactive seizures are an abnormal reaction of a normal brain to physiological stress or transient epileptic insult. Examples are the seizures that accompany meningitis or encephalitis, and reactive seizures should be distinguished from reflex epilepsy when epileptic seizures are triggered by a specific stimulating agent [23, pp. 3–21]. Triggering factors in reflex epilepsies are not epileptogenic in a nonpredisposed person: for example, photic stimuli in photogenic epilepsy, or hyperventilation in absence epilepsy.

III. CLASSIFICATION OF EPILEPTIC SEIZURES

A. Background

The International League Against Epilepsy (ILAE) has adopted two classifications: one for epileptic seizures and another for epilepsies and epileptic syndromes. Although there is a disagreement among experts, it has been proved to be an important means of communication between centers and presents a compromised framework for the study of epilepsy. Classification of seizures is based on their clinical symptomatology supplemented by EEG data.

The initial classification of epileptic seizures in 1969 was published by the International League Against Epilepsy. This classification presented two major categories of seizures (focal and generalized) and a third category of secondary generalization of partial seizures. The 1969 classification was revised in 1981.

Although this classification is intended to be clinically oriented, some seizures cannot be classified accurately based on their clinical features. As a result, the EEG has become an integral part of this classification [15,16]. Advances in the simultaneous recording of the EEG and the clinical event by closed-circuit television monitoring has further clarified and better defined the clinical variation of some seizures. This information was used in the last classification, which was proposed in 1981 and has remained unchanged until the time of this writing. In the 1981 classification, the previous term *focal seizure* was changed to *partial*. Also, the terms *akinetic*, meaning an arrest or freezing of activity, and *astatic*, referring to an incoordinated, staggering movement, were dropped [24].

The earlier classifications of epileptic seizures were aimed particularly at describing presenting symptoms and elucidating whether a seizure is based primarily on an organic or a hysterical basis [25]. The basic division of classification between generalized and partial seizures, while dating back to Jackson, did not become common usage until accepted by the Commission on Classification of the International League Against Epilepsy (ILAE) in 1969.

Initial classification of seizures was based on a description of the clinical presentation of the event, such as absence, grand mal, petit mal, focal, psychomotor, myoclonic, atonic, and so on. Later, advances in electroencephalography, and more recently, simultaneous video and EEG monitoring have made it possible to recognize several subtypes and variations of different forms of partial and generalized seizures. The 1969 classification distinguished between primary generalized epilepsy and secondary generalization from partial seizures. The other major distinction from previous versions was the division of partial seizures into simple partial and complex partial seizures. The term *complex* was referred to seizures involving intellectual function or interpretive cortex. In the 1981 revision, the term *complex* refers to the impairment of consciousness.

Epileptic seizures are classified into two major types. The first is *partial seizures*, when epileptic discharges and their clinical symptoms are confined to a part of one hemisphere. Depending on the presence or absence of alteration of consciousness, partial seizures are further divided into simple *partial* and *complex* partial seizures. The second is *generalized seizures*, in which the clinical changes indicate simultaneous involvement of both hemispheres.

The epileptic focus may not have a recognizable clinical presentation and may not be electrophysiologically detectable until it reaches neighboring areas or a synaptically related region of the brain with recognizable clinical function. Clinical symptoms may remain localized to the site of discharges or propagate to a larger region and become generalized (secondary generalization). Speed of generalization may be so fast that the initial focus goes unrecognized, both clinically and electroencephalographically.

In younger children and nonverbal patients, motor manifestation, severe autonomic changes, and automatism remain the major alerting symptoms for the caretaker. Inconsistency in terminology, imprecise definition, and confusion in the field of epilepsy arises out of the lack of easily recognizable and localizable clinical signatures for the ictal event in some epileptic seizures. This inconsistency is more noticeable in young children and nonverbal patients.

Although it is very important to distinguish between epileptic seizures and epileptic disorders, knowledge of some epileptic disorders is limited to their phenomenology (seizure type). Temporal lobe epilepsy, psychomotor seizures, limbic seizures, and complex partial seizures of the temporal region and extratemporal region are a few examples of epileptic seizures without a known epileptic disorder. In the 1981 classification of epileptic seizures the descriptive terms used in the 1969 classification, such as grand mal, petit mal, psychomotor, and focal seizures, were eliminated and replaced by concise and more accurate definitions. The main attention is directed to signs and symptoms of the initial presentation of the seizures and their cortical location. In clinical practice, differentiation of localization-related (focal) seizures from generalized seizures is the first step in classification of the patient's seizure. The next step is assessment of consciousness, whether it is intact or impaired. In difficult cases simultaneous evaluation of EEG and video recording has proven to be very helpful.

It should be kept in mind that the localization of seizure onset in a part of the brain does not necessarily mean that a pathologic lesion is in that area [26]. The present classification is based more on the functional aspect of the cortical site of discharges than on the localization of an anatomic change.

B. Brief Definition of Some Common Seizures and Their Salient Features

1. Generalized Seizures

a. Atonic Seizures. Ictal attacks are manifested by sudden loss of postural tone and falling. A fragmentary attack may cause segmental weakness such as a head or limb drop. The duration of these seizures is very short and the EEG shows a slow spike or a multiple spike and wave of 1 to 2.5 Hz. This type of seizure is frequently seen in childhood epileptic encephalopathy with diffuse slow spike–waves (Lennox–Gastaut syndrome).

b. Myoclonic Seizures. These seizures consist of involuntary contractions of limb and truncal muscles which are sudden, brief, and recurrent. They may be localized or generalized. Myoclonic jerks may have cortical, subcortical, brainstem, or spinal cord origin (see Chapter 9).

c. Tonic–Clonic Seizures. The ictal event is manifested by sudden onset of a high-pitched cry, caused by forcible expiration with involuntary contraction of respiratory and laryngeal muscles. These episodes are followed by stiffness of the body and tonic contraction of the axial and limb muscles. The legs extend, the arms flex, and respiration stops. At this stage, cyanosis is noted and the tonic stage is followed by clonic movement. At times, the tongue is bitten by contraction of masticatory muscles. Urinary incontinence may occur. Increased salivation and deep breathing cause frothing at the mouth. This stage is followed by diffuse relaxation, unconsciousness, and postictal sleep. Upon awakening, the patient is confused and sleepy and may show signs of autonomic dysfunction. The patient is amnestic for the entire event.

d. Simple Absence Seizures. Seizures are characterized by a short interruption of consciousness manifested by a blank stare lasting from 3 to 30 s. No auras or focal symptoms are noted. Flickering of the eyelids or eyebrows and upward deviation of the eyes are accompaniments.

e. Complex Absence Seizures. This term is used when absences are associated with postural changes, such as mild clonic movements, an atonic attack causing the patient to fall, or a tonic deviation of the head.

f. Atypical Absence Seizures. In atypical absence, the atonic component, autonomic changes, and automatisms are more pronounced. Onset and termination of seizures are less clear than in simple absence seizures. Complex and atypical absence seizures can be very similar.

2. Partial Seizures

a. Simple Partial Seizures. Simple partial seizures are characterized by a limited spread of the discharges and no loss of consciousness. There is clinical and EEG evidence of a localized onset.

1. *Simple motor seizures*. Any part of the body may be activated. Epileptic discharges may remain localized or become disseminated to adjacent areas; Jacksonian march.

2. *Sensory seizures*. Seizures may manifest by simple visual, auditory, olfactory, gustatory, or vertiginous feelings, flashing lights, buzzing, or unpleasant odors.

3. *Somatosensory seizures*. Consciousness is maintained and the patient complains of feeling numbness, deadness, and a pins-and-needles sensation. These types of seizures have to be differentiated from other paroxysmal nonepileptic events such as atypical migraine, paroxysmal vertigo, and emotional disorders. An electroencephalogram or video-EEG monitoring is helpful.

4. *Psychic seizures*. Psychic seizures consist of impairment of memory (dysmnesia) of various types, such as deja vu, jamais vu, flashback experiences of previous events, and forced thinking (thought or series of recollections intrude upon the mind). Affective symptoms presenting as fear or depression, smiling, laughter, or intense fear; objective autonomic signs such as pupillary dilatation, palpitation, perspiration, pallor, flushing, illusions, or distorted perceptions; and visual distortions such as change of size, distance, symmetry, or shape of objects are seen in simple or complex partial seizures. Distortion of

sounds, such as increased sensitivity or cyclic fluctuation of a sound or melody, a feeling of floating, or depersonalization are frequent in complex partial seizures of temporal lobe origin [12].

b. Complex Partial Seizures. Complex partial seizures of temporal lobe origin may begin with emotional, psychic, illusionary, hallucinatory, or unusual sensory symptoms. After this aura, the patient performs semipurposeful activity (automatism) such as picking at clothes, examining nearby objects, walking about, or more elaborate behavior. The patient is amnestic for these events and may resist efforts to be restrained. These episodes last 1 to 3 min and the patient remains unaware of his or her activities. Clouding of consciousness with automatic behavior and amnesia can be the initial symptom. Seizures originating from the frontal, parietal, or occipital region may produce identical symptoms (i.e., complex partial seizures). Frontal complex partial seizures usually begin with a blank stare and often occur in clusters. Seizures arising from occipital and posterior temporal are more likely to cause visual hallucinations. Anteromedial temporal seizures may be associated with a sense of an unpleasant odor and ictal automatic behavior. Automatisms may occur after epileptic discharges have propagated bilaterally. Automatisms are also seen in seizures of nonfocal origin.

IV. PATHOPHYSIOLOGY OF IDIOPATHIC SEIZURES

The pathophysiologic basis of the seizures of idiopathic (primary) generalized epilepsy has been studied by many investigators with contradictory results. The centrencephalic theory of primary generalized seizures promoted by Penfield and Jasper in 1954 [5] postulated the subcortical origin of seizure in a nonspecific rostral brainstem structure, especially the thalamus at the center of the encephalon, to be responsible for the sudden and generalized cortical discharges. Other investigators were unable to document thalamic discharges preceding cortical discharges. Thus they suggested that the brainstem plays no role and seizures start from the cortex and rapidly spread throughout both hemispheres via intra- and interhemispheric association pathways, rather than starting from deep midline structure. The present view of Gloor and co-workers presents the corticoreticular theory of primary generalized epilepsy, which suggests that the principal element is the diffuse hyperexcitability of the cortex. When the hyperexcitable zone is sufficiently great, it transforms the cortical spindles produced by the thalmocortical volleys into bursts of spike-and-wave complexes. The pathogenesis of the seizures of idiopathic (primary) partial epilepsies and the epileptic focus in the absence of any discernible lesion is now unclear. Gastaut and Gloor [5] believe that there is a localized increased hyperexcitability of neural aggregates and offer a hypothesis similar to primary generalized epilepsy, the only difference being that this hyperexcitability is limited to the part of the cortex causing partial seizures. Local abnormalities in amino acid metabolism, focal deefferentation resulting in hyperexcitability, and restricted corticoreticular dysfunction limited to a single corticothalamic sector have all been proposed as the possible pathogenesis of idiopathic (primary) focal epilepsies. Gastaut [5] has proposed a hypothesis based on local dysmetabolism caused by the structural and functional changes in an individual with genetic predisposition for epilepsy. An abnormal synaptogenesis, disorders of elimination of axonal collaterals, dysmaturation, and abnormal cortical efferentation also have been considered important factors for development of focal epileptogenic processes.

V. CLASSIFICATION OF EPILEPSIES

A. Background

In 1985, the proposal for classification of epilepsy and epileptic syndromes, as opposed to the classification of seizures, was published by ILAE. Despite some inconsistency and difficulty to apply this classification in daily practice, it is gaining popularity among epileptologists. The classification recognizes a dichotomy between disorders manifesting as generalized or partial seizures, and separates idiopathic and symptomatic epilepsies. Epileptic disorders are divided into two major classes of generalized and localization related epilepsies, and each class is subdivided into symptomatic (secondary to preceding diseases) and idiopathic (primary). Some syndromes may be assigned to either idiopathic or symptomatic, as there may not be sufficient evidence for their definitive categorization. The terms *primary* and *secondary* are replaced by *idiopathic* and *symptomatic*, respectively. The terms *focal*, *local*, and *partial* have been replaced by the term *localization-related epilepsies*. It is also recognized that some patients may have both generalized and localization-related seizures. The category of undetermined epilepsies is reserved for those disorders in which the type of seizure cannot be ascertained as to localization related or generalized. There also is a separate category for special syndromes. In practice, about one-fourth of epileptic syndromes cannot be classified, because they are atypical, rare, or because of insufficient information. Examples are patients with electrical status epilepticus during sleep and the Landau–Kleffner syndrome of acquired epileptic aphasia [5]. The 1985 classification was revised in 1989, which represents a consensus statement compatible with the view of the majority of international epileptologists [11].

B. Localization-Related Epilepsies and Syndromes

1. Benign Childhood Epilepsy with Centrotemporal Spikes (Benign Rolandic Epilepsy)

This condition was first described in 1958 by Nayrac and Beaussart [27]. It is a frequent childhood seizure with the age of onset in the first decade of life and with spontaneous resolution during the second decade. The onset of the disease is between the ages of 2 and 14 years, and more commonly between 5 and 10 years [28,29]. Seizures are usually nocturnal and manifested by unilateral facial twitches, cessation of speech, and excessive salivation. Cessation of speech should be distinguished from true aphasia. Frequently, parents are awakened by noises from the child's room and the child is found with drooling and twitching or jerking, usually of an arm and one side of the face. In benign rolandic seizures, the child cannot talk due to motor interference and involvement of the articulatory muscles during the seizure, not due to epileptic involvement of language centers in the cortex.

Consciousness remains intact and the patient can describe the event unless secondary generalization occurs. Sometimes attacks start with a somatosensory aura, usually involving the tongue, cheek, or gums. According to Loiseau [28], 50% of patients with benign rolandic epilepsy have fewer than 5 seizures and only 8% have 20 seizures or more. As its name implies, the prognosis is excellent [29a].

Benign rolandic epilepsy has been reported in several members of the same or successive generations, suggesting a genetic predisposition [30]. It is frequently seen in more than one member of the family and some siblings may never develop clinical symptoms despite the typical EEG abnormalities. This type of epilepsy has a very typical EEG pattern [31,28]. Computerized tomography (CT) scans in these children are always normal [32]. Seizures can be so infrequent, and limited to sleep, that therapy with anticonvulsants is not indicated.

The term *benign epilepsy* implies that no severe seizures capable of leaving residua occur and that there is no evidence of intellectual or neurological deterioration during the course of this epilepsy [29]. Given the frequency of the condition, benign rolandic epilepsy may occasionally occur in brain-damaged children, but the brain damage and the rolandic epilepsy are not related [29]. It is considered that midtemporal EEG foci are controlled by a single dominant gene with age-dependent penetrance [33]. Benign rolandic epilepsy also is seen in conjunction with other genetic epileptic propensities, particularly febrile seizure and generalized epilepsy. It is estimated that benign rolandic epilepsy constitutes 16% of epileptic patients in an epilepsy outpatient service [34]. The incidence of benign rolandic epilepsy is quite high. The prevalence of rolandic seizures is four to seven times that of petit mal epilepsy [35]. The disorder accounts for 11.5 to 25% of epilepsies of school-age children.

Variability of the total number of seizures may range from 1 in the entire course of the syndrome up to several daily seizures. Ninety-eight percent of patients are seizure-free by 12 years of age. If therapy is indicated, seizures are easy to control with antiepileptic drugs. Most antiepileptic drugs used in partial epilepsy are effective and one should chose one with the least likelihood of adversities.

Oropharyngeal involvement in benign rolandic seizures can be differentiated from the alimentary automatisms of complex partial seizures by absence of impairment of consciousness and the typical EEG changes of rolandic epilepsy [29]. Rarely, patients may have a combination of rolandic foci and bursts of 3-Hz spike-and-wave complexes during wakefulness with or without typical or atypical absences. A combination of this picture in cases with bilateral rolandic discharges should not be mistaken for Lennox–Gastaut syndrome [33].

Electroencephalographically, spike discharges are localized over the midtemporal- central region and may be unilateral or bilateral. Typically, these discharges become very abundant during sleep. Background activities of the electroencephalogram will remain normal and appropriate for the patient's age. The EEG tends to normalize and seizures tend to disappear around puberty. Occasionally, the epileptogenic foci arise from another area of the hemisphere (parietal, frontal, or occipital) [29]. The EEG abnormality persists for several years after the seizures are controlled. The EEG abnormality does not correlate with the severity of the clinical seizure disorder. Typically, the spikes increase in number during both non-rapid eye movement (REM) and REM sleep, but are more frequent during non-REM sleep [29]. The EEG may remain unchanged, even with effective treatment [35]. About 50 to 70% of children with rolandic spikes have an associated seizure disorder. Forty percent of patients with typical EEG changes of rolandic epilepsy never develop seizures in their life [36].

As rolandic discharges similar to those seen in benign rolandic epilepsy are seen in children with cerebral damage, there remains the question of neuroradiological workup in children with benign rolandic epilepsy. Blom and Heigbel [37] concluded that the clinical picture and neurological findings in each patient must be the decisive factor rather than the morphology of spikes, presentation of seizures, or localization of epileptic activities. In most patients the partial nature of seizures warrants imaging such as CT or magnetic resonance imaging (MRI) of the head [37].

2. Benign Occipital Epilepsy

This syndrome is recognized by the presence of continuous spike discharges arising from the occipital region which cease with eye opening [38]. There is also an occipital epilepsy with continuous spike–waves which is not necessarily benign [39]. Benign occipital epilepsy has a male predominance. Seizures start with visual symptoms (amaurosis, phosphenes, illusions, or hallucinations) and are often followed by hemiclonic seizures or automatisms [40]. In 25% of patients, seizures are followed by migrainous headaches (see Chapter 1). Seizures may propagate to the motor or temporal lobe and cause hemiclonic movement or complex partial seizures. Nausea and vomiting are not uncommon during the postictal period. The syndrome of benign occipital epilepsy usually starts at the age of 6 years with visual symptoms that may be followed by hemisensory, hemimotor, or complex partial phenomena. Temporal-occipital spikes also have been reported in adolescents who had vascular migraine and occasional focal or generalized seizures with an aura [41]. Typically, the EEG shows high-amplitude spike-and-wave discharges in the occipital region. At times, discharges are bilaterally synchronous with propagation toward the posterior temporal region.

Association of this syndrome with childhood absence epilepsy and benign rolandic epilepsy has been reported [42]. Occasionally, headaches are seen during the ictal event. In this situation this syndrome can be differentiated from vascular migraine because of the severe epileptic EEG abnormalities. Gastaut reports a 19% incidence of family history of migraines in children with benign occipital epilepsy. The exact prognosis of this condition is not known. Full remission of seizures has been reported in 92% of patients by the age of 19 years. In some patients with vascular migraine, interictal EEG abnormalities identical to benign occipital epilepsy are seen, which may suggest a relationship between the two conditions. A syndrome similar to the benign occipital epilepsy may be seen in children with lesional epilepsies [43, pp. 112–39].

3. Temporal Lobe Epilepsy

Partial seizures with complex symptomatology usually arises from the temporal lobe. The term *complex* implies impairment of consciousness. This term should not be used interchangeably with psychomotor seizures, as psychomotor symptoms are seen in other types of epilepsies. Complex partial seizures may have a temporal or extra temporal origin. *Simple partial seizures of temporal lobe origin* may evolve into complex partial seizures causing impairment of consciousness. Recognition of these early signs are important and difficult in children. Seizures arising from the temporal lobe are typically characterized by autonomic and/or psychic symptoms, and certain sensory phenomena, such as olfactory, auditory, oral, and alimentary automatism with postictal confusion and amnesia [11].

Recognition of complex partial seizures in the pediatric age group is difficult especially when the condition is caused by a secondary propagation of discharges to the hippocampal region and the initial simple partial phase has gone unnoticed. Identification of the initial simple partial phase is an important factor to distinguish complex partial seizure from generalized absence. The initial phase helps to localize or to lateralize the involved hemisphere. Aura, the onset of the seizure, may be vague gastrointestinal complaints or complex automatisms.

Automatisms, an ictal symptom, consist of behaviors that occur in association with a state of impaired consciousness and amnesia during or following a seizure. The individual fails to imprint memories. It may manifest by simple actions such as chewing, swallowing, licking, picking at and straightening one's clothes, walking from one room to another, rearranging objects on a desk, partial undressing, or walking out of a building into the street. This state of complete amnesia, depressed responsiveness, and automatic activity indicates bilateral dysfunction of brain. Mimetic, verbal, sexual, and ambulatory autom atism have been reported in complex partial seizures of temporal lobe origin. Reactive automatisms may not be stereotyped, as they are determined by environmental stimuli [23,pp.150–56].

Different types of automatism have been recognized by videotape studies of children with complex partial seizures [44]; among them, gestural, alimentary, verbal, and aimless motor activities are very frequent. The automatism usually happens after the child's consciousness has been impaired. Automatisms can also be seen during the postictal phase.

Autonomic symptoms, an unusual ictal symptom such as thirst, and desire to micturate are noted in some forms of seizures. Autonomic symptoms, sensory or motor phenomena, or psychic symptoms manifested by fear, dread, and apprehension are common in complex partial seizures. Alimentary symptoms such as tongue movement, swallowing, lip smacking, repetitive sucking, and chewing are more frequent in younger children. The most common behavioral changes in infants are cessation of activities and eye deviation.

It is not known what percentage of complex partial seizures have an identifiable etiology. A long list of etiological factors, such as birth asphyxia, head injury, neoplasm, infection, and malformation, has been reported in children with complex partial seizures. A prospective study has not supported the relationship between a history of febrile convulsions in infancy and complex partial seizures.

Engel [23, pp. 150–56] recognizes typical and atypical complex partial seizures. Some forms of atypical absence with focal or lateralized presentation may resemble complex partial seizures, and some partial seizures of extratemporal origin may be associated with impairment of consciousness without invading the temporal lobe.

Various EEG patterns have been reported which may show unilateral or bilateral interruption of background activity, low-amplitude fast activities, rhythmic spikes and rhythmic slow waves, or may not show any abnormality. Ictal discharges may propagate to the entire hemisphere or both hemispheres, giving a pattern of generalized tonic–clonic seizure (secondary generalization). Interictal discharges on the EEG may be seen over the temporal region. Discharges may be arising from the frontal or occipital regions. A normal EEG in children with complex partial seizures is not uncommon. The ictal EEG may remain unchanged during the simple partial phase of complex partial seizures. It may be associated with attenuation of background rhythm or focal paroxysmal rhythmic discharges. Depth electrode studies during complex partial seizures have revealed bilateral mesial temporal discharges as the most common electrophysiological correlate [23, pp. 150–56].

Hippocampal seizures (amygdalohippocampal) are the most common form of temporal lobe seizures causing complex partial symptomatology. Rising epigastric discomfort, nausea, pallor, flushing of the face, pupillary dilatation, fear, panic, and olfactory-gustatory hallucinations are frequent clinical warnings of an ictal event. The interictal scalp EEG may be normal or may manifest with unilateral or bilateral sharp or slow waves. Bilateral interictal discharges may be synchronous or asynchronous.

Complex partial seizures of temporal lobe origin is one of the most intractable and commonly encountered seizure type when all age groups are considered. In one study, 17% of children with complex partial seizures underwent spontaneous recovery [45]. It constitutes 42% of partial seizures and 26% of all seizures [46]. Forty-two percent of patients with temporal lobe epilepsy have an onset of some form of convulsive phenomena in the first decade of life [47]. In the Ounsted report on 100 children with temporal lobe epilepsy, approximately one-third were known to have preexisting brain insult of varying etiology, one-third had a history of status epilepticus in early life, and one-third had no definite cause [89,48]. Herniation of the medial and inferior parts of the temporal lobe secondary to brain edema caused by birth injury has been considered an important factor [49]. Hippocampal sclerosis is bilateral in more than 50% of patients [23, pp. 150–56]. Manifestation of the simple partial temporal lobe may go undetected or unreported by the patient, due to retrograde amnesia.

4. Lateral Temporal Epilepsy

Complex partial seizures originating in the lateral temporal lobe are frequently associated with auditory hallucinations, illusions, or a dreamy state. Lateral temporal discharges may propagate and clinical symptoms evolve to complex partial seizures if it affects the mesial temporal or extratemporal structures. Clinically, the patient may present complex motor automatism, fumbling, picking, repetitive activity, or motionless stare. Older children and adults may describe more complex perceptual disturbances, such as micropsia, macropsia, and complex visual hallucinations.

Dysmnesic phenomena, psychic, automatic manifestation, illusion, and hallucination are frequently seen in this condition. Auditory, visual, and vertiginous experience frequently are caused by lateral temporal or occipital cortex, which may or may not propagate into medial temporal structures. Ictal dysmnesic symptoms represent distorted memory experiences and inappropriate feelings of familiarity. Ictal cognitive disturbances consist of depersonalization, dream states, and distortion of time sense. Recognition of these symptoms is very difficult in childhood.

It is important to differentiate impairment of consciousness in complex partial seizures from postictal amnesia or other cognitive or psychic phenomena of unilateral hippocampal involvement. Impairment of consciousness will always suggest bilateral hippocampal involvement during the ictal event, which may or may not have bilateral expression on the EEG. At times, preexisting injury to one hippocampal region causes impairment of consciousness during unilateral ictal event in the hippocampus. Impairment of consciousness may be the only clinical manifestation of a complex partial seizure. Motionless stares are also very frequent [50].

Epileptic discharges arising from other areas of the cortex present with specific features. Epileptic discharges in the occipital lobe are frequently associated with ocular symptoms and visual disturbances but may propagate to the lateral temporal lobe. Complex partial seizures arising from the frontal lobe are frequently associated with postural or motor symptomatology. Behavioral and automatism, which are seen in patients with complex partial seizures, could be a postictal phenomenon. The relationship between behavior disorders and temporal lobe epilepsy remains controversial. Psychosocial disturbances are frequent in temporal lobe epilepsy.

In contrast to their relatively high incidence of medical intractability, temporal lobe epilepsies are more likely than other types of epilepsy to respond to surgical resection (see Chapter 14).

C. Epilepsies and Syndromes: Undetermined as Focal or Generalized Epilepsy

Acquired epileptic aphasia (Landau–Kleffner syndrome) is in the category of epilepsies and syndromes which are undetermined as to whether they are focal or generalized. It was first described by Landau and Kleffner [51] in 1957. Symptoms begin in early childhood after the development of language. There is gradual loss of language function and the appearance of interictal epileptiform discharges on the EEG. The electroencephalogram later demonstrates bilaterally synchronous diffuse spike-and-wave activities. The preponderance of discharges are over the temporal lobe and at times are localized only in the temporal region. As this disease progresses, the EEG abnormalities became more continuous. Generally, seizures are seen only several years after the loss of language. Some patients never develop an epileptic seizure. Seizures are mild and have a tendency to remit with or without treatment, but the aphasia usually persists. The etiology is unknown. Focal inflammatory changes resembling Rasmussen syndrome has been reported in a few cases [52]. This syndrome should be differentiated from (1) transient aphasia following partial epilepsies, (2) complex partial seizures, and (3) unilateral status epilepticus. Onset of seizures has been as early as 18 months and as late as 13 years. The usual age is between 4 and 7 years. Language disturbance will develop over a brief period of time [53]. Behavior disturbance is reported in 66% of patients. Seizures may also be the first manifestation of this syndrome. The type of seizure is nonspecific and could be partial motor, generalized, complex partial, or atypical absences with atonia or generalized tonic–clonic [43, pp. 176–82]. Present evidence, based on EEG and neuropsychological findings, suggests bilateral brain involvement. An unproven hypothesis is the possibility of functional exclusion of both temporal lobes in language processing due to repetitive electrographic discharges [43, pp. 176–82]. The majority of seizures are generalized or simple partial motor. Suggested etiologies are (1) subcortical dysfunction affecting cortical function by process of deefferentation, (2) low-grade focal inflammatory process, and (3) subacute inflammatory process with a self-limiting course [43, pp. 176–82;52;53]. Language dysfunction is predominantly the deficit of auditory comprehension, which is progressive over a period of weeks or months. An abrupt cessation of language function or sudden aggravation also has been reported [54]. Writing and visioverbal ability is relatively well preserved. Intellectual function of the patient is usually well preserved. EEG findings are quite variable and at times show multifocal discharges that resemble benign partial epilepsy of childhood [53]. Discharges may be more frequent in the right hemisphere. The discharges disappear by the age of 15 years [55,56].

Some investigators have reported a correlation between the abundance of spike discharges during sleep and language deterioration and have found that the presence of continuous spike–wave activity during slow sleep corresponds with regression of language function. The ultimate outcome is still unclear [43, pp. 176–82]. In one study, 33% of patients had normal language and 66% had some degree of residual deficit [57]. Treatment has little effect on language recovery. The CT scan is normal. Anticonvulsant therapy is recommended if seizures are a significant problem [48, pp. 153–80].

D. Generalized Epilepsy

1. Absence Epilepsy

In 1769, Tissot had used the term *petit* in describing a young girl whose attacks were characterized by "a momentary loss of consciousness, cutting short her speech and by slight trembling of the eyes" [58]. Esquirol has used this term for various minor seizures, including vertiginous attacks. Gowers has used *petit mal* and *minor seizures* interchangeably, and Jackson has used the term *petit mal* to describe "slight cases of epilepsy, beginning by loss of consciousness" [59]. Now the term *absence seizures* refer to a sudden interruption of activities with a bland stare. When spoken to, the patient is usually unresponsive. A momentary lapse of consciousness is also a common phenomenon in complex partial seizures. When a complex partial seizure is brief, it can mimic generalized absence epilepsies.

Klass and Daly were first to demonstrate that absence attacks may range from a simple momentary arrest to complicated automatic movements resembling those seen during seizures of temporal lobe origin, such as chewing, swallowing, and lip smacking. From a behavioral point of view, an observer cannot, with certainty, distinguish such seizures as arising in the temporal lobe or belonging to the group of absence attacks [59,60].

Childhood absence has an age of onset of 4 to 8 years. The absences are brief, usually less than 20 s, with a typical EEG spike-and-wave pattern of 2.5 to 3.5 Hz during the seizure. There is a strong genetic predisposition condition, and absences are seen more frequently in females. Hyperventilation is an effective procedure to reproduce typical clinical and electroencephalographic findings in patients with absence seizures. Untreated, they are easily provoked by hyperventilation. The prognosis of childhood absences is very good. Tonic–clonic seizures have been reported in about 40% of patients with absence seizures, but they usually appear in adolescence. When absence seizures begin in adolescence, the frequency of spells is less, but the possibility of generalized tonic–clonic seizures is much higher and may even begin prior to the onset of absences. A family history of epilepsy or febrile convulsions is noted in 15 to 25% of close relatives of patients with absence seizures [61,62].

In general, complex partial seizures with absences are preceded by an aura and their duration is longer than that of true absences. Postictal confusion and complex automatisms are also helpful to differentiate these two conditions. Interictal discharges are the main clue in cases that cannot be distinguished clinically.

The EEG cannot always differentiate these two conditions. Even in complex partial seizures, discharges may be generalized due to the location of the focus on the medial surface of the frontal region or bilateral inferior mesial temporal lobe and rapid generalization. Absences in primary generalized epilepsy are associated with (1) a normal background EEG, (2) lack of focal neurological signs or mental retardation, and (3) typical 3-Hz bursts of spikes and slow waves. Absences in secondary generalized epilepsy, complex partial seizures, are frequently associated with (1) focal seizures, usually of tonic or atonic type, (2) cognitive impairment, (3) diffuse slowing of the background electroencephalogram, and (4) bursts of spike–wave discharges at a frequency of 1.5 to 2.5 Hz.

The frequency of spells may range from a few to many per day. Rarely, absence may persist during adult life. Favorable prognostic factors in typical absence epilepsy are (1) absence of generalized tonic–clonic seizures, (2) normal intelligence, and (3) a negative family history of seizure disorders.

Juvenile absence epilepsy starts around puberty. The number of seizures are less than childhood absence, but generalized tonic–clonic seizures are more frequent. Spike discharges are often faster than 3 Hz. Occasionally, myoclonic seizures accompany this type of epilepsy.

The hallmark of the absence attack is a sudden onset, with interruption of ongoing activities, a blank stare, possibly a brief upward rotation of the eyes, and maintenance of postural tone. The patient is amnestic during the period of the attack. The attack may last from a few seconds to $\frac{1}{2}$ min and is always associated with impairment of consciousness. Mild clonic movement affecting the eyelids or facial muscles, and a reduction of muscle tone, when severe, may cause drop attacks. Tonic muscular contraction and automatism, such as aimless walking, swallowing, fumbling, or grunting, may be noted during the complex absence attack.

The characteristic EEG pattern of childhood absence was first described by Gibbs [63]. The detailed clinical manifestation of absence seizures, based on video recording, has been studied by Penry and co-workers. It involves fine clonic twitching movements and automatisms [64]. The susceptibility for developing or manifesting concurrent generalized tonic–clonic seizures is less in childhood absence than in the juvenile type [65].

Epidemiological data indicate that absence epilepsy is a genetic disease. Studies on typical absence seizures have revealed that monozygotic twins have a 75% concordance for clinical absence seizures and an 84% concordance for 3-Hz spike and wave trait on their EEGs [66]. Metrakos and Metrakos [8,67] concluded that a 3-Hz spike is inherited in an autosomal dominant mode with an age-dependent penetrance. Penetrance is low at birth, rise rapidly to a maximum of about 40% around the age of 10 years, and gradually declines to near zero after the age of 40. Only one-fifth of patients with the spike-and-wave trait will have clinical seizures. Andermann [68] postulated and provided evidence in support of the concept of multifactorial inheritance of generalized and focal epilepsies. In this view, clinical manifestations, EEG features, prognosis, and response to therapy will completely change, for example, when a patient with absence seizures demonstrates evidence of brain damage [19,69].

Absence seizures constitute 3 to 4% of all patients with epilepsy. Three-hertz spike-and-wave complexes are also prevalent in close relatives of probands with febrile convulsions or focal seizures. In 14% of patients with absence epilepsy, the illness starts with both petit mal and tonic–clonic convulsions. Siblings and offspring of patients with absence seizures are at a 50% risk of inheriting spike-and-wave abnormalities in their electroencephalograms but a 12% risk of having one of the generalized seizures and an 8% risk of having absence epilepsy [8].

Patients with classical absences may have as many as several hundred seizures per day. The term *pyknolepsy* is applied to this type of epilepsy (*pyknos* means "crowded clusters"). Automatism, which involves quasi-purposeful movement is seen in prolonged absence seizures. Eighty-eight percent of patients with atypical absence have been seen to have automatic behavior during video recording [64]. Autonomic dysfunctions such as pupillary dilation, color changes, and excessive salivation are also noted during absence seizures. Impairment of consciousness may go clinically undetected if the duration is brief (i.e., less than 3 s). However, neuropsychological testing, or activities that demand continuous performance tasks and response testing, may detect cognitive dysfunction even if discharge duration is less than 3 s. Postictal confusion is not seen in absence.

In atypical absence, postural changes such as tonic axial movement and atonic drops are frequent. Onset or cessation of attacks is not abrupt. Spike-and-wave discharges on the EEG are irregular and often asymmetrical. Background activities of the EEG are usually abnormal in atypical absence epilepsy. Many of these patients fit more in the category of secondary bilateral synchrony than primary generalized absence [70].

Epilepsy with myoclonic absence and juvenile myoclonic epilepsy are discussed in Chapter 9, as myoclonic jerks remains a prominent feature of these types of epilepsies. From an EEG point of view, epilepsy with myoclonic absence resembles absence seizures.

2. Lennox–Gastaut Syndrome

In the recent international classification of epilepsies, the Lennox–Gastaut syndrome appears in the category of generalized epilepsies and syndromes, the subtype of cryptogenic or symptomatic. This syndrome appears in preschool-age children and is manifested by mixed seizure types (i.e., tonic, atonic, and absences). Other types of seizures, such as myoclonic and generalized tonic–clonic, can also occur. A history of a previous encephalopathy, either intrauterine or acquired postnatal, is seen in 60% of the cases. This syndrome was originally described by Lennox and Davis [71,72]. Later, Gastaut gave a full description of the clinical and EEG presentation of this syndrome [70]. The typical clinical symptoms can be summarized in a triad of multiple seizure types, mental retardation, and slow spike and waves in the EEG [73]. The peak age of onset is between 3 and 5 years, but the condition can start as early as 1 year of age. Seizures may be more frequent during sleep.

Atonic attacks cause frequent falls or may be limited to brief head nods. Patients may have frequent absence attacks in which the onset and termination of the attack are less obvious than in typical absence seizures. Lennox–Gastaut syndrome is slightly more frequent in males.

The interictal EEG shows slowing of the background activities with generalized slow spike-and-wave bursts of 1.5 to 2.5 Hz. During tonic seizures, bursts of 10- to 20-Hz rhythmic high-voltage fast frequency are seen in all leads. Historically, the term *petit mal variant* was coined by Gibbs in patients with EEG discharges of slow rhythmic spike–waves and was differentiated from typical 3-Hz spike waves in petit mal seizures [72,74,75]. In 1945, Lennox differentiated this syndrome from typical petit [71]. The full clinical presentation of the disease was described first by Sorel in 1964 and by Gastaut in 1966 [74,76]. It was Gastaut who under the heading "Childhood Epileptic Encephalopathy with Diffuse Slow Spike-Waves," discussed the EEG and clinical picture and proposed the term *Lennox syndrome* [74,76,77]. Initially, the terms *petit mal variant*, *myokinetic epilepsy*, and *petit mal akinetique* were used until extensive review by several investigators characterized this condition as a syndrome with a triad of mixed epileptic seizures, EEG abnormalities, and mental retardation.

The prevalence of Lennox–Gastaut syndrome is about 3 to 10.7% of the epilepsies based on conclusive criteria by several authors [78]. The first seizure may be focal or generalized, and can be brief or prolonged. The etiology of the preexisting encephalopathies, when known, is heterogeneous. In 20 to 30% of the cases the etiology remains unknown. Onset of the disease after the age of 10 years is uncommon.

Tonic seizures are the most common type of seizure in the Lennox–Gastaut syndrome. Tonic seizures may be global or axial. The tonic activity may spread to the proximal upper limbs with elevations of the shoulders and abduction of the arms [43, pp. 39–65]. Atonic seizures are the most frequent cause of drop attacks in this syndrome. It may not be associated with alteration of consciousness, and patients stand up immediately after a fall. Myoclonic jerks may precede an atonic attack or may involve the upper extremity while the lower extremity undergoes atonic seizures. Absences may be associated with tonic or atonic postural changes. Automatism and autonomic phenomena are frequent. Generalized tonic–clonic attacks are not uncommon. Mental retardation is seen in 20 to 60% of patients with Lennox–Gastaut syndrome before the onset of a seizure, and this may increase to 75 to 93% of patients 5 years after onset [79]. The etiology of progressive intellectual deterioration is unknown. Several factors might contribute, including cessation of learning, multiple antiepileptic drugs, the effect of repeated seizures themselves, and the presence of an ongoing process [43, pp. 39–65]. Approximately 80% of patients will continue to have seizures all their lives. Atypical absences usually do not begin until the age of 4 years [23,pp.3–21]. Regardless of etiology, even in the cryptogenic form, diffuse cortical and subcortical dysfunction is necessary for development of this syndrome [80].

Ictal manifestation may be associated with a short period of flattening of the background rhythm or generalized slow spike–wave activities. Loss of consciousness during absence attacks in this syndrome is less complete than in typical absence epilepsies. Frequently, loss of tone is associated with excessive salivation. Sometimes it is difficult to differentiate on the EEG ictal from interictal discharges. During the absence attack the EEG may continue to show continuous rhythmic 2- to 2.5-Hz discharges. Massive myoclonic attacks may also be seen as another ictal pattern, with an EEG pattern of polyspikes and waves or diffuse slow waves. Status epilepticus is not uncommon in patients with Lennox–Gastaut syndrome and may manifest as a repeated tonic seizures or myoclonic–atonic attacks. Status epilepticus can last for several days or weeks and become refractory to treatment. This syndrome has a chronic course and usually, after a few years, becomes less active. However, the intellectual condition of the patient does not show improvement. A complete seizure-free recovery is exceptional; only 6.7% of Gastaut's 1973 series became seizure-free. In general, the prognosis for normal development is poor [78].

The main indicators of a poor prognosis are (1) symptomatic character of the syndrome, such as Lennox–Gastaut in patients with a previous history of infantile myoclonic spasms or developmental delay; (2) early onset, less than 3 years of age; (3) frequent and intractable seizures and repeated status epilepticus; (4) slowing of background activity on the EEG; and (5) the presence of a localized abnormality on the EEG [78].

Doose has described a syndrome similar to the Lennox–Gastaut syndrome but with normal psychointellectual development. Seizures are more myoclonic or myoclonic–astatic in type. A family history of seizures is more frequent [81,82]. A number of authors have questioned the existence of this entity [83,84]. At times it is called centrencephalic myoclonic–astatic petit mal of Doose. The EEG has a pattern of 4- to 7-Hz theta activity and fast spike–wave discharges.

The treatment of Lennox–Gastaut syndrome is difficult and disappointing [85] (see Chapter 9). Sectioning of the corpus callosum is now being recommended for Lennox–Gastaut patients with medically intractable generalized seizures [43, pp. 39–65].

3. Juvenile Epilepsy with Generalized Tonic–Clonic Seizures

As its name implies, this type of epilepsy is manifested by generalized tonic–clonic seizures, and the usual age of onset is between 14 and 18 years. This form of epilepsy is slightly more predominant in males, some patients have a history of absence seizures at an earlier age, and some may have concomitant absence and generalized tonic–clonic seizures. Distribution of seizures is equal between day and night. A positive family history for febrile seizures or other types of primary generalized epilepsy is reported in 25% of cases. Interictal EEGs are normal and the patient's psychointellectual development is intact [73,86]. Two forms of generalized tonic–clonic epilepsy have been reported: (1) awakening clonic–tonic–clonic epilepsy and (2) primary generalized tonic–clonic epilepsy.

a. Awakening Clonic–Tonic–Clonic Epilepsy. Initial clonic jerks are followed by the tonic phase, when consciousness is lost. The tonic phase lasts only 10 to 20 s and terminates with a final phase of clonic jerks. The clinical hallmark is a stereotyped motor and automatic manifestation with loss of consciousness. Cyanosis and cessation of respiration happens during tonic contraction of diaphragm and intercostal muscles. Generalized tonic phase is terminated with vibratory tremor followed by clonic jerk, which progressively slows down. During this phase, expiratory grunts are noted and the tongue may be bitten during this stage. The clonic phase usually lasts about 1 min and is followed by diffuse muscle relaxation. Careful observation shows that there is a second phase of tonic contraction. Urinary or fecal incontinence is seen in 30% of cases. Other autonomic phenomena, including excessive bronchial secretions, are noted. Some generalized tonic–clonic seizures are immediately preceded by a series of myoclonic jerks [87]. Awakening grand mals start at puberty. This type of epilepsy may be linked to the phenotypes of the genetic substrate of Janz's "impulsive petit mal" [88].

b. Generalized Tonic–Clonic Epilepsy. This disorder is manifested by generalized tonic–clonic seizures. In general, it has a better prognosis than clonic–tonic–clonic seizures [86]. Primary generalized epilepsy of adolescence with generalized tonic–clonic seizures may have its onset as early as 8 to 9 years, but more than two-thirds of patients have their first attack before 19 years of age with peak frequency at 14 to 16 years [43, pp. 100–111]. Seizures usually happen 30 min following awakening, but they may also happen during sleep. Sleep deprivation and sometimes photic stimulation can activate seizures. They also occur 3 or 4 days preceding menstruation. This syndrome has a close relationship with benign juvenile myoclonic epilepsy and epilepsies with typical absence of onset in adolescence. Both type of epilepsies should be differentiated from secondary generalized tonic–clonic convulsions. O'Donohoe reports that 70% of all seizures in childhood are generalized tonic–clonic, but Gastaut [43, pp. 140–75] reports that only 9.5% of the classifiable epilepsies of childhood are primary generalized. Without extensive electrophysiological and video monitoring, it is difficult to separate the secondary generalized tonic–clonic from primary generalized epilepsy. Difficulty arises when the onset of partial seizures do not have clinical presentation until discharges become generalized or generalization from initial focus is very rapid.

REFERENCES

1. Willis T. A full view of all the diseases incident to children. London, 1742:130–31.
2. Underwood M. A treatise on the diseases of children. Philadelphia, 1743:12.
3. Matson RH. Classification of epileptic seizures and classification of epilepsies or epileptic syndromes. In: American academy of neurology. Annual Course 212. 1986:4–8.
4. Babb TL, Brown WJ. Pathological findings in epilepsy. In: Engel J Jr, ed. Surgical treatment of the epilepsies. New York: Raven Press, 1987:511–40.
5. Gastaut H, Zifkin BG. Classification of the epilepsies. Clin Neurophysiol 1985; 2(4):313–26.
6. Gastaut H. Classification of the epilepsies. Proposal for an international classification. Epilepsia 1969; 6:10(Suppl):S14–S21.
7. Merlis JK. Proposal for an international classification of the epilepsies. Epilepsia 1970; 11:114–19.
8. Metrakos K, Metrakos J. Genetics of convulsive disorders. Neurology (Cleve) 1961; 11:474–83.

9. Gloor P. Generalized epilepsy with spike and wave discharge, a reinterpretation of its electrographic and clinical manifestation. Epilepsia 1979; 20:571–88.
10. Andermann E. (1980). Genetic aspects of epilepsy. In: Robb P. ed. Epilepsy updated: causes and treatment. Chicago: Year Book Medical Publishers, Inc., 1980:11–24.
11. Commission on Classification and Terminology of the International League Against Epilepsy. Proposal for classification of epilepsies and epileptic syndromes. Epilepsia 1989; 30(4):389–99.
12. Commission of Classification and Terminology of the International League Against Epilepsy. Proposal for revised clinical and electroencephalographic classification of epileptic seizures. Epilepsia 1981; 22:489–501.
13. Berkovic SF, Andermann F, Andermann E, Gloor P. Concepts of absence epilepsies: discrete syndromes or biological continuum. Neurology 1987; 37:993–1000.
14. Rodin EA. An assessment of current views on epilepsy. Epilepsia 1987; 28(3):267–71.
15. Rodin EA. Some relationships of induced seizure patterns to clinical findings in epileptic patients. Epilepsia 1964; 5:21–32.
16. Gastaut H, Gastaut JL, Goncalves E, Silva GE, Fernandez-Sanches GR. (1975). Relative frequency of different types of epilepsy: a study employing the classification of the International League Against Epilepsy. Epilepsia 1975; 16:456–61.
17. Joshi V, Katiyar BC, Mohan PK, Misra S, Shukla GD. Profile of epilepsy in a developing country: a study of 1,000 patients based on the international classification. Epilepsia 1977; 18:549–54.
18. Granieri E, Rosati G, Tola G, Pavoni M, Paolino E, Pinna L, Monetti VC. A descriptive study of epilepsy in the district of Copparo, Italy, 1964–1978. Epilepsia 1983; 24:502–14.
19. Sata S, Dreifuss FE, Penry JK, Kirby DD, Palesch Y. Long term follow-up of absence seizures. Neurology 1983; 33:1590–95.
20. Keranen T, Sillanpaa M, Riekkinen PJ. Distribution of seizure types in an epileptic population. Epilepsia 1988; 29(11):1–7.
21. Alving J. Classification of epilepsies. An investigation of 1,508 consecutive adult patients. Acta Neurol Scand 1978; 58:205–12.
22. Jackson JH. Selected writings of J. Hughlings Jackson. In: Taylor JA, ed. Epilepsy and epileptiform convulsions. Vol. 1. London: Hodder and Stoughton, 1931.
23. Engel J Jr. Seizures and epilepsy. Philadelphia: FA Davis Company, 1989.
24. Commission of Classification and Terminology of the International League Against Epilepsy. Proposal for classification of epilepsies and epileptic syndromes. Epilepsia 1985; 26(3):268–78.
25. Commission of Classification and Terminology of the International League Against Epilepsy. Proposal for revised clinical and electroencephalographic classification of epileptic seizures. Epilepsia 1981; 22:489–501.
26. Porter RJ. Etiology and classification of epileptic seizures. In: Robb P, ed. Epilepsy updated: causes and treatment. Chicago: Year Book Medical Publishers, Inc., 1980.
27. Nayrac P, Beaussart M. LesPointes-Ondes prerolandiques: expression EEG treis particuliere. Etude electroclinique de 21 cas. Rev Neurol (Paris) 1958; 99:201.

28. Loiseau P, Beaussart M. The seizures of benign childhood epilepsy with rolandic paroxysmal discharges. Epilepsia 1973; 14:381.
29. Aicardi J. Benign rolandic epilepsy. Int Pediatr 1987; 12:176–81.
29a. Loiseau P. et al. Long term prognosis in two forms of childhood epilepsy: typical absence seizures and epilepsy with rolandic (centro temporal) EEG foci. Ann Neurol 1983; 13:642.
30. Aicardi J. The benign epilepsies of childhood. In: Clifford-Rose F, ed. Research progress in epilepsy. London: Pitman Books Ltd., 1983; 231–39.
31. Lombroso CT. Sylvian seizures and midtemporal spike foci in children. Arch Neurol 1967; 17:52.
32. Gastaut HG, Gastaut JL. (1977). Computerized axial tomography in epilepsy. In: Penry JK, ed. Epilepsy. 8th International symposium. New York: Raven Press, 1977:5–15.
33. Aicardi J, Chevrie JJ. Atypical benign epilepsy of childhood. Dev Med Child Neurol 1982; 24:281–92.
34. Heijbel J, Blom S, Bergfors PG. Benign epilepsy with rolandic paroxysmal foci: a study of 324 cases. Epilepsia 1978; 19:337.
35. Loiseau P, Beaussart M. The seizures of benign childhood epilepsy with rolandic paroxysmal discharges. Epilepsia 1973; 14:381–89.
36. Lerman P, Kivity S. The benign focal epilepsies of childhood. In Pedley TA, Meldrum BS, eds. Recent advances in epilepsy. Vol. 3. Edinburgh: Churchill Livingstone, 1986:137–56.
37. Blom S, Heigbel JM. Benign epilepsy of children with centrotemporal EEG foci; a follow-up study in adulthood of patients initially studied as children. Epilepsia 1982; 23:629–32.
38. Gastaut H. A new type of epilepsy: benign partial epilepsy of childhood with occipital spike–waves. Clin Electroencephalogr 1982; 13:13–22.
39. Newton R, Aicardi J. Clinical findings in children with occipital spike–wave complexes suppressed by eye opening. Neurology 1983; 33:1526–29.
40. Dreifuss FE. Pediatric epilepsy syndromes: an overview. Cleve Clin J Med 1989; 56:S166–71.
41. Camfield PR, Metrakos K, Andermann F. Basilar migraine, seizures, and severe epileptiform EEG abnormalities. Neurology 1978; 28:584–88.
42. Gastaut H, Zifkin BG. Benign epilepsy of childhood with occipital spike and wave complexes. In: Andermann F, Lugaresi E, eds. Migraine and epilepsy. Boston: Butterworth 1987:47–81.
43. Aicardi J. Epilepsy in children. New York: Raven Press, 1986.
44. Holmes GL. Partial seizures in children. Pediatrics 1986; 77:725–31.
45. Kotagol P, Rothner AD, Erenberg G, et al. Complex partial seizures of childhood-onset: a five year follow-up study. Arch Neurol 1987; 44:1177–80.
46. Hauser WA, Kurland LT. The epidemiology of epilepsy in Rochester, Minnesota, 1935 through 1967. Epilepsia 1975; 16:1–66.
47. Aird RB, Venturini AM, Spielman PM. Antecedents of temporal lobe epilepsy. Arch Neurol 1967; 16:67–73.
48. O'Donahoe NV. (1985) Epilepsies of childhood. London: Butterworth & Company (Publishers) Ltd., 1985:92–105.

49. Wallace SJ. Neurological and intellectual deficits, convulsions with fever viewed as acute indications of life-long developmental defects. In Brazier MAB, Coceani F, eds. Brain dysfunctions in infantile febrile convulsions. New York: Raven Press, 1976:259–77.
50. Wieser HG. Electroclinical features of psychomotor seizures: stereo-electroencephalographic seizure patterns including clinical effects of intracerebral stimulation. London: Butterworth & Company (Publishers) Ltd., 1983:242.
51. Landau WM, Kleffner FR. Syndrome of acquired aphasia with convulsive disorder in children. Neurology 1957; 7:523–30.
52. Cole AJ, Andermann F, Taylor L, Olivier A, Rasmussen T, Robitaille Y, Spire JP. The Landau–Kleffner syndrome of acquired epileptic aphasia: unusual clinical outcome, surgical experience and absence of encephalitis. Neurology 1988; 38:31–38.
53. Beaumanoir A. The Landau–Kleffner syndrome. In: Roger J, Dravet C, Bureau M, Dreifuss FE, Wolf P, eds. Epileptic syndrome in infancy, childhood and adolescence. London: John Libbey Eurotext Ltd., 1985:181–91.
54. Shoumaker RD, Bennett DR, Bray PE, Curless RG. Clinical and EEG manifestations of an unusual aphasic syndrome in children. Neurology (Minneap) 1974; 24:10–16.
55. Gascon G, Victor D, Lombroso CT, Goodglass H. Language disorders, convulsive disorders, and electroencephalographic abnormalities: acquired syndrome in children. Arch Neurol 1973; 28:156–62.
56. Worster-Drought C. An unusual form of acquired aphasia in children. Dev Med Child Neurol 1971; 13:563–71.
57. Mantovani JF, Landau WM. Acquired aphasia with convulsive disorder: course and prognosis. Neurology 1980; 30:524–29.
58. Tempkin O. The falling sickness. A history of epilepsy from the Greeks to the beginnings of modern neurology. 2d ed. Baltimore: The Johns Hopkins University Press, 1971.
59. Klass D, Daly DD. Petit mal seizures. Electroencephalogr Clin Neurophysiol 1961; 13:824.
60. Daly DD. Reflections on the concept of petit mal. Epilepsia 1968; 9:175–78.
61. Currier RD, Koci KA, Seifman LJ. Prognosis of pure petit mal. A follow-up study. Neurology 1963; 13:959–67.
62. Livingston S, Torres I, Pauli LL, Rider RV. Petit mal epilepsy: result of a prolonged follow-up study of 117 patients. JAMA 1965; 194:113–18.
63. Gibbs FA, Davis H, Lennox MR. The EEG in epilepsy and in conditions of impaired consciousness. Arch Neurol Psychiatry 1935; 34:1134–48.
64. Penry JK, Porter RJ, Dreifuss FE. Simultaneous recording of absence seizures with video tape and electroencephalography: a study of 374 seizures in 84 patients. Brain 1975; 98:427–40.
65. Loiseau P. Epileptic syndromes in infancy, childhood and adolescence. In: Roger J, Dravet C, Bureau M, eds. Childhood absence epilepsy. London: John Libbey Eurotext Ltd, 1985:106–20.
66. Lennox WG, Lennox MA. Epilepsy and related disorders. Boston: Little, Brown and Company, 1960:548–74.

67. Metrakos K, Metrakos JD. Genetics of epilepsy. In: Vinken PJ, Bruyn GW, eds. Handbook of clinical neurology. Vol. 15. Amsterdam: North-Holland Publishing Company, 1974:429–39.
68. Andermann E. Multifactorial inheritance of generalized and focal epilepsy. In: Anderson VE, Hauser WA, Penry JK, Sing CF, eds. Genetic basis of the epilepsies. New York: Raven Press, 1982:355–74.
69. Holowach J, Thurston DL, O'Leary JL. Petit mal epilepsy. Pediatrics 1962; 60:893–901.
70. Sato S, Dreifuss FE, Penry JK. Long term follow-up of absence seizures. Neurology 1983; 33:1590–95.
71. Lennox WG, Davis JP. Clinical correlates of the fast and the slow spike–wave electroencephalogram. Trans Am Neurol Assoc 1949; 74:194–97.
72. Lennox WG. The slow-spike–wave EEG and its clinical correlates. In Lennox WG, ed. Epilepsy and related disorders. Vol. 1. Boston: Little, Brown and Company, 1960:156–70.
73. Ogunyemi AO, Dreifuss FE. Syndromes of epilepsy in childhood and adolescence. J Child Neurol 1988; 3:214–24.
74. Gastaut H, Roger J, Soulayrol R, Tassinari CA, Regis H, Dravet C. Childhood epileptic encephalopathy with diffuse slow spike–waves (otherwise known as "petit mal variant") or Lennox syndrome. Epilepsia 1966; 7:139–79.
75. Madsen JA, Bray PF. The coincidence of diffuse electroencephalographic spike–wave paroxysms and brain tumors. Neurology 1966; 16:546–55.
76. Schneider H, Vassellia F, Karbowski K. The Lennox syndrome. A clinical study of 40 children. Eur Neurol 1970; 4:289–300.
77. Gastaut H, Regis H. On the subject of Lennox's akinetic petit mal. Epilepsia 1961; 2:298–305.
78. Beaumanoir A. (1985). The Lennox–Gastaut syndrome. In: Roger J, Dravet C, Bureau M, Dreifuss FE, Wolf P, eds. Epileptic syndromes in infancy, childhood and adolescence. London: John Libbey Eurotext Ltd., 1985:89–99.
79. Chevrie JJ, Aicardi J. (1972). Childhood epileptic encephalopathy with slow spike–wave. A statistical study of 80 cases. Epilepsia 1972; 13:259–71.
80. Blume WT. (1987). Lennox–Gastaut syndrome. In: Luders H, Lesser RP, eds. Epilepsy: electroclinical syndromes. London: Springer-Verlag, 1987:73–92.
81. Doose M. (1985). Myoclonic astatic epilepsy of early childhood. In: Roger J, Dravet C, Bureau M, Dreifuss FE, Wolf P, eds. London: John Libbey Eurotext Ltd., 1985:100–104.
82. Doose H, Gerken H, Leonhardt R, Volzke E, Volz C. Centrencephalic myoclonic–astatic petit mal. Neuro pediatrics 1970; 2:59–78.
83. Hendriksen O. Discussion of myoclonic epilepsies and Lennox–Gastaut syndrome. In: Roger J, Dravet C, Bureau M, Dreifuss FE, Wolf P, eds. Epileptic syndromes in infancy, childhood and adolescence. London: John Libbey Eurotext Ltd., 1985:100–104.
84. Gastaut H. The Lennox–Gastaut syndrome: comments on the syndrome's terminology and nosological position amongst the secondary generalized epilepsies of childhood. Electroencephalogr Clin Neurophysiol 1982; (Suppl 35):71–84.

85. Roger J, Dravet C, Bureau M. The Lennox–Gastaut syndrome. Cleve Clin Med 1988; S-56. Part 2:172–80.
86. Delgado-Escueta AV, Treiman DM, Walsh GO. The treatable epilepsies. N Engl J Med 1983; 308(25):1508–14.
87. Delgado-Escueta AV. Epileptogenic paroxysms. Modern approaches and clinical correlations. Neurology 1979; 29:1014–22.
88. Delgado-Escueta AV, Treiman DM, Enrile Bacsal F. Genetic basis of the epilepsies. In: Anderson VE, Hauser WA, Penry JK, Sing CF, eds. Phenotypic variations of seizures in adolescents and adults. New York: Raven Press, 1982:49–81.
89. Ounsted C, Lindsay J, Norman R. Biological factors in temporal lobe epilepsy. Clinic in developmental medicine (1966) No. 22 London. Spastic international/ Heinemann Medical.

4

Treatment of Generalized Seizures: Absence, Generalized Tonic–Clonic, and Atonic

JEROME V. MURPHY
University of Missouri
and Children's Mercy Hospital
Kansas City, Missouri

I. ABSENCE SEIZURES

The pediatric epilepsies that have absence seizures as a clinical feature are not the most common pediatric epilepsies, but they are the easiest to diagnose and treat. The electroencephalogram (EEG) has a typical pattern, prerequisite for the diagnosis, they can be provoked during the medical evaluation by hyperventilation (HV), they typically appear in children with otherwise normal neurologic examinations, and they are responsive to ethosuximide or valproic acid. Of all the pediatric epilepsies, uncomplicated absence seizures are the least likely ones to need evaluation by a neurologic specialist.

A. Definition and Types

The former term, *petit mal*, is a French vestige. In 1815, before the invention of the EEG, prolonged seizures were termed grand mal, and those of brief duration were often called petit mal [1]. Livingston used the term *petit mal* more specifically to describe seizures accompanied by the classic 3-per-second spike-and-wave discharge on EEG [2].

In the modern nomenclature *absence seizure* is clinically a brief period of loss of awareness, with staring and retention of postural tone but without convulsive movements. In other words, the patients suddenly stops, stares, and then returns to the former activity (see Chapter 3).

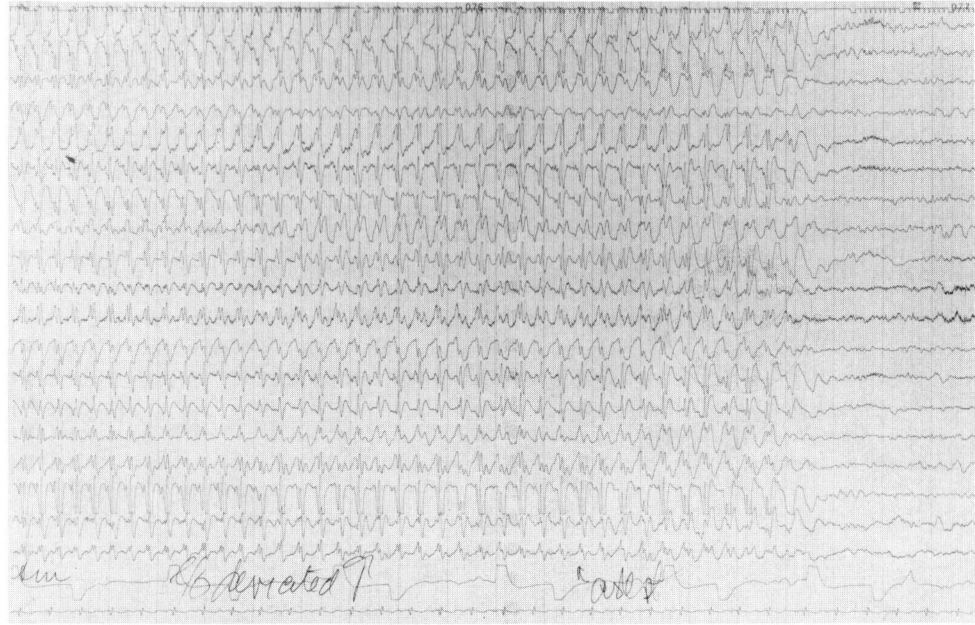

Figure 1 Typical EEG changes seen in absence epilepsy. With the patient awake and hyperventilating, rhythmic and synchronous, 3-per-second spike/slow-wave discharges are observed.

The accompanying EEG pattern is a specific, rhythmic, and generalized 3-per-second spike-and-wave discharge that is difficult to misdiagnose. Otherwise, the awake EEG is normal (Fig. 1). These seizures are not noted during sleep, and at that time, the generalized, or symmetrical, spike-wave discharges in the awake EEG may degenerate to irregular spike-and-wave discharge.

During the medical evaluation a typical seizure can be provoked by less than 2 min of high voltage. In younger children a tissue is held just in front of the nose and the patient is asked to keep it in the air, or horizontal, by blowing. Generally, it helps to time the hyperventilation. When a seizure is seen, the hyperventilation will cease briefly and will resume thereafter.

At the onset of an observed spell the loss of awareness can be demonstrated if the examiner counts starting at 1, recites the alphabet, or recites a rhyme. When the patient recovers, he or she will remember only the numbers or letters recited when the seizure stopped. Sometimes the seizure is accompanied by fluttering of the eyelids or minimal eye movements. Other seizures may be provoked by hyperventilation so that testing alone is not necessarily diagnostic unless the typical EEG changes are also present. The patient is immediately alert after an ab- sence seizure.

The absence seizure itself is classified as typical absence, complex absence, or atypical absence (see Chapter 3). The typical absence seizure as described above consists of stop, stare briefly, and then return to the prior activity. Complex absence seizures are accompanied by other generalized activities, such as myoclonic jerks, loss of postural tone or atonia, clonic jerks, or automatisms. The differential between complex absence seizures and partial complex seizures is important and difficult and may require a video EEG (Chapter 13) to capture an event and its EEG equivalent. The differentiation is important, as the etiologies, diagnostic workup, and effective antiepileptic drugs (AEDs) differ for these two types of seizures.

In atypical absence the seizure is less distinct and the rhythmic EEG discharge is slower [3]. Myoclonic jerks and falls are more frequently a part of these seizures, and the patient generally has a severe neurologic deficit. See Chapter 9 for a more complete description of myoclonic seizures. In general, a typical absence seizure is easy to identify, but complex and atypical absence seizures are somewhat more difficult to separate. The EEG will show the typical 3-per-second spike-and-wave changes in the typical and complex absence seizure, and it will demonstrate a slower spike-and-wave discharge in the atypical absence seizure. Given the frequency of other seizure types in children with one of the absence epilepsies, these epilepsies might well be considered as part of a continuum in the spectrum of epilepsies with primary generalized seizures [4].

1.Typical Absence Seizures

a. Childhood Absence Epilepsy. Typical absence epilepsy of childhood begins between the ages of 4 and 8 years. Dozens to hundreds of absence seizures may occur daily, but most are not recognized [5]. According to one report from a referral center, about 90% of absence seizures are accompanied by automatisms or minimal movement (i.e., they are complex). About 40% of patients with this epilepsy will have generalized tonic–clonic seizures [6–8]. Save for the seizures, patients with this epilepsy are generally normal, and imaging procedures [i.e., computerized tomography (CT) scans or magnetic resonance images] are unnecessary.

As a whole these children have no prior neurologic illness save for a positive history of febrile seizures [6,9]. The febril seizure is probably an early manifestation of the underlying epilepsy rather than an etiologic factor or an expression of an associated and distinct illness. Childhood absence epilepsy resolves in about 80% of patients. The prognosis is more favorable in normal males [7].

b. Juvenile Absence Epilepsy. Besides childhood absence epilepsy, there are two other pediatric epilepsies whose symptoms include absence seizures. A juvenile absence epilepsy has been described with the same seizures and EEG features. The absence seizures are much less frequent than the childhood onset, and generalized tonic–clonic seizures occur in about 80% of these patients. They are less likely to resolve with time. The frequency with which other generalized seizures occur at this age suggests that juvenile absence epilepsy is a generalized epilepsy occurring in adolescence which has variable and mixed expressions [10, pp. 79–99].

c. Juvenile Myoclonic Epilepsy. A third epilepsy with absence seizures is juvenile myoclonic epilepsy. In this category, myoclonic and generalized tonic–clonic seizures, on arising, are far more frequent than absence seizures [11]. See Chapter 9 for a further description of this epilepsy.

2. Complex Absence Seizures

Although typical absence seizures are the classically described model of this category of seizures, only about 10% of absence seizures are typical [8]. The large majority are accompanied by other movements, such as automatisms, mild clonic activities, changes in postural tone, eye blinking, or a combination of these activities. If the EEG consists of ictal 3-per-second spike-and-wave discharges, these are considered for prognostic and therapeutic purposes as absence seizures and should be classified into the categories of epilepsies with absence seizures described above.

3. Atypical Absence Seizures

These are perhaps the most difficult absence seizures to classify. They overlap electrically and clinically with many other epilepsies. Atypical absence seizures generally have a different accompaniment: that is, regular spike-and-wave discharges have a $\leq$ 2.5 per second frequency, or the spike and wave discharge is irregular. Atypical absence seizures are different statistically from typical absence seizures. They last $\geq$ 30 s or longer, are more frequently associated with other seizure types in the same person, and more frequently occur in those with cerebral palsy or mental retardation [3]. However, when taken on an individual basis it can be very difficult to distinguish atypical from typical (including complex) absence seizures without a video-EEG study of the event in question.

B. Etiology

The etiology of absence seizures is unknown, but it is a subject that has given rise to many theories to explain the very unusual phenomenon of all cortical neurones being simultaneously and instantaneously involved in seizure activity. In the mid-twentieth century the term *centrencephalic seizure* was used, implying that deep central structures, with diffuse connections throughout the cerebral hemispheres contained the triggering mechanism for absence seizures [12]. Subsequent depth electrode studies demonstrated a cortical origin for the spike-and-wave discharge, with no activation of the deeper central nuclei of the brain [13].

There is some suggestion that typical and complex absence seizures can be produced by focal cortical lesions, but these lesions are uncommon causes of absence seizures [14]. Electrical stimulation of the orbital frontal cortex has produced such seizures [15], and they can be seen in patients with acquired cerebral damage producing mental retardation [10, pp. 79–100;16]. Most patients with absence seizures do not have acquired brain lesions, suggesting an alternate etiology. There is one report of 3-per-second spike-and-wave pattern in patients with a 12p trisomy syndrome [17].

Most reported series of patients with absence seizures show a preponderance of females [6,7], which remains unexplained. Studies have shown an 80% concordance for absence seizures in monozygotic twins and a zero concordance in dizygotic twins [1]. Further support for a genetic etiology is found in the frequency of a positive family history for epilepsy, although relatives generally do not have absence seizures [6]. Although the etiology may be genetic, how this produces a self-maintaining and immediately generalized involvement of all cerebral cortex is still not clear.

C. Differential Diagnosis

The diagnosis of typical absence epilepsy is generally easily made, based on the clinical history, the typical changes on EEG, and the provocation by hyperventilation. An EEG with a 3-per-second spike and slow-wave bursts is prerequisite for the diagnosis, but the EEG changes themselves are not diagnostic without the clinical event, or seizure.

With the increased public awareness of this kind of epilepsy, and the education of teachers on this subject, the most common differential involves the child who is daydreaming in school. Helpful features in this situation are: (1) absence seizures are random events occurring at home and at school, whereas daydreaming is usually associated with specific environments, such as a classroom setting, and (2) absence seizures generally interrupt a normal activity, such as eating, speaking, writing, and so on, whereas students generally slip into a daydream. A child who appears unresponsive to a simulation is not one who is having an absence seizure unless that state is observed to have a sudden onset, interrupting an activity as described above.

The more difficult situation is the child who is not attentive at school, whose scholastic performance is deteriorating, and who has an abnormal EEG, demonstrating spike-and-wave discharges (see Fig. 2 of Chapter 1 for an example of such a patient). These children may be diagnosed as having epilepsy, based primarily on the EEG findings, and treatment is initiated in the expectation that grades will improve. Unless specific repetitive events can be demonstrated, such AED treatment will not help the child with poor scholastic performance. If the child does not have repetitive events suggestive of epilepsy, an EEG is not part of the evaluation of the child with learning difficulties.

The last differential diagnosis to be remembered is partial complex seizures. Automatisms can accompany absence seizures, and they are the mainstay of partial complex seizures. Features of complex partial seizures that help in their differentiation are the onset is not as sudden and may be accompanied by an aura, and the complex partial seizure generally has a longer duration. Finally, complex seizures very rarely have the electrical accompaniment of regular and generalized 3-per-second spike and slow-wave discharges at their onset. If confusion between these two seizure types exist, a video EEG should resolve the issue.

D. Prognosis

Childhood absence epilepsy generally has a very good prognosis. Significant prognostic features are the presence of a normal EEG in between the epileptic discharges and normal intelligence. Almost 90% of patients with both features will have resolution of their seizures, whereas only 15% of patients with neither feature will have resolution of the problem 5 years after onset. The overall rate for resolution of all seizures in patients with absence seizures is about 50% [6,7]. These figures do not hold true for juvenile absence epilepsy in which the absence seizures are more difficult to control.

E. Effective Drugs

The three most effective AEDs for the control of absence seizures are ethosuximide, valproic acid, and clonazepam. As clonazepam is the least tolerated, the choice of AED generally rests between the first two. In controlled studies ethosuximide and valproic acid are equally effective and provide complete seizure control in more than 80% of patients with childhood absence epilepsy [18–20]. The cost of the two AEDs is roughly similar (see Table 3 of Chapter 2).

Considering that ethosuximide will not control generalized tonic–clonic seizures and may even aggravate them [21], its use is not recommended in children with absence and generalized tonic–clonic seizures. Valproic acid would be the drug of choice on such a patient, rather than using polypharmacy (e.g., ethosuccimide and phenytoin). To reduce the remote risk of inducing the fatal hepatotoxicity associated with the use of valproic acid in children less than 10 years of age, ethosuximide is the treatment of choice if the child has only absence seizures. If a combination of ethosuximide and another AED becomes necessary, it must be remembered that both phenobarbital and carbamazepine have been reported to exacerbate absence seizures [21,22].

If the patient does not respond to either ethosuximide or valproic acid, the two in combination may be an effective therapy [24]. If that fails, clonazepam, in slowly incrementing doses (see Chapter 2, Section IV) is the treatment of choice. Tolerance is a problem with this benzodiazepine [23]. Nitrazepam and clobazam may be better tolerated, but these benzodiazepines are not available in this country.

Acetazolamide may have transient benefit in patients with intractable absence seizures [24]. The other popular AEDs are of dubious benefit in this epilepsy. If ethosuximide or valproic acid control all observed seizures, there will probably be a dramatic improvement in the EEG and hyperventilation will no longer provoke a seizure. Of all epilepsy-associated EEG abnormalities, the 3-per-second spike-and-wave discharge of childhood absence epilepsy seems the most sensitive to either ethosuximide or valproic acid.

In the patient with idiopathic absence seizures and no other neurologic abnormality, successful AED therapy can be slowly eliminated after 2 years of seizure control. Patients with associated neurologic abnormalities generally need longer therapy.

II. GENERALIZED TONIC–CLONIC SEIZURES

This is the classic seizure, the convulsion. Absence and partial seizures may go unnoticed to the unsuspecting observer, but the generalized tonic–clonic seizure is so striking and frightening as to create fears to impending death in an observer. This fear is in the eye of the beholder, as the child will be puzzled at the great concern demonstrated when he or she recovers and will only recognize that he or she is very tired and sore.

In the older literature the name *grand mal* was used to classify this type of seizure [25]. Petit mal seizures were generally absence seizures, and grand mal included tonic–clonic, tonic, and clonic seizures, whether they were focal or generalized. Concurrent with the introduction of procedures for accurately imaging brain, this terminology has been replaced with the international classification (see Chapter 3).

A. Definition and Types

The seizure itself starts with a sudden onset of rigidity, and the patient will frequently fall to the ground. There may be a transient phase of flexion preceding this. The patient lies rigidly extended, but not opisthotonic. After less than a minute, there occurs generalized clonic jerks of the body of varying force, frequently accompanied by expiratory grunts, with oral frothing. The tongue can be bitten during this phase. Respiration is irregular and cyanosis is frequently noted. Urinary and fecal incontinence can accompany the convulsion [10, pp. 100–112].

There is some variability in the expression of this seizure, giving rise to descriptive names such as tonic–clonic–tonic or generalized tonic seizures. In the latter the clonic activity is absent or minimal. This may be confused with opisthotonic posturing, and care must be taken to distinguish the two. Opisthotonic posturing posturing commonly occurs with uncal herniation in patients with severely increased intracranial pressure. Treatment with AEDs does not help.

1. Primary Generalized Tonic–Clonic Seizures

The two general classifications of generalized tonic–clonic seizures are primary generalized tonic–clonic seizures and secondary generalized tonic–clonic seizures. If the patient does not have another generalized seizure, such as absence, it may be very difficult to distinguish if the seizure is primary generalized or if the generalization is secondary to spread from an epileptogenic focus.

a. Reflex Epilepsies. Primary generalized tonic–clonic seizures are seen in what may be termed reflex epilepsies and in idiopathic epilepsies. The term *reflex epilepsy* might be a misnomer, as epilepsy is defined as unprovoked seizures, and clearly a reflex seizure is a provoked event. In the reflex epilepsies a stimulus provokes the convulsion, which is ages and electrically generalized at its onset. The commonest example of a reflex epilepsy is the *febrile seizure*. Fever alone can provoke a convulsion in a child between the ages of several months and 5 years. These are noted in 1 to 3% of the population. This subject is discussed in Chapter 8.

The second reflex epilepsy is *photosensitive epilepsy*. In this epilepsy the repetitive flashing of light at certain frequencies provokes a generalized tonic–clonic seizure. Classic environmental provocations include flashing lights at a dance floor, a gleaming white picket fence as one drives by in a car or truck, or the decelerating rotors of a helicopter with sun shining through. In England this will occur while watching television closely, as the image flashes at rates of 50 and 25 times a second. The frequency in this country is 60 per second, a rate apparently too rapid to precipitate such a reaction [26].

Photic stimulation can produce any of three generalized epilepsies: absence, generalized tonic–clonic, and myoclonic [27]. This photosensitive epilepsy can easily be demonstrated on EEG. Standard provocations on EEG are hyperventilation and photic stimulation. In the latter a repetitively flashing light at frequencies of 10 or more provokes the response in susceptible persons. Buildup of the electrical abnormality can easily be detected on the EEG, and the stimulus removed before a convulsion occurs.

This EEG phenomenon can be seen in patients with no other suggestion of a seizure disorder [27] and does not, per se, make a diagnosis of epilepsy (i.e., epilepsy is an observed clinical event, not an abnormality on EEG). Contrariwise, such a sensitivity can also be observed in children with spontaneous, unprovoked seizures. The phenomenon of photosensitivity can be significantly reduced or eliminated with valproate.

A third reflex epilepsy is *reading epilepsy*, a rare genetic pediatric epilepsy [28]. These generalized tonic–clonic seizures occur with prolonged reading and are preceded by quivering of the chin [29]. Epileptic changes can be seen on EEG, but only after prolonged reading. Clonazapam and valproate are effective therapies [30,31].

b. Generalized Tonic–Clonic Epilepsy of Adolescence. This epilepsy has been reported in adolescent patients who otherwise exhibit no neurologic abnormalities. It can start as early as 9 years of age. Seizures are generally observed on arising and are infrequent. The interictal EEG is normal or displays generalized epileptic changes during lethargy or sleep. Most patients respond favorably to a single AED [10, pp. 100–112]. The clinical overlap between this epilepsy and juvenile absence epilepsy suggests that they might be two manifestations of the same genetic epilepsy, as mentioned earlier.

c. Generalized Tonic–Clonic Epilepsy After Febrile Seizures. One to 3% of patients with febrile seizures will subsequently demonstrate generalized tonic–clonic seizures without fever [32]. As in most children with febrile seizures they are generally neurologically normal. Patients with generalized tonic–clonic seizures more commonly have a history of febrile seizures than controls. Undoubtedly, this represents an early manifestation of their epilepsy rather than a cause of the generalized epilepsy as stated for absence seizures [33].

2. Secondary Generalized Tonic–Clonic Seizures

Secondary generalized tonic–clonic seizures need to be identified, as they carry a higher risk for a focal abnormality of brain from which the epileptic discharge originates. Therefore, patients with secondary generalization will more frequently require imaging procedures than will patients with primary generalized tonic–clonic seizures. The prognosis and treatment for idiopathic, primary and secondary, generalized tonic–clonic seizures are the same (i.e., these two distinct seizure respond to the same AEDs, and the prognosis for control in at least one series seems no different) [34,35]. Treatment of secondary generalized epilepsy is described in Chapter 5.

The rapid and secondary generalized seizure may appear identical save that the interictal EEG frequently demonstrates a focal epileptogenic change (e.g., a localized spike or a spike and slow wave that recurs during the tracing). This is usually enough evidence to indicate that the generalized tonic–clonic seizure is secondary generalized. Classification becomes difficult when the EEG demonstrates both generalized spike-and-wave discharges as well as focal changes [36].

The presence of an aura, or warning, is another clue that the seizure is secondarily generalized. Clearly, focal warnings are weakness or altered sensation in a limb. Vaguer warning may not have clinical value [37].

When one considers that large portions of the cerebral cortex are distant from the recording electrodes of the routine scalp EEG, focal electrical changes in these portions of cerebral cortex may not be recorded on the EEG. Examples of such hidden cortex are the mesial cortex of the cerebral hemispheres above the corpus callosum, the cortex under the frontal lobes, and the mesial temporal cortex. Therefore, some focal seizures that secondarily generalize may not have a localizing change on EEG unless unique EEG montages are used. In that situation the warning or aura that the patient describes is more important than the EEG in indicating that the patient has a secondary generalized seizure disorder.

B. Etiology

The etiology of primary generalized tonic–clonic seizures is poorly understood. In animals this kind of seizure can be produced by pentylenetetrazol. When that is done, recording electrodes in the animal's reticular activating system of the brainstem demonstrate continuous activity during the tonic phase of the convulsion, and periodic fast activity during the clonic phase, synchronous with the animal's motor activity [10, pp. 100–112].

Bancaud reported that stimulation of frontal cortex of patients with generalized tonic–clonic seizures produced generalized tonic–clonic seizures. (As described above, such an intervention can also provoke absence seizure in patients with an absence epilepsy [15].) Therefore, based on these observations of animals and humans, generalized tonic–clonic seizures can have either a brainstem or a cortical origin.

Toxic factors that may produce generalized tonic–clonic seizures include hypoglycemia, alcohol withdrawal after habitual exposure, and severe hypoxic damage. Factors that are associated with the later development of generalized tonic–clonic seizures are a prior history of febrile seizures, a history of seizures in the patient's mother, and head trauma severe enough to produce either amnesia for the event, skull fracture, or loss of consciousness. Important factors that are *not* associated with generalized tonic–clonic seizures are symptoms of mild asphyxia in the newborn infant [33]. If intrapartum asphyxia is severe enough to cause a seizure disorder, it is also severe enough to lead to mental retardation and cerebral palsy. Basically, mild intrapartum asphyxia does not relate to subsequent epilepsy.

Regarding causation, primary generalized tonic–clonic seizures in persons who are otherwise neurologically normal probably have a genetic origin, and brain imaging procedures are not diagnostically useful. As these seizures are studied, many may be found to have secondary generalizations from presently unrecognized foci.

C. Differential Diagnosis

These are generally the easiest of the epilepsies to recognize and the only kind of seizure for which the word *convulsion* is used. They rarely go unnoticed if observers are available, but may be unrecognized during sleep. In that situation the patient frequently recognizes that he or she had a seizure during the night, by a generalized muscular ache, confusion, a bitten lip or tongue, or evidence of incontinence.

1. Syncopal Attacks

Asystole or acute hypotension can provoke opisthotonus with arching of the back and rigid extension of the extremities with external rotation of the hands. This can be mistaken for a tonic seizure, and the differential is important.

Children with the prolonged QT syndrome will have episodic loss of consciousness due to cerebral ischemia [38]. It has been mistaken for epilepsy, and treated with AEDs. The concurrent EEG, during a syncopal event, will show generalized slowing during the ischemia and opisthotonus, without evident epileptic activity. If the syncopal event is prolonged, death occurs. For this reason it is very important to record the EKG on an extra channel of the EEG. The abnormal and variable QT interval is obvious.

2. Pseudoseizures

As a sole event, pseudoseizures are rare in children and more frequent in adolescence. Unfortunately, they can occur in patients with bona fide epilepsy, thereby making correct diagnosis difficult. Helpful features in the pseudoseizure are several: These will not occur during sleep; the limb movements are usually flailing of the extremities rather than clonic, rhythmic jerks, and the head will move vigorously from side to side [39,40]. A normal EEG during the event in question rules out a seizure disorder. A normal EEG at other times is not helpful.

Due to the variable manifestation of seizures, distinction can be very difficult and may require the use of a video EEG with a recorded spell. Sometimes the spell can be provoked during the EEG by suggestion (e.g., injecting saline while claiming that the agent will provoke a spell, or having the EEG technicians misinform the patient that the electrical pattern is building up to a seizure).

3. Other Seizure Disorders

Generalized tonic–clonic seizures may appear in other epilepsies. As stated earlier, a significant number of patients with absence epilepsy in childhood or adolescence also will have generalized convulsions. The distinction is important in the selection of AED and can usually be made by the interictal EEG pattern. If the two kinds of seizures are equally frequent, treatment with an AED controlling both seizure types (i.e., valproic acid) is indicated.

Generalized myoclonic seizures (Chapter 9) may also be accompanied by generalized tonic–clonic seizures. In general, the tonic–clonic are easier to control than the myoclonic seizures. There is some overlap in effective AEDs in these two seizure disorders.

As discussed above, secondary generalized tonic–clonic seizures are distinguished from the primary seizure on any of several features. These include the presence of a focal onset of the observed seizures, focal changes on the interictal EEG, or the presence of an aura or warning to the convulsion.

D. Prognosis

In large series of patients with primary generalized tonic–clonic seizures, the outlook was excellent, with almost two-thirds having complete control, or less than one seizure annually, on therapy [41]. In one long-term study 85% of patients were in remission 20 years following diagnosis [38]. Unfortunately, most such series include adults and children, and most are reported from epilepsy centers, where more difficult epilepsies tend to be referred.

If a patient is seizure-free for several years, a trial withdrawal of AEDs is warranted. In one series of 186 patients with grand mal seizures (see above for definition) who were seizure-free for 3 years, 88% remained seizure-free following withdrawal of medications [41]. Relapses with drug withdrawal were more likely if the seizures had their onset at less than 3 years of age. The EEG was not predictive of recurrence, but this was not uniformly done on all 186 patients.

E. Effective Drugs

Primary generalized tonic–clonic seizures respond equally favorably to any of several AEDs. These include phenytoin, valproic acid, carbamazepine, phenobarbital, and primidone [42]. The selection involves factors other than the diagnosed epilepsy, and these are discussed in Chapter 2. In our clinic there is probably equal use of phenytoin, valproic acid, and carbamazepine in such patients.

Phenobarbital and primidone are used when satisfactory control is not obtained with the first three AEDs. Control of the seizures can generally be obtained with monotherapy with any one of these AEDs.

REFERENCES

1. Lennox WG, Lennox MA. Epilepsy and related disorders. Boston: Little, Brown and Company, 1960: 66–174.
2. Livingston S. Comprehensive management of epilepsy in infancy, childhood, and adolescence. Springfield, IL: Charles C Thomas, 1729: 47–95.
3. Holmes GL, McKeever M, Adamson M. Absence seizures in children: clinical and electrographic features. Ann Neurol 1989; 21:268–73.
4. Berkovic SF, Andermann F, Andermann E, Gloor P. Concepts of absence epilepsies: discrete syndromes or biologic continuum? Neurology 1987; 37:993–1000.
5. Keilson MJ, Hauser WA, Magrill JP, Tepperberg J. Ambulatory cassette EEG in absence epilepsy. Pediatr Neurol 1987; 3:273–76.

6. Sato S, Dreifuss FE, Penry JK. Prognostic factors in absence seizures. Neurology 1976; 26:788–96.
7. Sato S, Dreifuss FE, Penry JK, Kirby DD, Palesch Y. Long-term followup of absence seizures. Neurology 1983; 33:1590–95.
8. Loiseau P, Pestre M, Dartigues JF, Commenges D, Barberger-Gateau C, Cohadon S. Long-term prognosis in two forms of childhood epilepsy: typical absence seizures and epilepsy with rolandic (centrotemporal) EEG foci. Ann Neurol 1983; 3:642–48.
9. Rocca WA, Sharbrough FW, Hauser WA, Annegers JF, Schoenberg BS. Risk factors for absence seizures: a population-based case-control study in Rochester, Minnesota. Neurology 1987; 37:1309–14.
10. Aicardi J. Epilepsy in children. New York: Raven Press, 1986.
11. Asconape J, Penry JK. Some clinical and EEG aspects of benign myoclonic epilepsy. Epilepsia 1984; 25:108–14.
12. Penfield W. Epileptic automatism and the centrencephalic integrating system. Res Publ Assoc Nerv Ment Dis Proc 1950; 30:513–28.
13. Niedermeyer E, Laws ER Jr, Walter AE. Depth EEG findings in epileptics with generalized spike-wave complexes. Arch Neurol 1969; 21:51–58.
14. Farwell JR, Stuntz JT. Frontoparietal astrocytoma causing absence seizures and bilaterally synchronous epileptiform discharges. Epilepsia 1984; 25:695–98.
15. Bancaud J, Talairach J, Morel P, Bresson M, Bonis A, Geier S, Hemon E, Buser P. "Generalized" epileptic seizures elicited by electrical stimulation of the frontal lobe in man. Electroencephalogr Clin Neurophysiol 1974; 37:275–82.
16. Dalby MA. Epilepsy and 3 per second spike wave rhythms. A clinical, EEG, and prognostic analysis of 346 patients. Acta Neurol Scand 1969; 40(Suppl):1–183.
17. Guerrini R, Bureau M, Mattei M-G, Battaglia A, Galland M-C, Roger J. Trisomy 12p syndrome: a chromosomal disorder associated with generalized 3-Hz spike and wave discharge. Epilepsia 1990; 31:557–66.
18. Callaghan N, O'Hare J, O'Driscoll, O'Neill, Daly N. Comparative study of ethosuximide and sodium valproate in the treatment of typical absence seizures (petit mal). Dev Med Child Neurol 1982; 24:830–36.
19. Sato S, White BG, Penry JK, Dreifuss FE, Sackellares JC, Kupferberg HJ. Valproic acid versus ethosuximide in the treatment of absence seizures. Neurology 1982; 32:157–63.
20. Santavouri P. Absence seizures: valproate or ethosuximide? Acta Neurol Scand 1974; 68(Suppl 97):41–48.
21. Penry JK, So E. Refractoriness of absence seizures and phenobarbital. Neurology 1981; 31(Suppl):158.
22. Rowan AJ, Meijer JW, de Beer-Pawlikowski N, Van Der Geest, Mieinardi H. Valproate–ethosuximide combination therapy for refractory absence seizures. Arch Neurol 1983; 40:797–802.
23. Sherwin AL. Absence seizures. In: Morselli PL, Pipenger CE, Penry JK, eds. Antiepileptic drug therapy in children. New York: Raven Press, 1983:153–61.
24. Lombroso CT, Forsythe I. A long-term follow-up of acetazolamide (Diamox) in the treatment of epilepsy. Epilepsia 1960; 1:493–500.
25. Livingston, Term Grand Mal

26. Holmes G. Diagnosis and management of seizures in children. Philadelphia: WB Saunders Company, 19:162–72.
27. Gastaut H, Trevisan C, Naquet R. Diagnostic value of electroencephalographic abnormalities provoked by intermittent stimulation. Electroencephalogr Clin Neurophysiol 1958; 10:194–95.
28. Daly RF, Forster RM. Inheritance of reading epilepsy. Neurology 1975; 25:1051–54.
29. Ramani V. Primary reading epilepsy. Arch Neurol 1983; 40:39–41.
30. Login IS, Kolakovich TM. Successful treatment of primary reading epilepsy with clonazepam. Ann Neurol 1978; 1:55–56.
31. Vanderzant DO, Fitz R, Holmes G, Greenberg HS, Sackellares JC. Treatment of primary reading epilepsy with valproic acid. Arch Neurol 1982; 35:452–53.
32. Nelson K. Febriles to ep
33. Rocca WA, Sharbrough FW, Hauser WA, Annegers JF, Schoenberg BS. Risk factors for generalized tonic–clonic seizures: a population-based case-control study in Rochester, Minnesota. Neurology 1987; 37:1315–22.
34. Sofijanov NG. Clinical evolution and prognosis of childhood epilepsies. Epilepsia 1982; 23:61–69.
35. D'Alessandro, Pazzaglia P, Tinuper R, Ferrara R, Fabbri R, Lugaresi E. Prognostic and electroclinical features of grand mal epilepsies. Eur Neurol 1986; 25:339–45.
36. O'Brien JL, Goldensohn ES, Hoefer PF. EEG abnormalities in addition to bilateral synchronous 3 per second and wave activity in petit mal. Electroencephalogr Clin Neurophysiol 1959; 11:747–76.
37. Van Donselaar CA, Geerts AT, Schimsheimer R-J. Usefulness of an aura for classification of a first generalized seizure. Epilepsia 1990; 31:529–35.
38. Weintraub RG, Gow RM, Wilkinson JL. The congenital long QT syndromes in childhood. J Am Coll Cardiol 1990; 16:674–80.
39. Holmes GL, Sackellares JC, McKiernan J, Ragland M, Dreifuss FE. Evaluation of childhood pseudoseizures using EEG telemetry and video tape monitoring. J Pediatr 1980; 97:554–58.
40. Gates JR, Ramani V, Whalen S, Loewson R. Ictal characteristics of pseudoseizures. Arch Neurol 1985; 42:1183–1187.
41. Ehrhardt P, Forsythe WI. Prognosis after a grand mal seizure: a study of 187 children with three year remissions. Dev Med Child Neurol 1989; 31:633–39.
42. de Silva M, McArdle B, McGowan M, Reynolds EH, Neville B, Johnson AL. Monotherapy for newly diagnosed childhood epilepsy: a comparative trial and prognostic evaluation (abstr). Epilepsia 1989; 30:662.

5

Treatment of Partial Seizures

JEROME V. MURPHY
University of Missouri
and Children's Mercy Hospital
Kansas City, Missouri

I. DEFINITION

Partial seizures are seizures whose symptoms or electroencephalographic associations indicate that they start from, or predominantly involve, a focal area of brain. The evidence that a seizure arises from a specific area of brain is based on one or more of the following observations: the focal nature of the aura or warning, localized expression of the seizure according to the patient or a witness, or focal interictal changes on the electroencephalogram (EEG). The video-EEG recording of a seizure is particularly helpful in documenting the partial or focal nature of the seizure.

Partial seizures can be easy or difficult to diagnose. If the patient or his or her family describes recurrent clonic activity of a specific limb, with retention of awareness, the patient has simple partial seizures. On the other hand, the observers may be called to the patient's side only by the disruption that accompanies the secondary generalization from a simple partial seizure. The partial seizure may go unnoticed, being forgotten by the patient and unobserved by others. In such a secondary generalized seizure, if the interictal EEG is normal, the mistaken diagnosis of a primary generalized epilepsy could persist. As most AEDs (antiepileptic drugs) are equally effective in generalized tonic-clonic or partial seizures, the correct categorization will not affect treatment. The proper classification of the seizure may make a difference in (1) the need for an imaging procedure of brain, (2) prognosis, and (3) the consideration of the patient as a candidate for therapeutic neurosurgical intervention.

In the international classification of seizures (Chapter 3) partial seizures are divided into simple partial seizures and complex partial seizures. In the *simple partial seizure*, there are motor or sensory changes in a part of the body which correlates with abnormal neuronal discharges associated with the area of the brain which represents that function. The electrical abnormality can spread contiguously to involve adjacent areas of brain, as in a jacksonian march, or it can spread in a saltatory fashion by connection fibers to involve distal sites. In this way a seizure that starts in one arm may spread via the corpus callosum to involve the other arm before convulsive movements are observed in the face or leg of the original side. The electrical abnormality producing a simple partial seizure can rapidly extend to produce either a complex partial seizure, a multifocal seizure, or a generalized motor seizure. Secondary generalization to produce typical absence seizures, with 3-per-second spike/slow-wave discharges, has not been observed.

A *complex partial seizure* is defined as a partial seizure with impairment of consciousness (Chapter 3). Generally, this category has replaced what were formerly referred to as psychomotor or temporal lobe seizures. In theory it would still be possible to have an epileptic discharge orignating in the temporal lobe which produces a seizure with psychic, motor, cognitive, or behavioral abnormalities without a disturbance of consciousness. In the international classification of seizures this seizure of temporal lobe origin would be a simple partial seizure when consciousness is retained, and a complex partial seizure when the same seizure progresses to impair consciousness.

Although most complex partial seizures originate in the temporal lobe of the brain, epileptic foci originating elsewhere can also produce partial seizures with impairment of consciousness [1–4]. Complex partial seizures are deserving of particular attention, as they are probably the most difficult to control, and they most often lead to consideration for seizure surgery when available AEDs fail (see Chapter 14). Most adults with complex partial seizures have had the onset of their epilepsy in childhood [2,5]. Hopefully, appropriate therapy at their onset will improve outcome.

II. SIMPLE PARTIAL SEIZURES

A. Nonlesional Epilepsies

1. Benign Rolandic Epilepsy

This epilepsy is the most common of the pediatric epilepsies. In a Swedish study 16% of the patients attending a pediatric epilepsy clinic had this epilepsy. It was four times more common than absence seizures [6]. The features of benign ro-

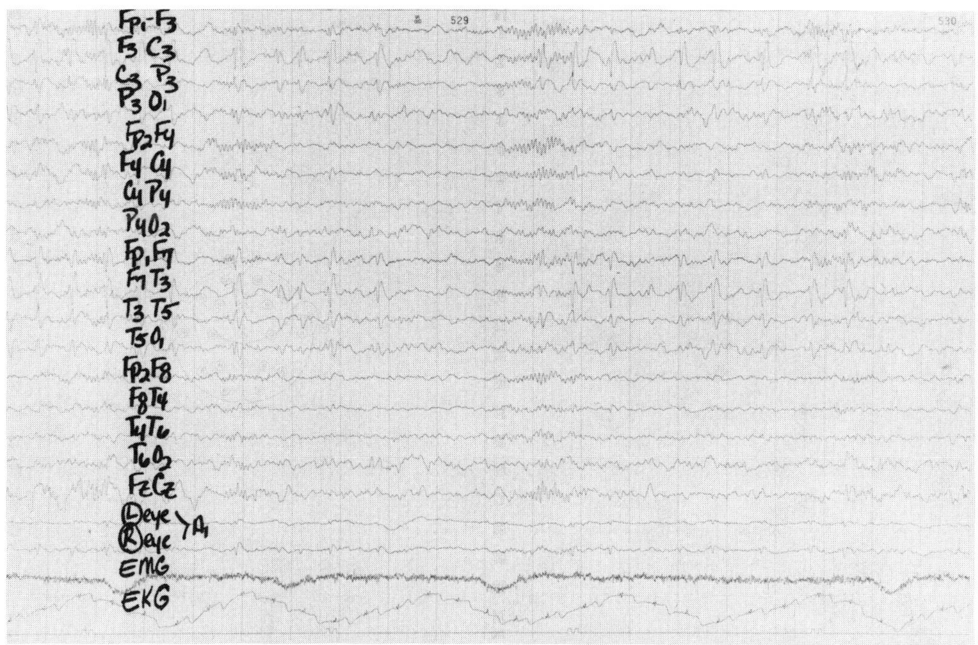

Figure 1 Typical EEG changes in benign rolandic epilepsy. During the drowsy state of this recording a sharp and slow-wave complex is noted in leads T4 and T6, overlying the right temporal lobe. Except for these changes during drowsiness and sleep, the EEG is normal.

landic epilepsy are (1) recurrent sleep-related, typical partial motor seizures involving face and accompanied by aphasia, (2) onset between 4 and 10 years of age, (3) typical changes on EEG, and (4) absence of a neurologic deficit related to the epilepsy. Secondary generalization of the seizure can occur. The key feature of this epilepsy is the EEG, which demonstrates a prominent sharp and slow-wave focus over one temporal or rolandic area, which, like the seizure, is most active during drowsiness or sleep. The slow-wave focus originates from the rolandic area, not the temporal lobe [7, 8]. (A typical EEG is demonstrated in Figure 1.) Otherwise, the EEG is normal.

This same EEG change has been demonstrated in one-half of the siblings of patients with benign rolandic epilepsy [9] and in about 1% of healthy children [10]. (The study cited [10] utilized only awake tracings. The frequency in the normal population might be a lot higher if the recording were continued during sleep [9].) This EEG abnormality is identical in interictal EEGs whether or not the patient has epilepsy [7], and therefore the findings of such changes on an

EEG does not mean that the patient has, or will have, epilepsy. This EEG abnormality may be a genetic marker of the epilepsy, but the penetrance or expression of the gene(s) is not complete. This is a prime example that an epileptiform change in the EEG is not by itself diagnostic of epilepsy.

The ictal event consists of unilateral clonic activity of the face and the arm on the same side, generally during sleep. He or she is aware of the event but is unable to speak while it is occurring. The seizure is brief, less than 5 min., and the patient rapidly returns to sleep without sequelae. If the seizure is prolonged, there will be a postictal weakness of the involved limb. Secondary generalization has been reported.

This epilepsy usually remits by 16 years of age, for which reason it is called benign. Even if the seizures are severe, difficult to control, or followed by a hemiplegia, the prognosis is very favorable [11,12]. If a diagnosis is secure, based on the symptoms, lack of other neurologic abnormalities, and the typical EEG changes, imaging procedures of brain are unnecessary.

The presence of typical benign rolandic seizures are rarely an indication for chronic treatment with AEDs, and such therapy has not been proven to affect the epilepsy or its outcome [13]. If the seizures are expressed only at night, assurance to the family about the benign nature of the illness, not the chronic use of AEDs, is the optimal treatment. We would disagree with Aicardi's statement that "treatment should be regularly advised" [14, p. 124].

If the seizures are diurnal, the patient and the family may prefer AED therapy. In the few children who need therapeutic intervention phenytoin, valproic acid, carbamazepine, or phenobarbital are effective AEDs. As these seizures rarely cause any sequelae, it is essential that therapy, if it is used, not produce adversity.

In children who do not have epilepsy, an erroneous interpretation of the EEG may lead to the conclusion that certain undesirable behaviors are really uncontrolled seizures. Diagnostic neuroimaging and prolonged AED therapy might be recommended. As an example, we were recently asked to give a second opinion on a child who had periodic rages. An EEG, done as part of the psychiatric evaluation, showed rolandic sharp and slow-wave complexes during sleep. The neurologist who interpreted the EEG diagnosed epilepsy and recommended AED therapy. The patient's mother was referred to protective services, as she refused this recommendation. We were able to convince this protective governmental agency, the neurologist who interpreted the EEG, the psychiatrist who ordered the EEG, and the mother that the findings on EEG were coincidental and not related to the periodic rages.

2. Benign Occipital Epilepsy

This epilepsy shares features with migraine headaches. Patients will frequently experience incapacitating headaches associated with visual distortions. The diagnostic features are absence of neurologic abnormalities save for seizures, and a strikingly abnormal EEG with the irregular expression of posterior spikes and slow waves only when the patient's eyes are closed. They promptly disappear with eye opening. The EEG changes are the hallmark of the entity [15,16].

In a typical event the patient has the onset of nocturnal seizures around age 5 years. The seizure, generally nocturnal, is preceded by visual phenomena with tonic deviation of the eyes, followed by vomiting and headaches. Onset is before the age of 8 years, females predominate, and seizures resolve by age 12 years. A smaller subgroup has a later onset, and the prognosis is not as good. In the absence of other neurologic abnormalities, imaging procedures of brain are unnecessary.

There are also patients with visual changes and severe headaches who have similarly abnormal EEGs. This syndrome has been called epileptiform EEG changes and basilar migraine and may be the same as benign occipital epilepsy, except that seizures do not occur. Others suggest that it is a subgroup of benign rolandic epilepsy with migration of the epileptic focus to the occipital lobe [17].

As in other epilepsies, consideration of the frequency and severity of the occipital seizure must be taken into account before concluding that chronic treatment with AEDs is needed. As most of these seizures are nocturnal, they seldom interfere with diurnal activities. Almost all AEDs are effective in controlling seizures, and the benzodiazepines appear to be the most effective AED [15].

3. Epileptic Aphasia

Epileptic aphasia, or the Landau–Kleffner syndrome [18], might better be considered as an encephalopathy with spike discharges on the EEG rather than as an epilepsy. The reason for this is that only 70% of patients will have recognized seizures. Epileptic aphasia starts in the first few years of life. A child with previously normal language skills will become aphasic with loss of comprehension and use of language. Seizures are absent or infrequent and easy to control. Nonlanguage skills are relatively preserved. Behavioral disturbances are common. For this diagnosis the EEG must display paroxysmal epileptiform changes at least during sleep [19]. Treatment with AEDs can control the infrequent seizures but rarely provides significant resolution of the lost verbal skills [20].

These patients have an auditory agnosia, but its pathogenesis is unclear [21]. As epilepsy in a patient with acquired deafness could produce identical symptoms, tests of auditory acuity are mandatory in patients presenting with acquired aphasia. By definition, patients with epileptic aphasia have normal auditory acuities. The outcome of the Landau–Kleffner syndrome is variable, with some patients recovering language and going on to lead useful and independent lives. Even recovered patients have mild to severe verbal difficulties with associated impairments in social development [22,23].

Although epileptic aphasia is not associated with a cerebral lesion, positron emission tomography (PET) and single photon emission computed tomography (SPECT) have demonstrated focal abnormalities [24,25]. Four patients have had complete resolution of the EEG abnormalities and recovery of speech following subpial intracortical resection [24]. Another three successive patients have demonstrated resolution of their aphasia and normalization of the EEG following treatment with corticosteroids [25]. Further studies of the involved areas of brain are necessary to elucidate the pathogenesis of this intriguing epilepsy.

There are other localization-related epilepsies that are nonlesional and appear benign. The interested reader is referred elsewhere for their description [26].

B. Lesional Epilepsies

1. Cortical

Seizures produced by cortical lesions are very variable in their expression, depending on the cortical origin of the event and the subsequent spread of the electrical abnormality. Complex partial seizures in temporal lobe epilepsy are the most common of these seizures and are discussed later in this chapter as a specific entity. Seizures that originate in the frontal lobe of brain generally have a strong motor or postural component. This may help in differentiating complex partial seizures of frontal lobe origin from those of temporal lobe origin [3].

Strongly forced and consistent lateral head and eye movement is a frequent accompaniment of a partial seizure, and several studies have been published examining the value of this movement as a localizing feature [27,28]. A recent study suggests that forced head turning, involving head and neck, has localizing value. In a seizure of frontal lobe origin the focus is contralateral to the direction of the head movements, whereas a complex partial seizure, from the temporal lobe, induces movement toward the focus. This simplistic theory becomes confusing when simple partial seizures progress to become complex partial seizures, or vice versa.

2. Epilepsia Partialis Continua

A less frequently encountered seizure in children is epilepsy partialis continua (EPC). This is a partial seizure with continual clonic activity that can last for hours, days, or months and which is not frequently responsive to standard AED therapy. It usually involves a part of a limb (e.g., a toe or a finger) with periodic spread to involve more of that limb. It may be secondary to a static atrophic brain lesion or an inflammatory lesion, complicating the course of a viral encephalitis. The patient's alertness is appropriate for the underlying neuropathology [29,30].

The EEG demonstrates an electric abnormality appropriate to the involved part of the body. The seizure activity generally remits on its own. The recovery from the seizure is not necessarily associated with improvement in neurologic function.

Treatment of EPC with available AEDs is generally unsatisfactory. Phenytoin, carbamazepine, valproate, or phenobarbital may suppress, but will not relieve, the symptoms without producing excessive sedation [29]. In one series of 26 children with EPC, two groups could be recognized. Eleven children had a static encephalopathy and EPC which resolved during sleep. Six of these 11 children could be controlled with AEDs. Another 11 had a progressive neurodegeneration, continuous seizures, and a failure to respond to AEDs. Four patients defied classification [30].

3. Hypothalamic Lesions

Leisons of the hypothalamus can produce a unique seizure, referred to as a gelastic seizure. These are seen in young preschool children with hamartomatous malformations of this area [31,32]. The random seizures consist of peculiar laughter, for which it is named, accompanied by complex behaviors, such as circular walking, staring, eye deviation, and so on. Loss of postural tone with subsequent injury may occur. These harmartomas generally are seen in previously normal infants, whose delay becomes more evident as they grow older. Complex partial seizures may produce unusual laughter, but they are distinguished from these harmartomatous malformations by imaging procedures of brain as well as the ictal EEG.

These seizures are unusual for the following reasons. They do not respond favorably to standard AED therapy, and the EEG during a spell attenuates to somewhat regular slow waves. Neither spikes nor sharp waves accompany the slowing [32]. The lack of sharp waves or spikes probably relates to the fact that the recording electrodes on the scalp are at a significant distance from the site of seizure activity (i.e., in the hypothalamus).

It is important to recognize these seizures for several reasons. The failure to diagnose the periodic symptoms as epilepsy correctly will lead to the conclusion that the seizures are behaviors, and they will be treated as such. Imaging procedures are necessary to diagnose the hypothalamic tumor. In the long run, referral to a tertiary care center is probably necessary for the appropriate evaluation and to decide whether or not surgical intervention is appropriate. In at least one patient, partial surgical resection was associated with a marked and prolonged improvement in seizure control and patient development [33].

II. COMPLEX PARTIAL SEIZURES

A. Definition

By definition, complex partial seizures are differentiated from simple partial seizures only by the accompanying impairment of consciousness. Despite the focal nature of the seizure, the patient's awareness is impaired or eliminated. In the past this category of seizures was generally called temporal lobe or psychomotor seizures. They generally presented with complex behaviors (e.g., walking, feeling) or complex sensations (e.g., jamais vu, fear).

This classification of partial seizures is meant primarily for epilepsies in the adult, where (1) temporal lobe functions are well differentiated, and (2) retention or impairment of consciousness can be ascertained. In the infant and the very young child localization of specific functions to one temporal lobe has not occurred, and therefore a simple and a complex partial seizure can be unnecessarily difficult to differentiate [14, pp. 140–75]. Considering that children frequently have difficulty recounting the events occurring in a seizure, the required impairment of consciousness necessary for specific classification can be hard to prove.

In infants complex partial seizures differ from those seen in older children and adults. Behavioral arrest is followed by forced lateralization of gaze and facial automatisms. One upper extremity may be extended and the hand is fisted and flexed forward. The posture resembles a tonic neck reflex. Convulsive movements can accompany these activities. Most patients have evidence of neurologic impairment [35–38].

In the older child the complex partial seizure may be preceded by a recognized aura of visceral, gustatory, or olfactory nature, or by an unusual and difficult to describe sensation. They generally start with a blank stare or with an activity. The activity may be the perseveration of a prior behavior (e.g., continuing to walk when everyone else in line has stopped) or it may be a new onset automatism. Examples of the complex and inappropriate behaviors, or automatisms, are picking at imaginary objects, playing with clothing, climbing onto the dining room table during a meal, chewing, yelling (generally incomprehensibly), and walking in a circle repetitively. The seizure is frequently accompanied by convulsive movements. Fatigue usually follows the seizure [1,34]. Obviously, these unrecognized seizures may be treated as inappropriate behaviors unless they secondarily generalize.

In between seizures most children have no focal abnormalities on neurologic examination. However, behavioral abnormalities and intellectual delay are not uncommon accompaniments [39]. Recent publications suggest that these behavioral findings relate to the presence of chronic illness, not the electrical disturbance in the temporal lobe [39]. In one study of children with complex partial seizures, half the children had persistent behavioral, scholastic, or employment difficulties on follow-up [40]. Patients rarely outgrow the need for AED therapy, save for the few whose seizures resolve concurrent with temporal lobe resections [40,41].

B. Differential Diagnosis

1. Other Seizures

Complex partial seizures should be differentiated both from other seizures and from nonepileptic events. As children are unable to describe the event in detail, the presence or absence of awareness can be difficult to determine. An example of this is benign rolandic epilepsy. In the nocturnal seizures accompanying this epilepsy the patient is unable to speak, but he or she is aware of the environment. Consciousness is preserved, but it may be difficult to prove this due to the patient's inability to speak, and the uneven recall of the nocturnal event the following morning.

Absence seizures may be accompanied by facial or limb automatisms, again making the distinction from partial complex seizures difficult. The EEG is particularly helpful, as it will demonstrate generalized 3-per-second spike-and-wave discharges in absence seizures, which are not seen in partial complex seizures. In addition, patients generally recover promptly from an absence seizure without postictal depression [42].

2. Pseudoseizures

Pseudoseizures are also difficult to distinguish from partial complex seizures, especially when pseudoseizures occur in a patient who is known to have complex partial seizures [43–44]. Thrashing and amnesia for the event are common accompaniments of pediatric pseudoseizures [43]. Differential factors described in Chapter 1 and video EEGs may be useful in separating the two events.

Simple partial seizures may be confused with complex partial when a simple seizure is embellished [46]. In this situation unusual behaviors accompany a simple partial seizures, or occur after the partial seizure has electrically ceased. Such embellishments have thus far only been reported in adults.

3. Behaviors

Rages or other behaviors may be mistaken for seizures, especially if the patient has an abnormal EEG. The difference here is that generally rages, or episodic dyscontrol, are provoked events, even though the provocation is minimal and the reaction is severely destructive [47]. Save for hyperventilation, photic stimulation, or sleep deprivation, seizures are not provoked events. In addition, a rage is usually goal directed, with the patient attacking an individual or destroying an object. A seizure will never lead to such coordinated and directed behaviors unless the patient is frightened or restrained upon recovery from a seizure.

In the same sense, criminal behaviors have occasionally been attributed to a seizure. In one such case a mother's imprisonment for the murder of her child was dismissed on the basis of an epileptogenic EEG and an observed convulsion [48]. The court accepted the plea of an "abnormality of mind induced by disease" in this 19 year-old woman. Obviously, this does not constitute scientific proof that the murder and the epilepsy were associated events. In a through study of ictal aggression in adults, the ictal aggressive acts always occurred early in the seizure and were very brief, lasting an average of 29 s. The acts were stereotyped, simple, unsustained, and nonpurposeful, as opposed to a criminal act [49].

4. Abdominal Distress

Vague and nonspecific abdominal distress can precede a complex partial seizure, and such aura can occur in the absence of a following seizure. On the other hand, *abdominal epilepsy* is a term that has been used and abused in the past to describe children who have abdominal pain and an abnormal EEG [50]. The coincidence of an abnormal interictal EEG and periodic abdominal pain is never sufficient to diagnose abdominal epilepsy, and one follow-up study failed to find the development of more typical features of epilepsy [51].

To diagnose abdominal epilepsy, epileptic EEG changes have to occur concurrent with the clinical event. If the event is too infrequent to capture on video or ambulatory EEG, the diagnosis of partial seizures can be made only if the abdominal distress is followed on occasion by a typical complex partial seizure. Even then the diagnosis is suspect. Lacking this kind of documentation for the diagnosis of epilepsy, the diagnosis of abdominal epilepsy is always suspect. A prompt and persistent response to an AED can be diagnostically helpful and eventually misleading.

Cyclic vomiting, occurring without more typical epileptic events, is never a seizure. It has been associated with migraine [52], and psychiatric intervention has been beneficial [53]. In Hammond's 1974 report of 35 patients hospitalized with cyclic vomiting, 12 were available for long-term follow-up. None had developed epilepsy, 8 developed migraine headaches, and 8 had significant psychological disorders [54].

5. Migraine

Migraine may be difficult to distinguish from seizures when migranous events are not accompanied by the typical disabling headache and when the patient with migraine has an abnormal EEG. Migranous events that suggest partial seizures are acute confusional migraine [55] and migraine with micropsia [56]. Helpful distinguishing associations are the positive family history of migraine and the presence of typical disabling headaches in patients with migraine headaches.

6. Cardiogenic Syncope

Various disorders of cardiac conduction can produce periodic loss of consciousness, preceded by an aura of light-headedness. The loss of consciousness may be accompanied by postural changes suggestive of a seizure and followed by postictal lethargy. Considering the aura and the atypical posturing, a diagnosis of complex partial seizures might be made.

The EEG of a child recently seen in our neurophysiology laboratory demonstrates this problem. The boy had 2-per-month spells consisting of an aura of fright, followed by loss of consciousness with decorticate posturing. Diagnoses were constipation and epilepsy. Adequate phenytoin therapy failed to alleviate these symptoms. The EEG recorded during an event is demonstrated in Fig. 2.

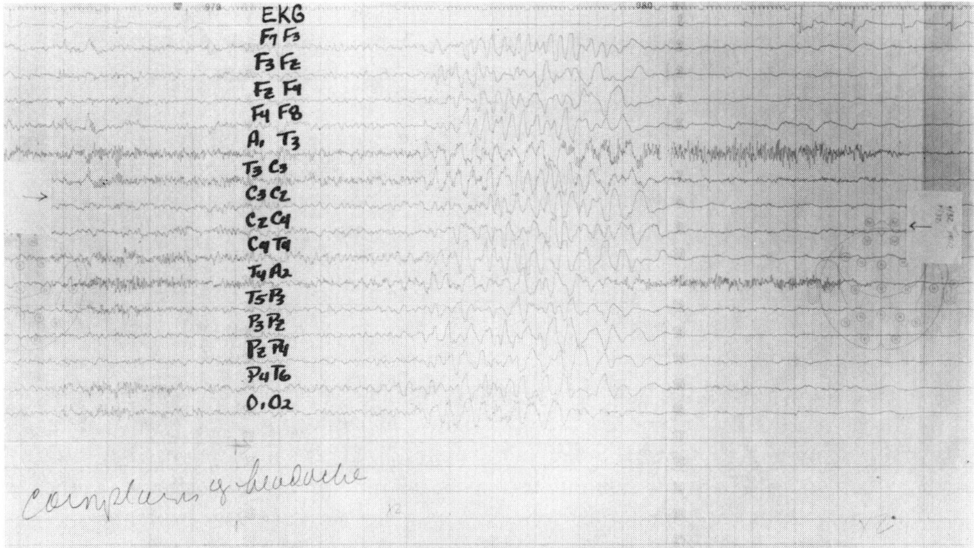

Figure 2 EEG from a boy who had bimonthly spells consisting of a scream, elbow and wrist flexion across his abdomen, upward eye deviation, loss of awareness, falling, and postictal lethargy. A diagnosis of complex partial seizures was based on the nature of the seizures and mild unilateral slowing on EEG. Phenytoin therapy was ineffective. The EEG during the event is isoelectric, and the EKG, in the first or top lead, demonstrates asystole. With this record it is obvious that the event is cardiac, not cerebral, in origin.

C. Etiologies

Any of the numerous focal lesions that occur in brain can produce focal seizures, and the location of this anatomic abnormality relates to the type of seizure seen. Even in patients with a long history of intractable seizures, the finding of intracerebral masses, including tumors, is not uncommon [57]. Their frequency will probably diminish with the increasing diagnostic use of magnetic resonance imaging (MRI).

Most patients with complex partial seizures have seizure foci originating in a temporal lobe, but frontal and occipital lobe foci have also been reported in patients with partial complex seizures [3,4]. The underlying lesion in the temporal lobe most commonly is mesial temporal sclerosis (MTS) or scarring and neuronal loss in a specific areas of the hippocampus [58,59].

More important than the glial scarring is the absence of neurones in Sommer's sector of the hippocampus. It appears that these changes cause a synaptic reorganization which becomes epileptogenic. Other abnormalities in the temporal lobe causing complex partial seizures include low-grade tumors, hamartomatous malformations, or heterotopias. Some patients have been noted to have double pathologies in the temporal lobe (e.g., mesial temporal lobe sclerosis and a temporal lobe hamartoma) [5,59].

The pathology in infants with complex partial seizures is different from that seen in older children. In one recent study of infants with complex partial seizures, 90% of 50 infants had an underlying etiology for their seizures, and the most common etiology was birth asphyxia. Other etiologies reflected neurologic diseases common in this age group (e.g., prematurity, meningitis, jaundice) [36].

Whether MTS is a cause or an effect (i.e., the chicken or the egg) of complex partial seizures is frequently argued [60]. Supporting the proposal that the MTS is secondary to the seizures is the observation that patients with seizures secondary to tumors of the temporal lobe have hippocampal cell loss (i.e., minimal evidence of MTS) [5,59]. On the other hand, the following three observations make it more likely that MTS causes the epilepsy: (1) frank (as opposed to minimal change) MTS is the commonest lesion in complex partial seizures; (2) the electrical focus for complex partial seizures generally correlates with the specific temporal lobe demonstrating MST; and (3) surgical removal of temporal lobes with this lesion is frequently followed by resolution of, or remarkable improvement in, the patient's complex partial seizures [61].

If MTS causes complex partial seizures, what in turn causes MTS? The frequency of perinatal problems in patients who demonstrate this lesion suggested that MTS occurred secondary to intrapartum injury, with mesial herniation of the temporal lobe during a difficult delivery [62]. Later studies have failed to support this hypothesis. Children with severe birth asphyxia may have partial seizures, but these are not the children with isolated MTS. Given their generally severe neurologic handicaps, surgical intervention is not indicated for seizure control [63]. Neither obstetric complications nor Apgar scores are predictive for epilepsy. [64,65].

A second and more plausible theory is that MTS is related to febrile seizures. Falconer concluded that ferbrile seizures were an etiology when he recognized their high frequency in patients observed to have MTS in resected surgical specimens [5]. Prospective studies, mostly involving short-term follow-up, have not supported this association [66–68]. Retrospective studies of febrile seizures indicate that the febrile seizures associated with subsequent partial seizures have atypical features. They occur very early in life and are unduly prolonged [69,70].

Two retrospective studies have been able to associate the degree of hippocampal neuronal loss with the presence of prolonged seizures in childhood [58,59]. Although more data are necessary, it is probable that either (1) atypical febrile seizures or prolonged convulsions in infants produce excitotoxic changes in the developing hippocampus that can lead to neuronal death, synaptic reorganization, and partial seizures, or (2) that atypical or prolonged seizures occur in infants already with developing MTS and therefore at risk for subsequent development of partial seizures. Prospective follow-up studies of infants with prolonged convulsions or atypical febrile seizures are necessary [3,4] to determine definitively the etiology of partial complex seizures of temporal lobe origin. Armed with this information, a program for the prevention of the initial event may then be explored.

IV. EVALUATION

Based on the information above, it is obvious that the evaluation of a patient with partial seizures demands a through description of the event to determine that the patient has partial seizures, a careful history looking for genetic or physical causation, a complete neurologic assessment looking for localizing features that might indicate the anatomic origin of the partial seizures, and an EEG. If all this information indicates that the patient has a benign partial epilepsy, no further workup is necessary, and the merits of observation or intervention with AEDs can be considered.

If the information provided and the EEG are not sufficient to establish a diagnosis, a video EEG, to capture and record the event simultaneously on EEG and videotape, can be extremely helpful. Its value diminishes if the event in question is not captured during the recording.

When a partial epilepsy is diagnosed, based on the initial evaluation above, and the patient's features are not those of a benign epilepsy, an imaging procedure is mandatory. Initially, a CT (computerized tomography) scan of the head is sufficient. If a more detailed image of the epileptic focus is desirable, a magnetic resonance image (MRI) is the next logical step [71–73].

Positron emission tomography (PET) will measure the rates of glucose utilization in different areas of the brain by measuring cerebral concentrations of the injected, radioactive, deoxyfluoroglucose. If the patient has a seizure after injection of the deoxyfluoroglucose and before the imaging procedure, the active epileptic focus will have a high metabolic rate and increased uptake of the radioactive compound. An inactive epileptic focus generally has a low metabolic rate and low concentration of the radioactive compound [74,75].

Single photon emission computed tomography (SPECT) measures variations in blood flow in areas of brain. Active epileptic foci frequently have increased blood flow [76]. Both PET and SPECT are available in large metropolitan medical centers, and there use is usually limited to intensively studied patients with intractable epilepsies who are being considered for surgery.

V. EFFICACIOUS ANTIEPILEPTIC DRUGS

Once it is concluded that the patient has partial seizures and that they warrant prophylactic AED therapy, drug therapy can be initiated concurrent with the ongoing evaluation of the seizure focus. If a video EEG is indicated, it may be necessary to withdraw AEDs temporarily to provoke a seizure. In this situation, care must be taken to have the patient in a center where a prolonged seizure can be appropriately managed, as in a hospital.

As described in Chapter 2, there are five AEDs which are equally effective in controlling partial seizures: carbamazepine, phenobarbital, phenytoin, primidone, and valproic acid divalproex sodium. Therefore, factors other than the specific nature of the epilepsy are used in AED selection. (This observation does not lessen the importance in diagnosing the epilepsy and its etiology correctly. The correct diagnosis is essential for providing a prognosis and the potential benefit from surgery [40,63].)

The other factors that are useful in AED selection include age of patient, potential drug adversities, cost, and estimated ability of the patient and family to comply with a complex or simple AED regimen. The reader is referred to Chapter 2 for a description of how these factors relate to AED selection. In our comprehensive epilepsy center we tend to avoid initiating treatment with primidone or phenobarbital due to their frequently detrimental effects on performance.

Whatever AED regimen is employed, it is essential that the regimen be limited to the fewest drugs that will provide control for the seizures and will least impair the child's performance. Monotherapy with an effective AED that is well tolerated is the goal of therapy.

REFERENCES

1. Yamamoto N, Watanabe K, Negoro T, Takaesu E, Aso K, Furune S, Takahashi I. Complex partial seizures in children: ictal manifestations and their clinical course. Neurology 1987; 37:1379–82.
2. Wylie E, Rothner AD, Luders H. Partial seizures in children: clinical features, medical treatment and surgical considerations. Pediatr Clin North Am 1989; 36:343–64.
3. Williamson PD, Spencer DD, Spencer SS, Novelly RA, Mattson RH. Complex partial seizures of frontal lobe origin. Ann Neurol 1985; 18:497–504.
4. Williamson PD, Spencer SS, Spencer DD. Complex partial seizures with occipital lobe onset (abstr). Epilepsia 1981; 22:247–48.
5. Falconer MA, Serafetinides EA, Corsellis JAN. Etiology and pathogenesis of temporal lobe epilepsy. Arch Neurol 1964; 10:233–48.
6. Cavazzutti GB. Epidemiology of different types of epilepsy in school-age children of Modena, Italy. Epilepsia 1980; 21:57–62.
7. Gregory DL, Wong PK. (1984). Topographical analysis of the centrotemporal discharges in benign rolandic epilepsy of childhood. Epilepsia 1984; 25:705–11.
8. Gutierrez AR, Brick JF, Bodensteiner J. Dipole reversal: an ictal feature of benign partial epilepsy with centrotemporal spikes. Epilepsia 1990; 31:544–48.
9. Degen D, Degen H-E. Some genetic aspects of rolandic epilepsy. Epilepsia 1990; 31:795–802.

10. Eeg-Olofsson O, Petersen I, Sellden U. The development of the electroencephalogram in normal children from the age of 1 through 15 years. Paroxysmal activity. Neuropadiatrie 1971; 2:375–404.
11. Blom S, Heijbel J. Benign epilepsy of childhood with centrotemporal EEG foci: a followup study in an adulthood of patients initially studied as children. Epilepsia 1982; 23:629–32.
12. Loisseau P, Pestre M, Dartigues JF, Commenges D, Barberger-Gateau C, Cohadon S. Long-term prognosis in two forms of childhood epilepsy: typical absence seizures and epilepsu with rolandic (centrotemporal) EEG foci. Ann Neurol 1983; 13:642–48.
13. Ambrosetto G, Tassinari CA. Antiepileptic drug treatment of benign childhood epilepsy with rolandic spikes: is it necessary? Epilepsia 1990; 31:802–5.
14. Aicardi J. Epilepsy in children. New York: Raven Press, 1986.
15. Gastaut H. A new type of epilepsy: benign partial epilepsy of childhood with occipital spike waves. Clin Electroencephalogr 1982; 13:13–22.
16. Panayiotopoulos CP. Benign childhood epilepsy with occipital paroxysms: a 15-year prospective study. Ann Neurol 1989; 26:51–56.
17. Luders H, Lesser RP, Dinner DS, Morris HH III. Benign focal epilepsy of childhood. In: Luders H and Lesser RP, eds. Epilepsy: electroclinical syndromes. Berlin: Springer-Verlag, 1987:303–46.
18. Landau W, Kleffner F. Syndrome of acquired aphasia with convulsive disorder in children. Neurology 1957; 7:523–30.
19. Hirsch E, Marescaux C, Maquet P, Metz-lotz MN, Kiesmann M, Salmon E, Franck G, Kurtz D. Landau-Kleffner syndrome: a clinical and EEG study of five cases. Epilepsia 1990; 31:756–68.
20. Marescaux C, Hirsch E, Finck S, Maquet P, Schlumberger E, Sellal F, Metz-lutz MN, Alembik Y, Salmon E, Franck G, Kurtz D. Landau-Kleffner syndrome: a pharmacologic study of five cases. Epilepsia 1990; 31:768–77.
21. Rapin I, Mattis S, Rowan AJ, Golden GC. Verbal auditory agnosia in children. Dev Med Child Neurol 1977; 19:192–207.
22. Deonna T, Beaumanoir A, Gaillard F, Assal G. Acquired aphasia in childhood with seizure disorder: a heterogeneous syndrome. Neuropadiatrie 1977; 8:263–73.
23. Mantovani J, Landau W. Acquired aphasia with convulsive disorder: course and prognosis. Neurology 1980; 30:524–29.
24. Morrell F, Cooper M, Ali A, Smith MC, Pierre-Louis SJC, Whisler WW. Landau Kleffner syndrome: metabolic, blood flow, and electrophysiologic studies (abstr). Epilepsia 1990; 31:672.
25. Maquet P, Hirsch E, Dive D, Salmon E, Marescaux C, Franck G. Cerebral glucose utilization during sleep in Landau-Kleffner syndrome: a PET study. Epilepsia 1990; 31:778–83.
26. Doose H, Baier WK. Benign partial epilepsy and related conditions: multifactorial pathogenesis with hereditary impairment of brain muturation. Eur J Pediatr 1989; 149:152–58.
27. Wyllie E, Luders H, Morris HH, Lesser RP, Dinner DS. The lateralizing significance of versive head and eye movements during epileptic seizures. Neurology 1986; 36:606–11.

28. McLachlan RS. The significance of head and eye turning in seizures. Neurology 1987; 37:1617–19.
29. Thomas JE, Reggan TJ, Klass DW. Epilepsia partialis continua. Arch Neurol 1977; 34:266–75.
30. Dulac O, Dravet C, Plouin P, Bureau M, Ponsot G, Gerbaut L, Roger J, Arthuis M. Aspects nosologiques des épilepsies partielles continues chez l'enfant. Arch Fr Pediatr 1983; 40:687–704.
31. Gascon GG, Lombroso CT. Epileptic (gelastic) laughter. Epilepsia 1971; 12:63–76.
32. Berkovic SF, Andermann F, Melanson D, Ethier RE, Feindel W, Gloor P. Hypothalamic hamartomas and ictal laughter: evolution of a characteristic epileptic syndrome and diagnostic value of magnetic resonance imaging. Ann Neurol 1988; 23:429–39.
33. Malik S, Cruse RP, Wyllie E. Surgical cure of gelastic seizures and hypsarrhythmia due to a hypothalamic hamartoma: a unique case (abstract). Epilepsia 1990; 31:663–64.
34. Holmes GL. (1984). Partial complex seizures in children: an analysis of 69 seizures in 24 patients using EEG FM radiotelemetry and videotape recording. Electroencephalogr Clin Neurophysiol 1984; 57:13–20.
35. Duchowny MS. Complex partial seizures of infancy. Arch Neurol 1987; 44:911–14.
36. Pratap RC, Gururaj AK. Clinical and electroencephalographic features of partial complex seizures in infants. Acta Neurol Scand 1989; 79:123–27.
37. Blume WT. Clinical profile of partial seizures beginning at less than four years of age. Epilepsia 1989; 30:813–19.
38. Luna D, Dulac O, Plouin P. Ictal characteristics of cryptogenic partial epilepsies in infancy. Epilepsia 1989; 30:827–32.
39. Kaminer Y, Apter A, Aviv A, Lerman P, Tyano S. Psychopathology and temporal lobe epilepsy in adolescents. Acta Psychiatr Scand 1988; 77:640–44.
40. Lindsay J, Ounsted J, Richards P. Long-term outcome in children with temporal lobe seizures. IV. Genetic factors, febrile convulsions and the remission of seizures. Dev Med Child Neurol 1980; 22:429–39.
41. Kotagal P, Rothner AD, Erenberg G, Cruse RP, Wyllie E. Complex partial seizures of childhood onset. A five year followup. Arch Neurol 1987: 44:1177–80.
42. Holmes GL, McKeever M, Adamson M. Absence seizures in children: clinical and electroencephalographic features. Ann Neurol 1987; 21:268–73.
43. Wyllie E, Friedman D, Rothner AD, Luders H, Dinner D, Morris H III, Cruse R, Erenberg G, Kotagal P. (1990). Psychogenic seizures in children and adolescents: outcome after diagnosis by ictal video and electroencephalographic recording. Pediatrics 1990; 85:480–84.
44. Gates JR, Ramani V, Whalen SM, Whalen S, Loewenson R. Ictal characteristics of pseudoseizures. Arch Neurol 1985; 42:1183–87.
45. Holmes GL, Sackellares JC, McKiernan J, Ragland M, Dreifuss FE. Evaluation of childhood pseudoseizures using EEG telemetry and video tape monitoring. J Pediatr 1980; 97:554–58.
46. Smith DB, DeToledo J. Embellished simple partial seizures misdiagnosed as pseudoseizures (abstr). Epilepsia 1990; 31:647.

47. Elliot FA. The episodic dyscontrol syndrome and aggression. Neurol Clin 1984; 2: 113–25.
48. Hindler CG. Epilepsy and violence. Br J Psychiatry 1989; 155:246–49.
49. Delgado-Escueta AV, Mattson RH, King L, Goldensohn ES, Spiegel H, Madsen J, Crandall P, Dreifuss F, Porter RJ. The nature of aggression during epileptic seizures. N Engl J Med 1980; 305:711–16.
50. Douglas EF, White PT. Abdominal epilepsy: a reappraisal. J Pediatr 1971; 78:59–67.
51. Papatheophilou R, Jeavons PM, Disney ME. Recurrent abdominal pain: a clinical and electroencephalographic study. Dev Med Child Neurol 1972; 14:31–44.
52. Hoyt CS, Stickler GB. A study of 44 children with the syndrome of recurrent (cyclic) vomiting. Peidatrics 1960; 25:775–80.
53. Reinhart JB, Evans SL, McFadden DL. Cyclic vomiting in children: seen through the psychiatrist's eyes. Pediatrics 1977; 59:371–77.
54. Hammond J. The late sequelae of recurrent vomiting of childhood. Dev Med Child Neurol 1974; 16:15–22.
55. Gascon G, Barlow C. Juvenile migraine presenting as an acute confusional state. Pediatrics 1970; 45:628–35.
56. Hachinski VC, Porchawka J, Steele JC. Visual symptoms in the migraine syndrome. Neurology 1973; 23:570–79.
57. Spencer DD, Spencer SS, Mattson RH, Williamson PD. Intracerebral masses in patients with intractible partial epilepsy. Neurology 1984; 34:432–36.
58. Sagar HJ, Oxbury JM. Hippocampal neuron loss in temporal lobe epilepsy: correlation with early childhood convulsions. Ann Nuerol 1987; 23:334–40.
59. Babb TJ, Brown WJ. Pathological findings in epilepsy. In: Engel J Jr, ed. Surgical treatment of the epilepsies. New York: Raven Press, 1985:511–40.
60. Laxer KD. Introduction to symposium: mesial temporal lobe sclerosis (abstr). Epilepsia 1990; 31:673.
61. Lindsay J, Glaser G, Richards P, Ounsted C. Developmental aspects of focal epilepsies of childhood treated by neurosurgery. Dev Med Child Neurol 1984; 26:574–87.
62. Earle KM, Baldwin M, Penfield W. Incisural sclerosis and temporal lobe seizures produced by hippocampal herniation at birth. AMA Arch Neurol Psychiatry 1953; 69:27–42.
63. Lindsay J, Ounsted C, Richards P. Long-term outcome in children with temporal lobe seizures. V. Indications and contra-indications for neurosurgery. Dev Med Child Neurol 1984; 26:25–32.
64. Nelson KB, Ellenberg JH. Obstetric complications as risk factors for cerebral palsy or seizure disorders. JAMA 1984; 251:1843–48.
65. Rosen MG. Factors during labor and delivery that influence brain disorders. In: Freeman JM, ed. Prenatal and perinatal factors associated with brain disorders. NIH Publication 85–1149. 1985:237–61.
66. Lee K, Diaz M, Melchior. Temporal lobe epilepsy: not a consequence of childhood convulsions in Denmark. Acta Neurol Scand 1981: 63:231–36.
67. Annegers JF, Hauser WA, Elveback LR, Kurland LT. The risk of epilepsy following febrile convulsions. Neurology 1979; 29:297–303.

68. Wolf SM, Forsythe A. Epilepsy and mental retardation following febrile seizures in childhood. Acta Paediatr Scand 1989; 78:291–95.
69. Annegers JF, Hauser WA, Shirts SB, Kurland LT. Factors prognostic of unprovoked seizures after febrile convulsions. N Engl J Med 1987; 316:493–98.
70. Viani F, Beghi E, Romeo A, van Lierde A. Infantile febrile status epilepticus. Risk factors and outcome. Dev Med Child Neurol 1987; 29:495–501.
71. Conlon P, Trimble MR, Rogers D, Callicot C. Magnetic resonance imaging in epilepsy: a controlled study. Epilepsy Res 1988; 2:37–43.
72. Smith AS, Weinstein MA, Quencer RM, Muroff LR, Stonesifer KJ, Li FC, Wener L, Soloman MA, Cruse RP, Rosenberg LH. Association of heterotopic grey matter with seizures: MR imaging. Work in progress. Radiology 1988; 168:195–98.
73. Kendall BE. Magnetic resonance in diseases of the nervous system. Arch Dis Child 1988; 63:1301–4.
74. Council on Scientific Affairs. Position emission tomography: a new approach to brain chemistry. JAMA 1988; 260:2704–10.
75. Swartz BE, Halgren E, Delgado-Escueta AV, Mandelkern M, Gee M, Quinones N, Blahd WH, Repchan J. Neuroimaging in patients with seizures of probable frontal lobe origin. Epilepsia 1989; 30:547–48.
76. Denays R, Rubinstein M, Ham H, Piepsz, Noel P. Single photon emission computed tomography in seizures disorders. Arch Dis Child 1988; 63:1184–88.
77. Lindsay J, Ounsted C, Richards P. Long-term outcome in children with temporal lobe seizures. IV. Genetic factors, febrile convulsions and the remission of seizures. Dev Med Child Neurol 1980; 22:429–239.

6

Seizures in the First Week of Life

JEROME Y. YAGER
Royal University Hospital
Saskatoon, Saskatchewan, Canada

ROBERT C. VANNUCCI
Pennsylvania State University School of Medicine
The Milton S. Hershey Medical Center
Hershey, Pennsylvania

I. INTRODUCTION

Convulsive activity in the newborn infant is a common accompaniment to perinatal insults that affect the central nervous system [1–3]. Whereas in older infants, children, and adults, the majority of seizures are idiopathic (presumably genetic) in origin, convulsions that occur in the newborn infant almost invariably denote an underlying derangement of the brain that may be associated with permanent damage. Accordingly, it is important that the clinical manifestations and electroencephalographic (EEG) patterns that characterize seizures in the newborn infant are recognized early to ascertain the underlying etiology and to initiate appropriate medical therapy.

II. INCIDENCE

The incidence of seizures differs depending on the population of newborn infants under study. Craig [4] reported an incidence of 0.8% in an unselected group of newborn infants. Infants at "high risk" are more likely to exhibit seizure activity arising from an underlying, identifiable condition that prompts the infant's admission to a neonatal intensive care unit (NICU). Seay and Bray [5] reported an incidence of 20% in premature infants weighing less than 2500 g at birth, and Painter et al. [6] reported an incidence of 25% in infants weighing less than 1500 g at birth and surviving the newborn period. It is likely that the latter incidence figure would have been much higher if premature infants expiring in the newborn period had been included. Neonatal seizures are frequently associated with perinatal asphyxia, and the incidence approaches 50% in newborn infants who sustained fetal distress combined with clinical evidence of postnatal hypoxic-ischemic encephalopathy [3,7].

III. CLINICAL FEATURES

Owing to the morphologic and functional immaturity of the perinatal brain, newborn infants do not exhibit the generalized tonic-clonic seizures so typical of children and adults. Volpe [3,8,9] has characterized four specific types of seizures frequently encountered in the newborn period: subtle (fragmentary), tonic (focal or generalized), clonic (focal or multifocal), and myoclonic (focal, multifocal, or generalized).

A. Subtle (Fragmentary) Seizures

These seizures consist of tonic or jerking deviation of the eyes; abrupt eye opening or repetitive blinking of the eyelids; drooling, sucking, chewing, or buccal–lingual movements; stereotyped postures or movements of the extremities (pedaling, swimming, rowing); vasomotor instability; and abrupt changes in respiratory pattern or apnea. Subtle seizures occur in both full-term and premature infants and are often associated with one or other of the seizure types listed below. When exhibiting paroxysmal (epileptiform) discharges, the electroencephalogram (EEG) is characterized by 1- to 4-Hz high-voltage delta slow waves, sharp waves or spikes, a burst-suppression pattern (bursts of high voltage, slow and sharp wave activity, followed by an attentuation of the background pattern) or occasionally an 8- to 12-Hz alpha-like pattern.

B. Tonic Seizures

These seizures are characterized by tonic flexion or extension of the neck, trunk, and upper extremities, usually with extension of the lower extremities, and are occasionally focal but more commonly generalized. Such clinical episodes mimic closely the "decorticate" or "decerebrate" postures seen in older infants and children undergoing herniation of the brain secondary to cerebral hemispheric structural lesions or metabolic encephalopathy. Appoximately 70% of these seizures occur in infants weighing less than 2500 g. The EEG, when paroxysmal, is characterized by 1- to 4-Hz high-voltage delta slow waves, sharp waves, or spikes, a burst-suppression pattern or 8- to 12-Hz alpha-like activity. When tonic seizures are associated with epileptiform discharges on EEG, there is typically accompanying autonomic phenomena, including alterations in heart rate, blood pressure, cutaneous pallor, or flushing.

C. Clonic Seizures

Multifocal clonic seizures consist of jerking of one extremity, which then migrates randomly to other extremities. Upper limb and contralateral lower limb activitiy is frequently observed. Approximately 75% of these seizures occur in infants weighing more than 2500 g. The EEG is usually abnormal and is characterized by multifocal complexes of slow 1- to 4-Hz delta waves, spikes, or rhythmic theta- or alpha-like activity.

Focal clonic seizures consist of jerking limited to one or more extremities on the same side of the body with or without facial involvement. This seizure type is frequent in the newborn infant and often denotes an underlying structural lesion in the contralateral cerebral hemisphere. However, focal clonic seizures can also arise from a systemic metabolic derangement, such as hypoglycemia. The EEG typically is paroxysmal and is characterized by focal sharp wave or spike activity.

D. Myoclonic Seizures

Myoclonic seizures can be focal, multifocal, or generalized. Focal myoclonic seizures typically consist of single or multiple rapid contractions of the flexor muscles of an upper extremity, whereas multifocal myoclonic seizures are characterized by asynchronous twitching of several parts of the body. Generalized myoclonic seizures consist of single or multiple massive flexions of the head and trunk in association with flexion or extension of the extremities. These seizures are rare in the immediate newborn period, but when they occur they mimic ''infantile spasms'' seen in older infants.

All three forms of myoclonic seizures can also be seen during sleep in premature and full-term infants [10,11]. Labeled *benign neonatal sleep myoclonus*, these episodes typically resolve by 6 months of age. They are not associated with an underlying structural lesion in the brain or a metabolic derangement.

Seizure activity must be distinguished from clonus or jitteriness, neither of which is convulsive in nature nor responsive to anticonvulsant medication. Clonus is rhythmic in character, and the alternating movements (oscillations) are of equal velocity. The alternating (clonic) movements of seizures are of unequal velocity with rapid and slow components. Clonus can be precipitated or abolished by changes in position or by stimulation, whereas seizures are not altered by changes in posture, nor are they stimulus sensitive. Clonus is ablated by restraining limb movements; if this maneuver is attempted in seizure movements, underlying contractions will be felt. Finally, facial and occular movements are frequently present as a component of seizures but do not accompany clonus.

Attempts should also be made to distinguish between convulsive and nonconvulsive apnea. During convulsive apnea, the EEG demonstrates paroxysmal

Table 1 Frequency and Electrographic Correlation of Neonatal Seizures

Clinical seizure type	Frequency of seizure[a]	Electrographic correlation	
		Consistent	Inconsistent
Subtle (fragmentary)	30%		
Bicycling			+
Oral–buccal–lingual		+	
Tonic eye deviation		+	
Apnea			+
Complex purposeless movements			+
Clonic	25%	+	
Tonic	20%		+
Myoclonic	25%		
Focal, multifocal			+
Generalized		+	

Source: Data derived from Mizrahi and Kellaway (15), Legido et al. (16), and Sher et al. (17).
[a]Percentages denote relative prevalence of seizure types.

activity, most frequently an alpha-like rhythm [12]. Fenichel et al. [13] monitored the EEG and heart rate in newborn infants during apneic spells and found that bradycardia rarely occurred in conjunction with convulsive activity. Indeed, more recent studies have demonstrated an early increase in heart rate, often in association with an elevation in systemic blood pressure. Thus monitoring of the heart rate during apnea may be clinically useful in differentiating nonconvulsive from convulsive apnea. Prolonged apneic episodes without bradycardia would suggest the possibility of an underlying seizure disturbance. Fortunately, the vast majority of infants exhibiting convulsive apnea also display other subtle phenomena (occular or oral-facial movements), which together support the epileptiform nature of the episode [14].

IV. CLINICAL SEIZURES AND ELECTROGRAPHIC ABNORMALITIES

It must be emphasized that one or more of the four specific types of clinically manifest seizures as characterized by Volpe [3,8,9] are not necessarily epileptiform in nature. Using simultaneous continuous EEG and videotape monitoring, several investigators [15–17] have shown that newborn infants often exhibit clinically apparent ''seizure'' activity which is unaccompanied by paroxsymal (epileptiform) activity recorded on surface EEG (Table 1). The dissociation between clinically apparent seizures and electrical paroxsymal activity is common in infants exhibiting subtle (fragmentary) seizures and is especially common in generalized tonic seizures as well as focal and multifocal myoclonic seizures of prematurity [8,15]. It has been assumed that such seizures represent uninhibited reflex activiy originating in brainstem structures, which centers have been released physiologically or pathologically from higher inhibitory centers within the cerebral hemispheres. An alternative hypothesis is that such seizures are truly epileptic in nature but that the paroxsymal discharges are not propagated to the cortical surfaces of the cerebral hemispheres from their sites of origin in deep limbic structures, the diencephalon, or lower brainstem [8]. As a result, surface EEG electrodes do not detect the distant epileptiform activity.

Alternatively, even in those infants in whom clinical seizures have been diagnosed, many continue to exhibit electrographic seizures in the absence of associated clinical manifestations. Clancy et al. [18] conducted routine EEG examinations in 41 nonparalyzed sick neonates who displayed clinical features of seizure activity. Of 393 seizures recorded electrographically, only 21% were accompanied by distinct clinical features, the remaining 79% being occult. Similar results have been reported by Connell et al. [19], who recorded EEG seizure activity in the absence of clinical signs in 42% of neonatal seizures. The etiology of seizures in those infants in whom no clinical correlation occurs is predominantly cerebral hypoxia–ischemia or intraventricular hemorrhage.

V. ETIOLOGY

At no other time than during the newborn period is the brain more susceptible to injury. Although variable in expression, seizues in the newborn period are often the first indication of a neurologic affliction, be it acute or chronic [8,15]. As or more important than the seizures themselves are the underlying factors that herald their onset, as it is these predisposing factors upon which outcome primarily depends [20–23].

The relative contribution of the various etiologic factors related to neonatal seizures is shown in Fig. 1. Noteworthy is the shift in the percentages of the causative factors apparent in the 18 years between the first (1970) and the second (1987) studies. Whereas formerly, birth trauma and hypocalcemia accounted for 35% of neonatal seizures, the frequency of these conditions is now low, owing to improved obstetric management of distressed fetuses and to the introduction of infant formulas containing reduced amounts of phosphorus. Perinatal hypoxia–ischemia, intracranial hemorrhage, stroke, and meningitis have increased in relative importance, while the frequency of seizures arising from hypoglycemia and congenital malformations of the brain has remained relatively static.

The differential diagnosis of neonatal seizures is dependent in part on the maturity of the infant at birth, due to the existence of medical conditions peculiar

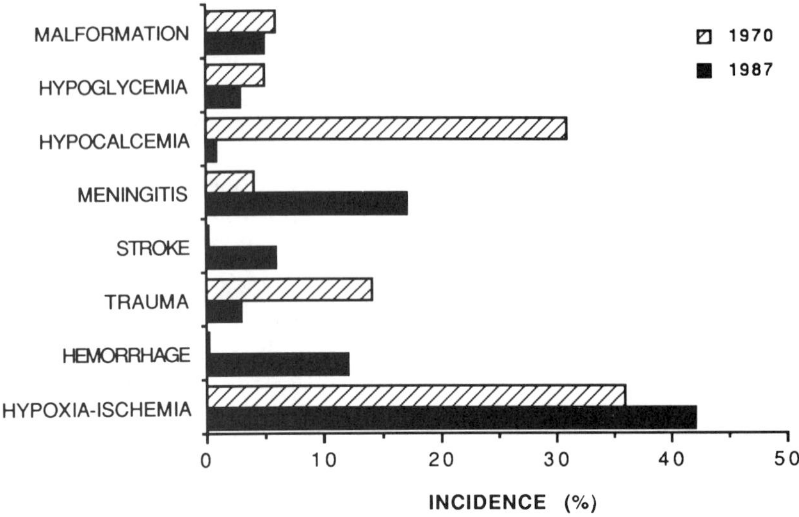

Figure 1 Comparison of prominent etiologic diagnoses of seizures in the newborn period. (Data modified from Refs. 1 and 15.)

to either premature or full-term infants. Intracranial hemorrhage and sepsis are frequent medical conditions in premature infants, whereas complications of cyanotic congenital heart disease, encephalitis, congenital malformations, andmiscellaneous conditions are encountered more commonly in full-term infants. A comprehensive list of possible etiological factors for any single newborn infant is shown in Table 2.

Hypoxic-ischemic encephalopathy continues to be the most frequent etiologic diagnosis, followed by sepsis, intracranial hemorrhage, and cerebral infarction. In this regard, prenatal or neonatal "stroke," previously mentioned rarely, is now frequently recognized as a cause of seizures in the newborn infant [15,24]. Metabolic derangements, particularly hypocalcemia and hypoglycemia, although important, no longer play a major contributory role, whereas the incidence of cerebral malformations have remained unchanged.

Both the timing of the seizure onset and the type of seizure can be important clues in the differential diagnosis. In general, etiologic factors that cause diffuse brain injury and result in lethargy or coma tend to be associated with subtle, tonic, or myoclonic seizures. As mentioned previously, these clinical events often have no or only variable electrographic correlation and are assumed to represent "brainstem release phenomena" [25,26]. Seizures due to metabolic disturbances, asphyxia, or intracranial hemorrhage result in the above-described clinical seizure types and usually occur within the first 72 h following birth.

Table 2 Differential Diagnosis of Neonatal Seizures

- Hypoxia–ischemia
  - Asphyxia
  - Occlusive vascular disease (stroke)
- CNS Infection
  - Meningitis
  - Encephalitis
  - Brain abscess
- Intracranial hemorrhage
  - Intraventricular
  - Intracerbral
  - Subarachnoid
  - Subdural
- CNS malformation
  - Neuronal migration
    - Schizencephaly
    - Lissencephaly
    - Microgyria
    - Agenesis of corpus callosum
  - Differentiation and cleavage
    - Holoprosencephaly
    - Encephalo/myelodysplasia
    - Hydranencephaly
    - Porencephaly
- Acute metabolic disorders
  - Hypocalcemia
  - Hypoglycemia
  - Hypomagnesemia
  - Hyponatremia
- Inborn errors of metabolism
  - Aminoacidopathies
    - Phenylketonuria
    - Maple syrup urine disease
    - Hyperglycinemia
  - Organic acidopathies
    - Propionic acidemia
    - Methylmalonic acidemia
- Peroxisomal disorders
  - Neonatal adrenoleukodystrophy
  - Zellweger syndrome
- Neurocutaneous disorders
  - Neurofibromatosis
  - Tuberous sclerosis
  - Sturge–Weber syndrome
- Toxins
  - Maternal drug ingestion
    - Cocaine
    - Heroin
    - Other narcotics
  - Local anesthetic injection
  - Bilirubin (kernicterus)
- Pyridoxine (B_6) dependency
- Benign seizures
  - Familial
  - Nonfamilial

Focal brain damage arising from perinatal stroke, infection, and malformation often leads to focal or multifocal clonic seizures in an otherwise alert infant at 3 to 5 days of postnatal age. EEG correlation is the rule with these events.

Several of the more common causes of neonatal seizures are discussed below.

A. Asphyxia (Hypoxia–Ischemia)

Hypoxic–ischemic encephalopathy remains the major cause of seizures within the first 72 h following birth. Most asphyxial insults are now recognized as having occurred prior to or during the onset of labor as opposed to resulting from postnatal events. Although not principally responsible for the seizures, associated metabolic findings may include hypoglycemia, hypocalcemia, and the syndrome of inappropriate antidiuretic hormone secretion resulting in hyponatremia. Inattention to these factors may contribute to the refractoriness of the seizures to treatment and may ultimately increase morbidity.

B. Intracranial Hemorrhage

Primary subarachnoid or subdural hemorrhages may occur in isolation, as a consequence of trauma or as a complication of asphyxia. When unassociated with other factors, the infant often appears remarkably well during the interictal period. Rarely, isoimmune thrombocytopenia, a disorder in which maternal antifetal platelet antibodies are formed, results in fetal thrombocytopenia and secondary intracranial hemorrhage, occasionally into the substance of the brain. Affected newborn infants exhibit severe thrombocytopenia and focal clonic seizures, ultimately with the formation of a porencephalic cyst, usually within one cerebral hemisphere [27,28].

C. Stroke

Not previously a well-recognized entity in the newborn infant, the advent of improved neuroradiologic techniques, including cranial ultrasonography and computed tomography, has allowed identification of focal cerebral vascular ischemia and consequent infarction as a common entity, particularly in the fetus ultimately delivered at term [15,24]. Newborn infants typically present with focal or multifocal clonic seizures combined with hypotonia, especially of the upper extremity contralateral to the cerebral infarction.

D. Central Nervous System Infection

Bacterial or viral infections of the central nervous system (meningitis or encephalitis) occur alone or in association with neonatal sepsis. The TORCH viruses, particularly herpes simplex, cause diffuse cerebral necrosis; infected infants often exhibit subtle, focal, or multifocal clonic seizures. Postnatal bacterial infections include group B β-*hemolytic streptococcus* and *Escherichia coli* as the most common agents causing meningitis. Early diagnosis and implementation of antibiotic therapy is essential.

E. CNS Malformations

Disturbances in neuronal induction, proliferation, or migration have consistently accounted for 5 to 10% of all seizures occuring in the first week of postnatal life. Phenotypically, these abnormalities may be associated with multiple congenital anomalies, including those of midline facial structures as well as facial dysmorphorism, as exemplified by holoprosencephaly, lissencephaly, and myelodysplasia. Alternatively, infants phenotypically may appear entirely normal despite major cerebral malformations; typical examples include hydranencephaly and schizencephaly. A presumptive cause for many of the abnormalities described above is occlusive vascular disease of the brain occurring in the first trimester of pregnancy, leading to destruction of primordial nerve cells.

The neurocutaneous syndromes (e.g., neurofibromatosis, tuberous sclerosis, Sturge–Weber syndrome), while not specifically central nervous system (CNS) malformations, occasionally present with seizures in the newborn period. Predominantly of the focal or multifocal clonic variety, these seizures are early manifestations of hamartomas, neurofibromas, or vascular malformations of the cerebral hemispheres. A thorough examination for the presence of café-au-lait spots of the skin and lisch nodules of the iris in neurofibromatosis, the depigmented skin lesions in tuberous sclerosis, or the facial port-wine stain of Sturge–Weber syndrome aid in the diagnosis.

F. Metabolic Derangements

Although a host of metabolic disturbances can cause seizures, the two most notable and treatable in the newborn infant are hypoglycemia and hypocalcemia. The onset of hypocalcemia is biphasic, occurring in the first 48 to 72 h of postnatal life and again between 4 and 7 days. Early hypocalcemia usually is manifest as a complication of maternal diabetes mellitus, maternal hyperparathyroidism, or Di George syndrome (hypoparathyroidism, aortic valve stenosis, thymic hypoplasia, and facial anomalies). Immature renal and parathyroid function, maternal vitamin D deficiency, and high-phosphate formulas result in hypocalcemia in the latter part of the first postnatal week. Increased awareness of the nutritional and metabolic requirements of the newborn infant have led to changes in infant formulas which have virtually eliminated hypocalcemia as a frequent cause of neonatal seizures.

Hypoglycemia, present when blood glucose concentrations decrease below 40 mg/dL in both full-term and premature infants, occurs as the sole metabolic derangement in offspring of diabetic mothers. Less frequently, hypoglycemia occurs in conjunction with inborn errors of metabolism, particularly organic acidemias and glycogen storage diseases. As mentioned previously, hypoglycemia also occurs as a complication of perinatal asphyxia, sepsis, and intrauterine growth retardation.

G. Drug Withdrawal Seizures

The increasing incidence of substance abuse among teenagers and young adults makes it imperative that physicians be aware of the potential perinatal complications resulting from drug withdrawal syndromes. Frequently associated with growth retardation, hypertonicity, and jitteriness, associated seizures tend to occur late in the course of the withdrawal. Herzlinger et al. [29] documented an incidence of neonatal seizures in 1.4% of newborn infants withdrawing from heroin and in 7.8% of infants following withdrawal of methadone. Clinical and experimental evidence also suggests a decreased threshold for seizures in newborn infants exposed to cocaine in utero [30,31].

H. Local Anesthetic Toxicity

Direct injection of local anesthetics into the fetus can occur inadvertently upon the induction of paracervical, pudendal, epidural, or vulvar anesthesia. Clinical manifestations of anesthetic toxicity in the newborn infant occur within the first 12 h following birth and are frequently mistaken as complications of asphyxia. Characteristically, affected infants display hypotonia, bradycardia, and hypoventilation or apnea. Seizures, usually tonic in nature, occur early. Two features help to distinguish these infants from those with hypoxic–ischemic encephalopathy. Local anesthetic intoxication results in widely dilated, fixed pupils and absent oculocephalic (doll's eye) reflexes, cranial nerve abnormalities that occur only in severely asphyxiated newborn infants. Treatment consists of supported measures and active diuresis [32,33].

I. Benign Neonatal Convulsions

1. Familial

A syndrome of autosomally dominant inherited seizures occurring in the newborn period has been well described [34,35]. Seizures occur between the second and third days of postnatal life and are characterized by frequent clonic activity, occasionally associated with apnea. The EEG is normal interictally [36]. Seizures are self-limited and generally disapper within 2 to 4 weeks. Neurologically, the disorder is benign and the affected infant develops normally. However, nonfebrile seizures occur later in childhood in 15% of affected newborn infants.

2. Nonfamilial ("Fifth-Day Fits")

Fifth-day fits occur typically in the latter part of the first week of life in an otherwise normal infant [37]. The seizures are of the clonic variety and generally multifocal in nature, occasionally lasting several hours. The EEG may be abnormal between seizures [36]. Episodes usually diminish within 24 h of onset and are followed by completely normal development. Although a metabolic cause for the disorder has been suspected, the etiology remains unknown [38].

J. Pyridoxine-Dependent Seizures

Seizures due to pyridoxine (vitamin B_6) dependency usually occur within the first day of postnatal life, although occasional cases have been described in which seizures begin in early childhood [39]. The rare disorder presumably results from a deficiency in the synthesis of the inhibitory neurotransmitter, γ-aminobutyric acid (GABA), the synthesis of which requires pyridoxine as a cofactor. Seizures are refractory to conventional anticonvulsant medication. Pyridoxine (50 to 100 mg), given intravenously, results in rapid normalization of the EEG and cessation of the seizures. The vitamin must be continued prophylactically in high doses to prevent seizure recurrence. Unfortunately, despite early intervention with pyridoxine, infants and children often exhibit subsequent mental retardation.

VI. DIAGNOSTIC INVESTIGATIONS

The diagnostic investigation of a newborn infant exhibiting seizure activity begins with a detailed review of pertinent historical (maternal and obstetric) and physical findings. Any of the following factors in a history are important: premature rupture of membranes, chorioamnionitis, maternal fever, or other evidence of either remote or recent systemic infection; difficult labor and deliver or evidence of fetal distress; family history of metabolic or endocrine disturbances, including diabetes and parathyroid disease; and maternal drug addiction. A family history of seizures restricted to the newborn period is occasionally elicited. Physical examination includes a search for signs of systemic or central nervous system infection, hypoxic or metabolic encephalopathy, or intracranial hemorrhage. In addition, a neurologic examination is performed to determine the functional status of the central nervous system and to uncover any focal abnormalities that might aid in localizing the origin of the seizures. Respiratory pattern, temperature, heart rate, and blood pressure are monitored closely to ascertain any diverse effect of seizures on these vital functions, and if such derangements occur they should be corrected promptly. A comprehensive list of laboratory studies indicated in a convulsing newborn infant is shown in Table 3.

VII. MANAGEMENT

Management of the convulsing infant has always been considered a medical emergency. First, a systemic metabolic derangement is sought and promptly treated if found. Blood should be collected for analysis of glucose, blood urea nitrogen, calcium, phosphorus, magnesium, and electrolytes. Arterial blood gases should also be obtained. A dextrostix examination is performed at cribside. Other immediately indicated studies are outlined in Table 3. A lumbar puncture is required to ascertain the presence or absence of intracranial hemorrhage, bacterial meningitis, or encephalitis. Other studies are performed as indicated when the investigations above do not establish the cause of the seizures.

Treatment of neonatal seizures is directed toward the correction of any underlying systemic metabolic derangement or structural lesion of the brain, if present, and toward the early control of the convulsive activity with antileptic

Table 3 Laboratory Studies to Evaluate Neonatal Seizures

A. Indicated
- Complete blood count, differential, platelet count; urinalysis
- Blood glucose (Dextrostix), BUN, Ca, P, Mg, electrolytes
- Blood oxygen and acid-base analysis
- Blood, CSF, and other bacterial cultures
- CSF analysis
- EEG

B. Upon clinical suspicion of specific disease
- Serum immunoglobulins, TORCH[a] antibody titers, and viral cultures
- Blood and urine metabolic studies (bilirubin, ammonia, lactate, $FeCl_3$, ammonia, reducing substance, etc.)
- Blood and urine toxic screen
- Blood and urine amino and organic acid screen
- CT or ultrasound scan

[a]TORCH = toxoplasmosis, rubella, cytomegalovirus, herpes simplex (consider also AIDS).

medications. Seizures of metabolic origin are treated by replacement of the deficient agent. Hypoglycemia is corrected by the intravenous injection of 10 to 15% glucose, 2 to 3 mL/kg, followed by an infusion of 5 to 10% glucose at a rate sufficient to maintain blood glucose above 50 mg/dL. Hypocalcemia is corrected by the slow intravenous administration of 5% calcium gluconate, 2 mL/kg, repeated as necessary to maintain serum calcium concentrations above 7 to 8 mg/dL, depending on the gestational age of the infant. The drug is best given with electrocardiographic monitoring. Hypomagnesemia (<1.0 mEq/L; 0.5 mmol/L) is corrected with 2 to 3% magnesium sulfate, 2 mL/kg, injected intravenously. Pyridoxine dependency seizures, although rare, are readily corrected with the intraveous injection of 50 to 100 mg of this vitamin.

Once it has been established that a metabolic derangement is not contributing to seizure activity in a newborn infant, an anticonvulsant medication is used in an attempt to control repetitive or continuous seizure activity (Table 4). If convulsions are subtle (fragmentary) or of short duration, phenobarbital or hydantoin (Dilantin), 20 mg/kg, is administered intravenously followed by 3 to 5 mg/kg per day with frequent monitoring of blood anticonvulsant levels [6,40,41]. Higher loading doses of phenobarbital are often required, as seizures especially of hypoxic–ischemic origin are often refractory to therapy [42,43].

Focal or generalized status epilepticus is a medical emergency and must be treated promptly. Status epilepticus is defined as continuous tonic or clonic convulsive activity lasting longer than 30 min or intermittent seizure activity lasting longer than 1 h. Several treatment modalities have been used to control status epilepticus in the newborn infant. We favor initial intravenous therapy with a short-acting anticonvulsant medication. Of the available drugs, diazepam (Val-

Table 4 Anticonvulsant Medications Used to Treat Neonatal Seizures

Major drugs
Phenobarbital: 20–60 mg/kg IV initially; 3–5 mg/kg per day thereafter
Hydantoin (Dilantin): 20 mg/kg IV initially; 3–5 mg/kg thereafter
Diazepam (Valium) or lorazepam (Ativan): 0.1–0.2 mg/kg IV for status epilepticus
Minor drugs
Paraldehyde: 0.1 mg/kg diluted 1:10 in 0.25 *N* saline IV or diluted 1:10 in mineral oil PR for status epilepticus
Valproic acid (Dapakene): 20–30 mg/kg PO initially; 20–30 mg/kg per day thereafter in three or four divided doses

ium) or lorazepam (Ativan) appear to be most useful, administered in doses of 0.1 to 0.2 mg/kg. Repeated doses can be given, but respiratory status must be carefully monitored, particularly if either of these agents is used in conjunction with phenobarbital. Another short-acting anticonvulsant medication of benefit is paraldehyde [44]. This medication generally is administered in a dose of 0.1 mL/kg diluted 1:10 in 0.25 *N* saline and given either rectally or intravenously. Because its metabolites are excreted through the lungs, this drug is contraindicated in infants with active pulmonary disease.

The anticonvulsant effects of both diazepam and paraldehyde are short-lived (minutes), thereby requiring the near-simultaneous administration of a longer-acting agent such as phenobarbital or hydantoin. Anticonvulsant blood levels must be monitored closely, and maintenance doses altered to achieve or maintain therapeutic levels (20 to 40 μg/mL). Because of difficulties in newborn infants of maintaining anticonvulsant levels with oral hydantoin as well as the problems of dispensing the oral suspension, we recommend use of this drug only when seizures are not well controlled with phenobarbital. Seizures of hypoxic, hemorrhagic, or infectious origin usually subside after 48 to 72 h, following which anticonvulsant drugs probably can be safely discontinued [8,15] (see below). However, some clinicians advocate maintaining anticonvulsant coverage during the first year of postnatal life.

VIII. DISCONTINUING ANTICONVULSANT MEDICATIONS

Several investigations have addressed the question of when to taper anticonvulsant medications following their initiation for control of seizures in the newborn period [9,45–47]. Unfortunately, many of these studies are flawed to the extent that selection bias predetermined which infants would be weaned from medication. Selection criteria included the underlying cause of the seizure, presence and severity of initial and subsequent EEG abnormalities, presence and extent of abnormalities on computerized tomography (CT) or ultrasound scan, and presence or absence of functional deficits on neurologic examination. In general, those infants in whom an acute insult to the brain had resolved, who exhibited normal initial and follow-up EEG recordings, whose CT or ultrasound scans were normal, and who were free of neurologic compromise were weaned from medication, usually successfully. What was not ascertained was whether or not those infants with a persistently abnormal EEG, CT or ultrasound scan, or neurologic examination also would have remained seizure free had they been weaned from medication, which usually they were not. One can conclude from these studies that anticonvulsant medications in most infants can be discontinued early (less than 3 months) with minimal to low risk of reoccurrence.

Over the past several years, we have approached the issue of discontinuing anticonvulsant medications in a specific manner. If a newborn infant (premature or full-term) has suffered an acute insult to the brain causing seizures (intracranial hemorrhage, infection or hypoxia–ischemia; metabolic encephalopathy), anticonvulsant medications are withdrawn prior to discharge if (1) the infant is stable neurologically and (2) one or more EEG recordings are normal or improving. Infants maintained on a single drug, usually phenobarbital, include those with congenital malformations of the brain, remote destructive lesions of the brain, unstable neurologic condition, or worsening EEG recordings over time. Such infants are reassessed at 1, 3, 6, and 12 months of age and later to determine the optimal age for drug withdrawal. Needless to say, newborn infants who exhibit recurrent seizures despite medication are considered epileptic, in whom drugs are manipulated as required for optimal seizure control. Frequently, such infants harbor congenital malformations of the brain, suffer a neurodegenerative or chronic metabolic disease, or evolve to experience infantile spasms (West syndrome) [45].

It is reasonable to discontinue anticonvulsant medication as early as possible following cessation of neonatal seizure activity given the recent notoriety especially of phenobarbital in producing adverse behavior and retarded development. It is common knowledge that phenobarbital leads to hyperactivity, irritability, and insomnia in up to one-third of older infants and children receiving the drug [48], and a recent investigation suggests a significant and possibly permanent delay in mental capacities in similarly aged infants and children [49]. Finally, experimental studies in animals have shown a deleterious effect of the long-term use of phenobarbital on brain growth and differentiation [50–52]. Our personal bias is that phenobarbital is safe when administered to newborn human infants over days to weeks but may be detrimental to functional neurologic maturation when administered over months to years.

IX. NEONATAL SEIZURES AND PERMANENT BRAIN DAMAGE

Despite the frequent occurrence of seizures in newborn infants, debate continues as to whether or not convulsive activity per se leads to permanent brain damage.

Data regarding a cause-and-effect relationship between seizures occurring in human infants and ultimate neurologic compromise are not available, owing largely to the fact that most seizures in the neonatal period occur as a consequence of developmental anomalies of or destructive insults to the immature brain. Such lesions of themselves are associated with a high incidence of retarded motor and mental development as well as chronic epilepsy.

Given the difficulties in ascribing acute or chronic brain damage to convulsive activity in the neonatal period, investigators have studied the effect of electrically or chemically induced seizures in developing experimental animals. In this regard, convulsions have been induced in immature animals of several species to ascertin the cerebral metabolic disturbances that occur during the course of continuous or repetitive seizure activity (for a review, see Ref. 53). In general, experimentally induced seizures are associated with a prompt increase in glucose consumption and glycolytic rate of the brain in an attempt to keep pace with the heightened metabolic activity produced by the seizures. Despite the increase in glucose utilization, major pertubations of the energy reserves in brain occur, although not to the extent of those that accompany hypoxic-ischemic brain damage. Thus it is not surprising that, to date, no investigator has been able to produce overt epileptic brain damage in the immature animal, including the rat, dog, or monkey. Whether prolonged convulsions (i.e., 1 or more hours) lead to a greater exhaustion of cerebral energy reserves and ultimate brain damage remains to be investigated.

Despite the fact that immature animals appear resistant to the acute brain damaging effect of repetitive or continuous seizure activity (status epilepticus), other animal investigations indicate that prolonged continuous or repetitive seizures can lead to long-lasting disturbances in brain growth and maturation [54–56] and may predispose the developing brain to epilepsy in later life [57]. Until more objective clinical evidence is available, it seems prudent to continue to treat vigorously all seizures occurring in the newborn infant.

Well-known complications of seizures not only in immature experimental animals but in human infants as well include concurrent alterations in systemic oxygen and acid-base status and in cardiovascular function [3,58]. Apnea occasionally accompanies seizure activity in newborn infants; which, if prolonged, leads to substantial systemic hypoxemia, acidosis, and hypotension secondary to cardiac depression. Cerebral hypoxia–ischemia is a well-known cause of acute brain damage. Equally concerning is an abrupt increase in systemic blood pressure which often accompanies neonatal seizures, including subtle seizures, even in paralyzed infants [3]. Such an increase in arterial blood pressure causes a concurrent increase in cerebral perfusion pressue in the face of immature or abolished cerebral blood flow autoregulation. In this regard, substantial increases in cerebral blood flow, and by inference, perfusion pressure, have been well documented in both immature experimental animals and newborn human infants

Table 5 Prognosis of Neonatal Seizures in Relation to Underlying Disease

Neurologic disease	Normal development (%)
Hypoxic–ischemic encephalopathy	50
Intraventricular hemorrhage	<10
Primary subarachnoid hemorrhage	90
Hypocalcemia	
Early onset	50
Late onset	100
Hypoglycemia	50
Bacterial meningitis	50
CNS malformation	0

Source: Volpe (3).

[59,60]. Such increases in cerebral blood flow and perfusion pressure may contribute to the occurrence of intraventricular hemorrhage or hemorrhagic infarction, especially in premature infants. In conclusion, the systemic oxygen and acid-base alterations and cardiovascular disturbances that accompany seizures may be equally if not more important to the pathogenesis of epileptic brain damage than the convulsive activity itself.

X. OUTCOME

The short-term prognosis for infants who have sustained seizures in the newborn period has improved over the past two decades [3]. Acute mortality has decreased from 39% to 15% in infants born prior to or after 1969; the declining mortality is probably a reflection of improved obstetric and neonatal care of sick newborn infants. Unfortunately, long-term morbidity, measured in the incidence of the neurologic sequelae of cerebral palsy, mental retardation, and epilepsy, has changed little or even increased (19 vs. 29%) since 1969 [3]. The unchanging or heightened neurologic morbidity of infants exhibiting neonatal seizures relates largely to the declining incidence of late-onset hypocalcemic seizures, a benign condition, combined with improved survival, especially of premature infants sustaining major destructive insults to their brains.

As mentioned previously, the long-term prognosis for infants sustaining neonatal seizures appears more dependent on the underlying cause than on the seizure per se. Volpe [3] has estimated the prognosis of neonatal seizures in relation to the precipitating neurologic condition. As can be seen in Table 5, seizures resulting from primary subarachnoid hemorrhage and late-onset hypocalcemia carry an excellent prognosis; from hypoxic-ischemic encephalopathy, meningitis, and hypoglycemia, an intermediate prognosis; and from intraventricular hemorrhage and congenital CNS anomaly, a poor prognosis. As Volpe [3] states, "the data indicate that the major task of the physician is to determine as precisely as possible the neurologic disease producing the seizures . . . in order that appropriate therapy can be instituted but also to ensure as meaningful a prognostic statement as possible."

The contribution of neonatal convulsive activity per se to mortality and ultimate neurologic morbidity remains unclear. The presence or absence of seizures, especially those associated with perinatal asphyxia, is believed by some investigators to be a strong discriminator of later normal or abnormal development [1,61,62]. Conversely, Finer et al. [63] found no relationship between the presence of postasphyxial seizures in full-term infants and ultimate outcome. However, seizures occurring within the first 24 h following birth in a previously asphyxiated infant did appear to correlate with a significantly increased incidence of neurologic handicap at follow-up when these infants were compared with infants in whom seizures occurred later. Late-onset (greater than 7 postnatal days) seizures also appear to be associated with increased neurologic morbidity, especially in small premature infants, related largely to postnatal cerebral hypoxia–ischemia and intraventricular hemorrhage [64]. Prolonged or repetitive seizures refractory to anticonvulsant medication as well as tonic or generalized myoclonic seizures also portend a poor prognosis [23,64,65]. Once again we conclude that the long-term prognosis of infants sustaining seizures in the newborn period appears to reflect predominantly the type and severity of the underlying insult to brain rather than the convulsive activity itself.

Acknowledgment

J.Y.Y. is the recipient of a grant from the Medical Research Council of Canada.

REFERENCES

1. Rose RL, Lombroso CT. Neonatal seizure status: a study of clinical, pathological and electroencephalographical features in 137 full-term babies with a long-term follow-up. Pediatrics 1970; 45:404–25.
2. Painter, MJ, Bergman I, Crumrine P. Neonatal seizures. Pediatr Clin North Am 1986; 33:91–109.
3. Volpe JJ, Neurology of the newborn II. Philadelphia: WB Saunders, 1987.
4. Craig WS. Convulsive movements occurring in the first 10 days of life. Arch Dis Child 1960; 35:336–39.
5. Seay AR, Bray PF. Significance of seizures in infants weighing less than 2500 grams. Arch Neurol 1977; 34:381–82.
6. Painter MJ, Pippenger C, MacDonald H, Piplick W. Phenobarbital and diphenylhydantoin levels in neonates with seizures. J Pediatr 1978; 92:315–19.

7. Vannucci RC. Acute perinatal brain injury: hypoxia–ischemia. In: Cohen WR, Acker DB, Friedman EA, eds. Management of labor. Rockville, MD: Aspen Publishers, 1989:183–244.
8. Volpe JJ. Neonatal seizures: current concepts and revised classification. Pediatrics 1989; 84:422–28.
9. Volpe JJ. Neonatal seizures: clinical overview. In: Wasterlain CG, Vert P, eds. Neonatal seizures. New York: Raven Press, 1990:27–40.
10. Blennow G. Benign infantile nocturnal myoclonus. Acta Pediatr Scand 1985; 74:505–7.
11. Coulter DL, Allen RJ. Benign neonatal sleep myoclonus. Arch Neurol 1982; 39:191–92.
12. Watanabe K, Hara K, Shuji M. Electroclinical studies of seizures in the newborn period. Folia Psychol Neurol Jpn 1977; 31:383–92.
13. Fenichel GM, Olson BJ, Fitzpatrick JE. Heart rate changes in convulsive and nonconvulsive apnea. Ann Neurol 1980; 7:577–82.
14. Watanabe K, Hara K, Miyazaki S. Apneic seizures in the newborn. Am J Dis Child 1982; 136:980–84.
15. Mizrahi EM, Kellaway P. Characterization and classification of neonatal seizures. Neurology 1987; 37:1837–44.
16. Legido A, Clancy RR, Verman PH. Recent advances in the diagnosis, treatment and prognosis of neonatal seizures. Pediatr Neurol 1988; 4:79–86.
17. Scher MS, Painter MJ, Bergman I, Barmada MA, Brunberg J. EEG diagnosis of neonatal seizures: clinical correlations and outcome. Pediatr Neurol 1989; 5:17–24.
18. Clancy RR, Legido A, Lewis D. Occult neonatal seizures. Epilepsia 1988; 29:256–61.
19. Connell J, Oozeer R, DeVries L, Dubowitz LMS, Dubowitz V. Continuous EEG monitoring of neonatal seizures: diagnostic and prognostic considerations. Arch Dis Child 1989; 64:452–58.
20. Keen JH, Lee D. Sequelae of neonatal convulsions. Arch Dis Child 1973; 48:542–46.
21. Dennis J. Neonatal convulsions: an etiology, late neonatal status and long-term outcome. Dev Med Child Neurol 1978; 20:153–58.
22. Holden KR, Mellits DE, Freeman JM. Neonatal seizures I. Correlation of prenatal and perinatal events with outcomes. Pediatrics 1982; 70:165–76.
23. Mellits DE, Holden KR, Freeman JM. Neonatal seizures II. A multivariate analysis of factors associated with outcome. Pediatrics 1982; 70:177–85.
24. Levy SR, Abrams IF, Marshall PC, and Rosqueti EE. Seizures and cerebral infarction in the full-term newborn. Ann Neurol 1985; 17:366–70.
25. Kellaway P, Hrachovy RA. Status epilepticus in newborns: a perspective. In Delgado-Escueta AV, Wasterlain CG, Treiman DM, Porter RJ, eds. New York: Raven Press, 1983:93–99.
26. Kellaway P, Mizrahi EM. Neonatal seizures. In: Luders H, Lesser RP, eds. Epilepsy: electrochemical syndromes. London: Springer-Verlag, 1987:13–47.
27. Naldo S, Messmore H, Caserta V, Fine M. CNS lesions in neonatal isoimmune thrombocytopenia. Arch Neurol 1983; 40:552–54.

28. Zalneraitis EL, Young RSK, Krisnamoorthy KS. Intracranial hemorrhage in utero as a complication of isoimmune thrombocytopenia. J Pediatr 1979; 95:611–14.
29. Herzlinger RA, Krandall RS, Vaughan HG. Neonatal seizures associated with narcotic withdrawal. J Pediatr 1977; 91:638.
30. Post RM, Kopanda RT. Cocaine, kindling and reverse tolerance. Lancet 1975; 1:409–10.
31. Fulroth R, Phillips B, Durand DJ. Perinatal outcome of infants exposed to cocaine and/or heroin in utero. Am J Dis Child 1989; 143:905–10.
32. Hillman GR, Hillman RE, Dodson WE. Diagnosis, treatment and follow-up of neonatal nepivacaine intoxication secondary to paracervical and pudendal blocker during labor. J Peditr 1979; 95:472.
33. Kim WY, Pomerance JJ, Miller AA. Lidocaine intoxication in a newborn following local anesthesia for episcotomy. Pediatrics 1979; 64:643.
34. Tibbles JAR. Dominant benign neonatal seizures. Dev Med Child Neurol 1980; 22:664–67.
35. Takebe Y, Chiba C, Kimura S. Benign familial neonatal convulsions. Brain Dev 1983; 5:319.
36. Plouin P. Benign neonatal convulsions. In: Dravet J, Bureau M, Driefuss FE, Wolf P, eds. Epileptic syndromes in infancey, childhood and adolescence. London: John Libbey Eurotext Ltd., 1985:2–11.
37. Pryor DS, Don N, Macourt DC. Fifth day fits: a syndrome of neonatal convulsions. Arch Dis Child 1981; 56:753–58.
38. Goldberg HJ, Sheeky EM. Fifth day fits: an acute zinc deficiency syndrome? Arch Dis Child 1983; 57:633–35.
39. Goutieres F, Aicardi J. Atypical presentations of pyridoxine-dependent seizures: a treatable cause of intractable epilepsy in infancy. Am Neurol 1985; 17:117–20.
40. Fischer JH, Lockman LA, Zaske D, Kriel R. Phenobarbital maintenance dose requirements in treating neonatal seizures. Neurology 1981; 31:1042–44.
41. Lockman LA, Kriel R, Zaske D, Thompson T, Virnig N. Phenobarbital dosage for control of neonatal seizures. Neurology 1979; 29:1445–49.
42. Gal P, Toback J, Boer H, Erkan N, Wells T. Efficacy of phenobarbital monotherapy in treatment of neonatal seizures: relationships to blood levels. Neurology 1982; 32:1401–4.
43. Gilman JT, Gal P, Duchowny MS. Rapid sequential phenobarbital treatment of neonatal seizures. Pediatrics 1989; 83:674–78.
44. Koren G, Butt W, Rajchgot P, Mayer J, Whyte H, Pape K, MacLeod SM. Intravenous paraldehyde for seizure control in newborn infants. Neurology 1986; 36:108–11.
45. Gal P, Boer HR. Early discontinuation of anticonvulsants after neonatal seizures: a preliminary report. South Med J 1982; 75:298–300.
46. Brod SA, Ment LR, Ehrenkrantz RA, Bridgers S. Predictors of success for drug discontinuation following neonatal seizures. Pediatr Neurol 1988; 4:13–17.
47. Ellison PH, Largent JA, Bahr JP. A scoring system to predict outcome following neonatal seizures. J Pediatr 1981; 99:455–59.
48. Camfield CS, Chaplin S, Doyle AB, Shapiro SH, Cummings C, Camfield PR. Side effects of phenobarbital in toddlers: behavioral and cognitive aspects. J Pediatr 1979; 95:361–65.

49. Farwell JR, Lee YJ, Hirtz DG, Sulzbacher SI, Ellenberg JH, Nelson KB. Phenobarbital for febrile seizures: effects on intelligence and on seizure recurrence. N Engl J Med 1990; 322:364–69.
50. Neale EA, Sher PK, Graubard BI. Differential toxicity of chronic exposure to phenytoin, phenobarbital or carbamazephine in cerebral cortical cell cultures. Pediatr Neurol 1985; 1:143–50.
51. Diaz J, Schain RJ, Bailey BG. Phenobarbital induced brain growth retardation in artifically reared rat pups. Biol Neonate 1977; 32:77–82.
52. Diaz J, Schain RJ. Phenobarbital: effects of long-term administration on behavior and brain on artifically reared rats. Science 1978; 199:90–95.
53. Vannucci RC, Fujikawa DG. Energy balance of the immature brain during status epilepticus. In: Wasterlain CG, Vert P, eds. Neonatal seizures. New York: Raven Press, 1990:99–112.
54. Wasterlain CG. Effects of neonatal status epilepticus on rat brain development. Neurology 1976; 26:975–86.
55. Wasterlain CG. Effects of neonatal seizures on ontogeny of reflexes and behavior. Eur Neurol 1977; 15:9–19.
56. Wasterlain CG, Plum F. Vulnerability of developing rat brain to electroconvulsive seizures. Arch Neurol 1973; 29:38–45.
57. Moshé SL, Albala BJ, Ackermann RF. Increased seizure susceptibility of the immature brain. Dev Brain Res 1983; 7:81–85.
58. Young RSK, Fripp RR, Yagel SK. Cardiac dysfunction during status epilepticus in the neonatal pig. Ann Neurol 1985; 18:291–97.
59. Young RSK, Osbakken MD, Briggs RW, Yagel SK, Rice DW, Goldberg S. ^{31}P NMR study of cerebral metabolism during prolonged seizures in the neonatal dog. Ann Neurol 1985; 18:14–20.
60. Perlman JM, Herscovitch P, Kreusser KL, Vopel JJ. Positron emission tomography in the newborn: effect of seizure on regional cerebral blood flow in an asphyxiated infant. Neurology 1985; 35:244–47.
61. Mulligan JC, Painter MJ, O'Donoughue PA, MacDonald HM, Allen AC, Taylor PM. Neonatal asphyxia. II. Neonatal mortality and long-term sequelae. J Pediatr 1980; 96:903–7.
62. Nelson KB, Broman RL. Perinatal risk factors in children with serious motor and mental handicaps. Ann Neurol 1977; 2:371–77.
63. Finer NN, Robertson CM, Richards RT, Pinnell LE, Petters KL. Hypoxic–ischemic encephalopathy in term neonates: perinatal factors and outcome. J Pediatr 1981; 98:112–17.
64. Bergman I, Painter MJ, Kirsch RP, Crumrine PK, David R. Outcome in neonates with convulsions treated in an intensive care unit. Ann Neurol 1983; 14:642–47.
65. Brown JK, Cockburn F, Forfar JO. Clinical and chemical correlates in convulsions of the newborn. Lancet 1972; 1:135–39.

7

Status Epilepticus

FEREYDOUN DEHKHARGHANI
University of Missouri
and Children's Mercy Hospital
Kansas City, Missouri

I. INTRODUCTION

It is estimated that 5% of all epileptic patients at some time in their lives experience an episode of status epilepticus. Each year about 8000 persons in the United States are hospitalized because of convulsive status epilepticus. Status epilepticus may be the first epileptic seizure in infants and children.

II. DEFINITION

Status epilepticus is continuous or rapidly recurrent seizure(s). It may be focal or generalized, depending on the type of status epilepticus; consciousness may be lost, impaired, or remain intact. The World Health Organization dictionary of epilepsy defines status epilepticus as "a condition characterized by an epileptic seizure that is sufficiently prolonged or repeated at sufficiently brief intervals so as to produce an unvarying and enduring epileptic condition" [1].

This definition is vague and has an unspecified length of time. Most authors have formulated their own definitions. Currently, a duration of 30 min is widely accepted; however, one can find various duration from 10 min to over an hour in literature. Thirty minutes' duration has gained more acceptance based on animal studies when it was found that in some species generalized convulsions lasting longer than 30 min, causing identifiable structural alterations in the central nervous system [2]. Repeated nonconvulsive seizures associated with impairment of consciousness should also be considered status epilepticus when the recurrence rate does not permit return of consciousness [3].

Serial seizures refer to convulsive seizures, lasting less than 30 min, with return of consciousness during the interictal state. Patients with serial seizures are at high risk to develop status epilepticus [4].

III. INCIDENCE OF STATUS EPILEPTICUS

The exact incidence of status epilepticus is not known. The proportion of patients with epilepsy who have experienced status epilepticus at some time ranges from 1.3 to 16% [5]. Between 0.5 and 1% of epileptic patients will have at least one episode of status epilepticus annually [6]. In the pediatric age group, status epilepticus or a history of status epilepticus is reported in 9.1% of children with seizures in the first year of life. Aicardi and Chevrie report that 16% of children with the diagnosis of epilepsy prior to age 15 years have experienced status epilepticus [7]. A higher proportion is reported in children in the first 2 years of life. One group reports that 12% of initial seizures last longer than 30 min [7a].

Status epilepticus as a first seizure in adults is rare, but 5% of children with febrile seizures may develop status epilepticus as their first seizure. This means that 125 to 250 cases of status epilepticus occur per 100,000 children [8]. In the total population it is estimated that each year, 60,000 to 160,000 persons in the United States will have at least one episode of convulsive status epilepticus [9]. Hauser reports that in about one-third of cases this is the first presenting seizure. One-third occur in patients who are known to have epilepsy, and the remaining one-third occur following acute central nervous system injury in previously normal individuals [6].

IV. CLASSIFICATION

Status epilepticus can be classified into two major categories: generalized and partial. Each category is further divided according to the international classification of epileptic seizures (see Chapter 3). Generalized status epilepticus is divided into two classes, convulsive and nonconvulsive. Partial status has two main classes, simple with elementary symptomatology and complex partial status. The cumulative changes caused by prolonged repeated seizures set off cascading events, resulting in either systemic or focal cerebral dysfunction. As duration of seizure is the most determining factor, by observation alone one cannot distinguish an isolated seizure from status epilepticus [10]. Although potentially, any type of epileptic seizure can evolve into status epilepticus, the tonic–clonic or convulsive status is a more common and serious one.

V. CONVULSIVE GENERALIZED STATUS EPILEPTICUS

1. *Tonic–clonic status epilepticus* may be generalized from the onset, but more frequently it is secondarily generalized, after an initial partial onset. Electroencephalogram recordings obtained during status epilepticus are very important for differentiating between partial and generalized convulsions in demonstrating localized or lateralized discharges. Most patients with generalized tonic–clonic status epilepticus have localized cerebral disturbances, and therefore, they have secondary generalized partial seizures [11]. If generalization is very rapid or if a partial seizure lacks motor components, initial partial symptoms may go undetected and the seizure may mistakenly be assumed to be generalized from the onset.

2. *Tonic status epilepticus* is more common in the pediatric age group and frequently is seen at the onset of tonic–clonic seizures in secondary generalized status. Seizures are manifested by slow, sustained muscle contraction. Tonic spasms may be focal, unilateral, or generalized; when duration of a tonic seizure is short, it may go undetected. Tonic status is commonly seen in children and adolescence with a previous history of epilepsy. Typically, the previous epilepsy is absence or Lennox–Gastaut syndrome (see Chapter 9). Tonic status has also been reported following intravenous injection of diazepam or clonazepam during treatment of absence status [12]. Tonic status may be associated with a mild to moderate degree of impairment of consciousness and confusional state. Autonomic dysfunction such as respiratory irregularities and excessive secretion is frequent in this type of status. Tonic status may last for several days and remain refractory to most antiepileptic drugs.

3. *Clonic status epilepticus* is manifested by rhythmic brief rapid, at times violent, muscle contraction. Clonic movement may be partial or generalized, bilaterally synchronous or asynchronous. When unilateral, they are not associated with loss of consciousness or autonomic dysfunction and are frequent in acute central nervous system injury, such as focal infection, vascular accident, and in neonates with severe hypoxic–ischemic encephalopathy.

4. *Myoclonic status epilepticus* is manifested by continuous or rapidly recurrent sudden, brief, shocklike muscle contraction. Myoclonic status epilepticus is seen in both primary generalized epilepsy, such as impulsive petit mal status and in children with epilepsy and chronic encephalopathy. An EEG is helpful to differentiate this type by showing rhythmical repeated spike–wave discharges superimposed on a background of diffuse slowing. At times, it is difficult to differentiate this type of status from nonepileptic myoclonic jerks of progressive degenerative central nervous system dysfunction.

VI. NONCONVULSIVE STATUS EPILEPTICUS

A. Absence Status

Absence status (spike–wave stupor) is a condition associated with continuous clouding of consciousness. This type of status has a characteristic EEG with bilaterally synchronous spike-and-wave discharges [13]. Absence status is seen more frequent in secondary generalized epilepsy, such as Lennox–Gastaut syndrome rather than with petit mal epilepsy (primary generalized epilepsy). However, these two conditions, clinically and electroencephalographically, cannot be distinguished during the actual ictus.

Significant controversies exist in nosological issues of absence status epilepticus, especially in the pediatric age group. In 75% of cases, absence status occurs before the age of 20 years, and most take place during the first decade [4]. Absence status is, in general, associated with simple or complex automatisms, but it may also be associated with minor motor manifestation such as head nodding, sagging of the knees, or minimal myoclonic movement of extremities. The psychic manifestations of *partial* nonconvulsive status epilepticus are indistinguishable from *generalized* nonconvulsive status [4].

Depression of mental state, automatisms, and confusional states are hallmarks of absence status. The exact incidents of absence status is unknown. Absence status has been reported after metrizamide myelography and amitriptyline therapy [14,15]. Due to its clinical presentation of confusional state and memory disturbance, absence status should be differentiated from acute psychiatric or toxic–metabolic disturbances. The EEG is very helpful in this differential.

B. Complex Partial Status Epilepticus

Complex partial status is manifested by prolonged and repeated episodes of complex partial seizures associated with impairment of consciousness, confusion, and memory disturbance. Memory deficit may persist for several weeks. The term *twilight state* has been applied to the clouding of consciousness seen in complex partial status epilepticus.

As in complex partial seizures, complex partial status can have its origin from either the temporal lobe or from extratemporal regions. Differentiation between complex partial status arising from the temporal lobe versus that arising from the frontal lobe is clinically and, at times, electroencephalographically, difficult. Associated focal neurological abnormality may help to differentiate these two conditions [4]. In typical complex partial status arising from the temporal lobe, discharges are seen independently or bilaterally synchronously from the temporal lobes.

Absence of generalized nonconvulsive status epilepticus is uncommonly associated with a focal EEG or focal clinical manifestation [16]. This feature can further complicate the differentiation of absence status of generalized epilepsy from a similarly appearing absence status of complex partial seizures. Complex partial status epilepticus is a rare condition in children [4]. Alternating discharges between two temporal lobes interrupted by bilaterally synchronous discharges is a typical pattern for complex partial nonconvulsive status epilepticus. This pattern is not rare in younger children with chronic epilepsy of temporal lobe origin. However, the clinical presentation is very variable, and an abnormal behavior with cycling variation may go undetected and only when bilateral dysfunction results in unresponsiveness may it be counted as a real ictal event. When clinically partial nonconvulsive status cannot be differentiated from generalized nonconvulsive status, the EEG is essential.

VII. EPILEPSIA PARTIALIS CONTINUA

The term *epilepsia partialis continua* or *Koshevnikoff syndrome* is referred to a condition associated with persistent localized seizures affecting the distal part of the extremities, generally lasting for days. At times, differentiation of this type of epilepsy with segmental myoclonus of noncortical origin is difficult. Epilepsia partialis continua is characterized by clonic movements, usually localized to the face or upper extremities that persist, either continuously or with only brief interruptions. This condition is seen in a variety of structural lesions, neoplastic, infectious, or vascular. It has also been reported in chronic focal encephalitis of Aguilar and Rasmussen [17,18].

VIII. ETIOLOGY

Status epilepticus has generally been categorized as either idiopathic or symptomatic. The symptomatic group may be secondary to an acute central nervous system (CNS) injury or a chronic long-standing central nervous system or systemic illness. In the Minneapolis study of status epilepticus [11], 16% of patients with status epilepticus had prior central nervous system insult, and 9% had newly diagnosed idiopathic epilepsy.

In Aicardi and Chevrie's series of 239 cases of status epilepticus in children, symptomatic and cryptogenic causes were evenly divided. In this study, one-half of the cryptogenic causes were associated with fever [7]. However, in other series, most patients had cerebral lesions [11].

Generalized convulsive status epilepticus may occur in patients with head injuries, fever, metabolic disturbances (e.g., hypoglycemia, hypocalcemia, and hyponatremia), central nervous system infection, vascular insult, brain tumors, toxic encephalopathy, and rapid anticonvulsant withdrawal.

Among precipitating factors, rapid antiepileptic drug withdrawal is believed to be very common [19]. Specific triggering factors may be sleep deprivation, intercurrent infection, and alcohol abuse. In children with convulsive status epilepticus, preexisting static or progressive encephalopathies are frequently present. There is a long list of drugs and potentially proconvulsant and environmental toxins such as DDT, lindane, and others which can cause combined toxic encephalopathy and status epilepticus [20]. Still the most common cause remains acute central nervous system or systemic insult. Patients with previously diagnosed epilepsy are the single largest group at risk [6]. In the pediatric age group, febrile convulsions and seizures complicating a central nervous system infection accounts for the majority of cases of status epilepticus. Twenty-five to 30% of cases remain idiopathic in children.

IX. PHYSIOLOGICAL CHANGES DURING STATUS EPILEPTICUS

Physiological changes during status epilepticus consist of an initial increase of cerebral blood flow due to decreased cerebral vascular resistance. Increase in blood pressure [21,22] is believed to be secondary to excessive sympathetic activity at the beginning of the convulsion. If status continues for a long period of time, blood pressure will drop and rise of cerebral venous pressure will cause increase intracranial pressure. Respiratory dysfunction is caused by multiple factors: involvement of the brainstem respiratory centers by abnormal electrical discharges, massive autonomic discharges causing bronchial hypersecretion [23], and medication used for treatment of status. All are important contributing causes to respiratory failure.

Wasterlain has shown that during status, glucose transport from the blood to the brain is impaired and blood glucose may not represent a fall in brain glucose level. In immature animals, depression of brain glucose can occur in the absence of hypoglycemia [24]. Marked initial rises in arterial and cerebral venous pressure, severe metabolic and respiratory acidosis, hypoglycemia, and reduced cerebral arteriovenous differences are noted in adolescent baboons during status epilepticus in the first 25 min of a seizure. After 25 min, severe hyperpyrexia, hyperkalemia, and hypoglycemia are noted [25]. The same investigator has shown dysfunction of several endocrine functions, autonomic activation at seizure onset, and spread of neuronal activity to the hypothalamus, leading to the liberation of releasing factors [26].

The increase in the cerebral metabolic rate during status epilepticus is due to an increase in cerebral oxygen and glucose consumption by excessive neuronal activity. Early physiological changes are referred to the systemic responses after 30 min of status epilepticus. Every attempt should be made to stop the seizure and correct these transient early physiological changes in order to prevent the later changes of status epilepticus, such as hypotension, increased central venous pressure, and increased cerebrospinal fluid pressure [27]. Reduction of mortalities and morbidity of status epilepticus in our time is due to the understanding of these physiological changes and rapid detection of the underlying cause of systemic changes. Hyperthermia, hypertension, and hypoxia are the most important factors. Experimental evidence suggests that brain injury starts after 25 to 30 min of prolonged status, and every attempt should be made to stop clinical and electrographic seizure in less than 30 min [21,28]. Anticonvulsant medication should be given intravenously to ensure effective blood and brain tissue concentrations. Once seizures are stopped, an adequate loading dose of long-acting maintenance anticonvulsant should be started. The child with status epilepticus should be positioned to avoid aspiration and facilitate a clearing of the airway.

X. CONSEQUENCES OF STATUS EPILEPTICUS

A. Direct Effect on the Brain

The most important factor in the outcome of status epilepticus is its underlying cause. Aicardi and Chevrie [7] found a mortality rate of 11% in a series of 239 children less than 15 years old with status epilepticus. A more recent study by Maytal et al. [29] showed only 3.6% mortality. In Aicardi's series 88 of 239 children had neurological sequelae (36%), whereas the study of Maytal showed a morbidity of only 9.1%. In both studies, morbidity was much higher in children under 3 years of age [4]. Twenty-five percent of children in Aicardi's series and 24% in Maytal's report of status epilepticus had idiopathic epilepsy.

There is no disagreement that the outcome of status epilepticus depends primarily on the underlying cause of status. Also, there is some agreement that many systemic changes take place during status epilepticus which can contribute to mortality and morbidity. These include alteration of blood pressure, respiratory and cardiac dysfunction, acidosis, and hypoglycemia. It is not known to what extent status epilepticus by and of itself, with its prolonged neuronal depolarization, can add to nerve cell injury. Some investigators strongly believe that prolonged seizures by themselves can damage nerve cells [30–32]. Others doubt that harmful events occur when the secondary complications of prolonged seizures are intensively managed [33]. In many reported cases of brain damage observed after status epilepticus, it is difficult to know if the seizure itself or a preexisting injury caused the damage. An important implication of this controversy is how aggressively one needs to treat status epilepticus. The possibility of an underlying cause must be investigated, and secondary complications of seizures (e.g., hypoxia, vascular collapse, and other systemic changes) must be avoided. If status otherwise does not harm the brain, extreme measures such as pentobarbital coma may not be necessary. Another unresolved issue is the effect of prolonged seizures on the brain at different ages [4].

Investigation of experimental models of status epilepticus using chemoconvulsant drugs supports the idea that prolonged epileptic discharges, per se, damage the brain. It is not just the metabolic demand of actively discharging neurons that makes a difference [21,28,30,33–36]. Deterioration of γ-aminobutyric acid

(GABA)-mediated inhibitors and formation of excitatory substances are considered an important factor. According to Lothman and colleagues, accumulation of calcium in neuronal cytoplasm during status epilepticus is caused by activation of glutamate receptors. Entry of calcium to cell cytoplasm unleashes a neurochemical cascade of nerve cell damage. These authors suggest the exotoxin-induced neuronal death during status epilepticus [2].

B. Risk of Subsequent Seizures

An important practical aspect in the long-term management of status epilepticus involves the risk of unprovoked seizures following status epilepticus. A study suggests that the risk of a further seizure (i.e., epilepsy) in a child who presents with status epilepticus is no different from the risk of recurrent seizure following the first seizure.

C. Age of Patient

The role of age in the outcome of status epilepticus is unclear in human subjects. Several authors [21,37] have concluded that the young brain had greater vulnerability to postconvulsive damage. In Maytal's series, neurologic sequelae was a function of age; neurologic sequelae occurred in 29% of infants younger than 1 year of age, 11% of children 1 to 3 years of age, and 6% of children older than 3 years of age [29]. It has been demonstrated that kindling, a phenomenon by which a normal neuron becomes epileptogenic by repeated stimulation [38,39], can be readily induced in rat pups when compared to adult rats [40]. This is in concordance with clinical observation of increased incidence of status epilepticus early in life [7]. If kindling occurs in humans, the infant would therefore be more at risk.

In a study of the outcome of convulsive disorders, Chevrie found that status epilepticus had a mortality rate of 26% in children of less than 6 months of age and 15% in children from 6 months to 1 year [41]. Dunn reports that the outcome is most closely associated with etiology and duration of status epilepticus, age being a minor factor [42].

Status epilepticus is a life-threatening emergency and must be intensely treated as such, with constant surveillance of vital functions and metabolic changes. The three major factors relating to outcome are (1) etiology, (2) duration of seizures, and (3) age of child [42,43].

XI. MANAGEMENT OF STATUS EPILEPTICUS

There are three important aspects in approaching the patient in status: (1) stabilization of the patient, (2) diagnostic evaluation, and (3) termination of the seizure.

A. Patient Stabilization

Management and correction of systemic disturbances by adequate respiration, perfusion, and correction of metabolic dysfunction and hyperthermia should remain the prime concern of physicians treating a child with status epilepticus. Priority should be given to airway patency, adequate ventilation, cardiovascular function, and blood pressure. If the patient's respiration is intact but there is evidence of hypoxia, oxygen can be administered by nasal cannula. If oxygen administration by inhalation is not adequate, intubation may become necessary. Intubation of the airway is not needed unless clinical condition or blood gases suggest hypoxia.

Animal studies have shown that irreversible neuronal damage occurs after $1\frac{1}{2}$ to 2 h of status epilepticus. Early in status, there is an increase in blood pressure and an increase in cerebral blood flow. Serum lactic concentration levels rise rapidly, serum glucose may initially decrease, but subsequently it is increased due to sympathetic activation. Within 30 min, cerebral autoregulation is lost and cerebral blood flow becomes pressure dependent. At the same time, metabolic acidosis continues and hyperthermia develops. Therefore, one needs to monitor and regulate blood pressure, glucose, electrolytes, and lactic acid concentration closely, and check rectal temperature frequently in a patient with status epilepticus. This is vitally important to avoid brain damage. Head injury and further bodily injury should be prevented during status epilepticus.

Vascular access, both venous and arterial, are needed. Treatment starts with the intravenous infusion of a isotonic saline or D 5% in $\frac{1}{2}N$ saline. Specimens of blood should be drawn for the determination of glucose, electrolytes, acid-base state, blood urea nitrogen (BUN), creatinine, calcium, magnesium, drug screen, and complete blood count. If the patient is a known epileptic, anticonvulsant serum levels should be performed at this stage. Although hypoglycemia is an uncommon cause of status epilepticus in children, an initial injection of glucose solution intravenously is recommended if immediate determination of glucose is not available. Treatment of hypoglycemia starts with a bolus dose of glucose of 0.5 to 1.0 g/kg (2 to 4 cc/kg D 25% or 1 to 2 cc/kg D 50% of glucose solution). Special attention should be paid to signs of increased intracranial pressure and decompensated cerebral edema with impending herniation, especially when the duration of the status is not known. The patient should be carefully monitored for secondary complications of major motor status epilepticus. These are metabolic disorders, cardiopulmonary failure, renal disorders, and autonomic dysfunction [44]. If the child is febrile, a spinal tap may be necessary to rule out meningitis. The patient in status needs continuous observation, frequent suctioning, maintenance of the patient's airway, recording of vital signs, and close monitoring of metabolic changes.

B. Diagnostic Evaluation

In most instances, status epilepticus occurs in a known epileptic patient as a result of poor compliance. In other patients, central nervous system infection, intracranial hemorrhage, hypoxic insult, acute vascular accident, metabolic dysfunction, intoxication, and hyperpyrexia must be considered as etiologies. Unless history and neurological examination have led to a specific diagnosis, such as history of rapid withdrawal of an anticonvulsant in a known epileptic patient, the initial workup has to exclude central nervous system infection, acute vascular accident with or without central nervous system hemorrhage, head injury, intoxication, and common metabolic disorder such as hypocalcemia and hypoglycemia.

An electroencephalogram is a very useful test in the management of status epilepticus. This will aid in the classification of the seizure type and may lead to a diagnosis of the underlying cause of the seizure. The EEG can be used to assess the effectiveness of therapy by looking for cessation of the electrographic signs of seizure activity. Every effort must be made to identify the precipitating factors of status epilepticus.

C. Termination of the Status Epilepticus

Children with generalized convulsive status epilepticus need admission to the hospital intensive care unit with close observation until status has stopped and the patient's vital signs are stable (Table 1).

A number of treatment protocols have been published for the management of status epilepticus. A formulated approach and step-by-step trial of anticonvulsant with knowledge of their pharmacodynamic properties, side effects, and interactions with other drugs is needed. Aicardi recommends a trial of a large intravenous dose (100 to 200 mg) of pyridoxine at the onset of treatment before long-acting anticonvulsants are given. We use pyridoxine only in selected children when no other etiology has been found, and status does not stop with conventional antiepileptic drugs. Pyridoxine dependency is much more common in infants. If withdrawal of an anticonvulsant has been considered the etiology of status epilepticus, the most logical approach is reestablishing a therapeutic blood level of the anticonvulsant withdrawn, if possible. Otherwise, the ideal drug for treatment of status epilepticus is one that enters the brain rapidly, has an immediate onset of anticonvulsant activity, does not significantly depress consciousness or respiratory function, has a long half-life so that therapeutic concentrations are maintained for hours, and can effectively block both the somatic manifestation of seizures and the neuronal discharges [10,45]. In reality, no single anticonvulsant has all these properties.

Regardless of the choice of anticonvulsant, continuous attention should be paid to the patient's systemic functions, including body temperature. Frequent

Table 1 Management of Prolonged Generalized Convulsions

Time after arrival in emergency room (min)	Support	Laboratory	Medications
0–10	Determine vital signs. Maintain airway. Nasal O_2 if needed. Check temperature. Obtain history and physical exam. Prevent aspiration. Maintain IV access with normal saline.	Check electrolytes, Mg, Ca, P, BUN, glucose, CBC. Obtain AED blood level of patient if known epileptic. Perform LP if child is febrile. Toxicology screen.	Rectal antipyretics if child is febrile. Correct hypoglycemia with bolus of 2 mL/kg of 50% glucose. Correct acidosis with bicarbonate if pH < 7.1.
10–20	Continue monitoring vital signs and oxygenation. Consider endotracheal intubation if needed.	Monitor ABGs. Correct abnormal laboratory values. Repeat blood glucose.	Diazepam 0.3 mg/kg IV or 0.4 mg/kg rectally or Lorazepam 0.1–0.2 mg/kg IV
20–30	Intubation Transfer to pediatric ICU if available.		Diazepam 0.3 mg/kg IV Phenytoin 20 mg/kg IV, loading dose (50 mg/min) undiluted or mixed in saline. Phenytoin precipitates when mixed with glucose containing solution.
30–40 (status epilepticus)	Support vital signs.	Check pertinent laboratory abnormalities. Obtain phenytoin level.	Phenobarbital Loading dose, 20 mg/kg IV, at rate of 100 mg/min.
40–50	Support vital signs.	AED levels.	Phenytoin Repeat $\frac{1}{2}$ loading dose to get level near 20–25 μg/mL.
50–60	Support vital signs.		Phenobarbital Repeat $\frac{1}{2}$ loading dose to get level near 40 μg/mL.
>60	Support vital signs. Observe for increased ICP. Monitor renal function. Watch for hyperthermia.	EEG. Blood gases.	Consider pentobarbital coma (see the text).

reassessment and documentation of the time period from onset of seizure is important. The physician should be aware that all anticonvulsants used for the treatment of status epilepticus can depress the patient's respiration and add to the preexisting compromised cerebral oxygenation.

Acute cerebral edema may develop following prolonged status, resulting in acute brain shifts and coning. Postural changes, such as decorticate or decerebrate rigidity during cerebral herniation, have to be differentiated from tonic seizure. At times, in status epilepticus, the diagnosis of this life-threatening condition is difficult and an EEG can be helpful.

As mortality and morbidity of status epilepticus relate directly to the underlying causes and duration of time before seizures stop, it is very important that every attempt be made to treat the underlying cause and stop generalized tonic–clonic seizures as soon as possible. Tonic, clonic, and myoclonic status epilepticus should be treated according to the same protocol as generalized tonic–clonic status epilepticus.

XII. ANTICONVULSANT DRUGS FREQUENTLY USED FOR TREATMENT OF STATUS EPILEPTICUS

A. Primary Drugs

1. Benzodiazepines

Diazepam (Valium) and lorazepam (Ativan) have both been used for treatment of status epilepticus.

a. Diazepam. *Diazepam* is very effective in grand mal, secondary generalized grand mal, focal motor, absence, myoclonic, and in partial complex and absence and hemiclonic status epilepticus [46]. It can be administered by the intravenous (IV) or rectal route. The mechanism of action of benzodiazepines is not exactly known. The enhancement of γ-aminobutyric acid (GABA)–mediated inhibitors has been demonstrated [47,48]. In most patients, status epilepticus stops 5 min after injection of IV diazepam (Valium) [49]. EEG recordings during status epilepticus have shown that rectal diazepam stops epileptic discharges within 1 to 9.5 min after its administration [50–54]. Diazepam is highly lipid soluble. Due to its rapid penetration to the brain and its effectiveness, diazepam has become the first drug of choice for rapid control of seizures. The toxicity of diazepam is low, and the main concern is respiratory depression [55]. Superimposition of diazepam on a previous dose of phenobarbital increases the likelihood of respiratory depression [56]. This side effect is less frequent in children than in adults. Due to its short duration of effectiveness and the redistribution of the drug from the brain to blood within 15 to 30 min, diazepam injection generally needs to be followed by a long-acting anticonvulsant to continue control of seizures. On this basis, some investigators have questioned the value of diazepam in the treatment of status epilepticus. They recommend long-acting anticonvulsants from the very beginning. However, as potentially a combination of these two medications may be more effective, many authors still recommend diazepam as the first drug of choice. The usual dose of diazepam is 0.25 to 0.5 mg/kg in infants and children [4,45].

b. Rectal Diazepam. Although the IV routes remain an ideal way, if an IV line is not easily available, rectal administration is easy and harmless to the mucosa. Using a dose of 0.3 to 0.5 mg/kg of IV formulation of diazepam instilled rectally, an effective blood level is reached in 5 to 10 min [45a]. Both absorption and elimination of the drug is longer when the rectal route has been used. Rectal administration of diazepam, using a dosage similar to the IV dosage, has shown to yield a similar blood level and is as effective as IV administration with less respiratory depression [57].

Rectal administration of diazepam, using the IV formulation at home by the caretaker, has also been found to be an effective way to treat prolonged seizures. This simple measure in patients with intractable seizures and periodic status epilepticus prevents frequent visits to the emergency room. The dose can be repeated once, if necessary. Diazepam is absorbed from the blood to the brain within seconds, and from the rectum to the brain within minutes.

Diazepam stops seizures successfully in the majority of cases of status epilepticus, but it is better against generalized rather than focal status epilepticus [46]. As a seizure may recur within 15 to 20 min, longer-acting antiepileptic drugs should be given shortly after the first dose of diazepam. Sedation after administration of IV diazepam is a disadvantage of this drug. Repeat dosage may be given in 20 to 30 minutes, if necessary. When status epilepticus responds to IV diazepam but recurs, diazepam can be used by continuous infusion of 50 mg in 250 mL of 5% dextrose in water run at 1 mL/kg per hour.

Tonic status is very resistant to diazepam therapy, and even paradoxically it can precipitate tonic status [24]. When the first treatment is a loading dose of phenytoin, diazepam can be used after half of the loading dose is infused.

c. Lorazepam. The effectiveness of lorazepam for treatment of status epilepticus has been shown in several studies [58–60]. The anticonvulsant effect of lorazepam becomes apparent within 5 min after injection. The advantage of lorazepam is that it has a longer duration of action than diazepam. Lorazepam is given intravenously at a rate of 2 mg/min or less, to a total dose of 0.1 mg/kg in an adult and 0.05 to 0.25 mg/kg in children [61]. It has been shown in adults that 4 mg of lorazepam has the same degree of effectiveness and side effect as 10 mg of diazepam [58]. Lorazepam has a three- to four fold longer half-life than diazepam, and it has been found effective in at least 75% of all types of status and 90% of cases with generalized convulsive status. This allows the option of attaining therapeutic levels of alternate anticonvulsants, such as carbamazepine and sodium valproate, if long-term antiepileptic therapy is indicated. Lorazepam can be administered by either a nasogastric tube or the rectal route [58]. Lorazepam has been used rectally to treat status epilepticus, but its peak concentration is low unless a dose two to four times higher than the IV dose is used. The recommended rectal dose of lorazepam is 0.05 to 0.1 mg/kg dose [62,63], but experience is limited in this route of administration.

2. Phenytoin

Some investigators recommend phenytoin (PHT) as the first drug of choice for treatment of status epilepticus. It has the disadvantage of a slower rate of action, but it has no sedative effect. This property of PHT is important to monitor the patient's mental status (e.g., in head injury). The loading dose of phenytoin is 20 mg/kg given intravenously with a speed of no more than 50 mg/min. An infusion rate exceeding 50 mg/min may significantly decrease blood pressure and heart rate. Some authorities recommend a slower rate of injection [64,65]. The patient's heart rate and blood pressure should be monitored during the administration of phenytoin. Diazepam infusion can be followed by IV phenytoin. The two can be given simultaneously.

Phenytoin should be used preferably as a direct intravenous injection followed by saline. Phenytoin is a highly basic substance, soluble in saline and not in dextrose solution. It also begins precipitation in saline after 10 to 15 min. Present phenytoin preparations may be diluted to 5 to 20 mg/cc in normal saline solution [8,66]. Intramuscular injection of phenytoin is unacceptable, as it causes muscle destruction [67] and has poor absorption from intramuscular sites.

Intravenous phenytoin is contraindicated in patients with a heart block, hypotension, and cardiac insufficiency [68]. Asystole may occur following bolus IV injection [8]. As a result, blood pressure and EKG must be monitored during phenytoin infusion. Although phenytoin's entry time to the brain is very rapid (1 min), its time to peak brain concentration is 15 to 30 min [45]. Phenytoin is effective for both partial and generalized convulsive status, but it is not recommended in treatment of generalized nonconvulsive status (petit mal status) [69,70]. If the seizure remains refractory to the initial loading dose half of this loading dose can be repeated [71], but blood levels need to be monitored. If seizures continue after a loading dose of phenytoin, other agents should be used because administration of more phenytoin may result in toxic levels, and possibly, this can lead to cerebellar damage and may precipitate more seizures [10]. Twenty-four hours after the loading dose, maintenance therapy can be started if this drug is effective. A loading dose will generally produce an adequate concentration of PHT in plasma for 24 h.

3. Phenobarbital

Penetration of phenobarbital into the central nervous system may take 6 min or more, but therapeutic blood concentration occurs 20 min after IV administration. In the human subject, a seizure is usually stopped with a peak serum concentration of phenobarbital below 15 μg/ml [4]. Sedation, respiratory depression, and hypotension are limiting factors in the use of phenobarbital in the treatment of status epilepticus. The drug may be useful in patients with anoxic encephalopathy because phenobarbital reduces the metabolic rate of the brain [4]. An IV loading dose of 20 mg/kg is recommended. The rate of administration should not exceed 60 mg/min. The recommended infusion rate in children is 30 mg/min [60]. Time to peak brain concentration is 30 min [45]. The disadvantages of phenobarbital are its relatively slow time to reach peak brain concentrations, prolonged unresponsiveness, and lethargy. Nevertheless, seizure control can be achieved within 10 to 15 min. Phenobarbital maintenance doses can be started at 24 h after the loading dose. Phenobarbital is recommended if the patient's seizures remain refractory to diazepam and phenytoin.

Phenobarbital is effective in generalized and partial status epilepticus. The depression of respiration is more profound if it is used at the same time with diazepam. A 20-mg/kg loading dose should cause a plasma concentration level of 20 μg/mL. Levels of about 15 μg/mL have been found effective for cessation of status. Phenobarbital is well absorbed in infants. Its effective blood level is 15 to 40 μg/mL. The median time of onset of cessation of seizure after injection of phenobarbital is 5.5 min [72]. In one random, nonblinded clinical trial in generalized convulsive status epilepticus, phenobarbital was as effective as a combination of diazepam and phenytoin [72].

B. Secondary Drugs

Other drugs, including paraldehyde, valproic acid, carbamazepine, lidocaine, and clonazepam, have been used in treatment of status epilepticus.

1. Paraldehyde

Paraldehyde has not been well studied in the management of status epilepticus. Rectal, intravenous, intramuscular, and nasogastric routes have been used. Paraldehyde reaches peak levels in the brain rapidly by IV administration. Its half-life is 6 h. The intravenous dose of paraldehyde is 0.1 to 0.3 mL/kg every 2 to 4 h or an IV drip of 4% solution at the rate of 3.75 mL/kg [73]. A 200-mg/kg loading dose given over 5 min followed by 20 mg/kg per hour can be expected to produce effective plasma levels above 10 mg/dL [74,75]. The intravenous administration of paraldehyde is done with a diluted solution, usually 4% of paraldehyde in normal saline. The intravenous dose of paraldehyde should be titrated [2]. The exact dose of paraldehyde has not been well established but ranges from 0.1 to 0.3 mL/kg given intravenously over 15 to 30 min [75,76]. Paraldehyde may decompose in some plastic syringes and the solution should be wrapped with paper or foil to prevent degradation by light. Sedation, respiratory depression, hypotension, and metabolic acidosis are the main side effects of treatment with paraldehyde. Paraldehyde is contraindicated in patients with pulmonary edema and hemorrhage.

Rectal administration is done by mixing paraldehyde with an equal volume of mineral oil. Recommended doses are 0.3 mL/kg or 1 to 1.5 mL per year of age (maximum of 7 mL) [3]. Nasogastric administration of paraldehyde is not recommended due to the risk of aspiration and causing pulmonary hemorrhage. Intramuscular injection should also be avoided. Paraldehyde can be used in patients who are in renal or hepatic failure because it is excreted through the lungs.

2. Clonazepam

Several reports [77–79] support the effectiveness of clonazepam in treatment of status epilepticus. Clonazepam has a longer duration of action than diazepam, with a half-life of 13 to 15 h. A longer duration of activity remains the only advantage of clonazepam to diazepam. Rectally, it has been used in children at a dose of 0.1 mg/kg [62].

3. Lidocaine

Lidocaine has been used with a bolus dose of 2 to 3 mg/kg followed by a slow infusion at 4 to 10 mg/kg per hour. It has a minimal sedative effect, but it can cause cardiovascular dysfunction. Antiepileptic action of lidocaine lasts 20 to 30 min. Therefore, a continuous infusion is usually necessary [73].

4. Valproic Acid

Valproic acid has been used rectally for the treatment of status epilepticus [80]. It has slow rate of absorption. Peak concentration is 0.5 to 2 h with a dose of 6 to 15 mg/kg of oral solution diluted with an equal volume of water [62].

5. Carbamazepine

Carbamazepine has been administered rectally. It has a slow rate of absorption and cathartic effect.

6. Thiopental
(sodium pentothal)

The thiopental loading dose is 30 mg/kg followed by a maintenance dose of 5 to 20 mg/kg per hour. The first 50 mg is given as a test dose to assess the patient's tolerance. The patient should be intubated [81].

7. Amobarbital

Sodium amytal recommended doses in adults and children over the age of 6 years are 65 to 500 mg. In younger children, a 125-mg/m^2 dose is recommended [82,83]. Amobarbital can act as a respiratory depressant; therefore, respiration of the patient should be closely monitored.

When the drug regimens outlined above fail, pentobarbital coma or general anesthesia may be required to minimize the metabolic sequelae of prolonged seizure activity and to suppress the process.

C. Pentobarbital Coma

When status epilepticus lasts longer than 60 min it is considered to be refractory. In animals, permanent neurological damage occurs after 60 min of convulsive status despite adequate ventilation. It is not known if this is true for humans. Possible protective effects of barbiturates include their roles in (1) reducing intracranial pressure and (2) reducing neuronal metabolic rate and need for oxygen. There are additional benefits of this short-acting barbiturate [84,86]. At what point of time the patient in status epilepticus should be subjected to barbiturate coma is controversial. In a well-prepared environment it takes at least 1 h to try the first round of conventional anticonvulsant drugs (diazepam, PHT, and PB), and some of these drugs could be tried for a second time, which would lengthen the duration of observation. Some authors recommend that only patients who fail to respond to the initial therapy for a minimum of 2 h should be subjected to treatment with pentobarbital coma. The current recommendation is that if seizures persist after 60 min, and if other drugs fail, barbiturate coma or generalized anesthesia be started [9]. Prior to the use of barbiturate coma, a search for potential underlying cause should have been completed, including a CT scan of the head, spinal tap, and blood culture.

The patient should undergo tracheal intubation with respiratory assistance. Blood pressure and cardiac monitoring is mandatory. The induction dose of pentobarbital is 10 mg/kg. If this does is ineffective, increments of 2.5 to 5 mg/kg every 2 to 5 min are added until burst suppression appears on EEG and a blood level of 20 to 40 μg/mL is achieved. This is followed with hourly doses of 3 mg/kg to maintain EEG at a burst suppression pattern. If the first 4 h of treatment in pentobarbital coma remains ineffective, the pentobarbital coma should be repeated. Every 12 h this barbiturate dose is reduced and an EEG is obtained for determination of seizure control. Treatment can be continued for days.

When pentobarbital coma is contemplated, an EEG recording is recommended. Pentobarbital is given until the EEG changes to a burst suppression pattern or becomes isoelectric. When burst suppression or an isoelectric pattern on EEG is established, treatment is continued for a minimum of 4 h and then the dose of pentobarbital is reduced until the EEG returns to a continuous pattern. Should generalized electrographic seizures remain present, the barbiturate coma is reinstituted. This procedure is then repeated as necessary [87]. If EEG findings are focal or clinically seizures are not generalized, pentobarbital is reduced and withdrawn over 12 to 24 h and maintenance treatment with conventional anticonvulsants is continued.

A very high dose of phenobarbital has also been successfully used in barbiturate coma [63,88]. Other short-acting barbiturates are also effective in the treatment of status epilepticus refractory to conventional antiepileptic therapy. Due to their generalized anesthetic effect, this medication should be used in an intensive care unit by a physician experienced in their use and prepared for management of their potential side effects such as hypotension. Short-acting barbiturates have rapid onset of action and a short half-life. In addition to anticonvulsant effect, they may have a protective value in cerebral hypoxia.

XIII. TREATMENT OF NONCONVULSIVE STATUS EPILEPTICUS

A. Generalized Nonconvulsive Status Epilepticus (Absence Status)

Diazepam IV or rectal is the drug of choice, with the same dose and precautions as mentioned above. Ethosuximide or valproate is needed for maintenance therapy, which can be started after the diazepam. Absence status in patients with Lennox–Gastaut syndrome is more refractory to diazepam than are absences in primary generalized epilepsy [79]. There are reports of patients with Lennox–Gastaut syndrome whose seizures have changed from the absence status to generalized tonic–clonic following the use of intravenous benzodiazepines [12,89,90].

B. Partial Nonconvulsive Status Epilepticus (Psychomotor Absence of Temporal or Extratemporal Origin)

Psychomotor absence is not a life-threatening event; however, many epileptologists believe that it should be treated aggressively to prevent permanent memory damage [3]. Phenytoin IV is the drug of choice for treatment of partial nonconvulsive status epilepticus. Precautions and doses are the same as in treatment of convulsive status epilepticus.

REFERENCES

1. Gastaut H. Dictionary of epilepsy, Part I, Definitions. Geneva: World Health Organization, 1973.
2. Lothman E. The biochemical basis and pathophysiology of status epilepticus. *Neurology* 1990; 40(Suppl 2): 13–23.
3. Engel J Jr. Seizures and epilepsy: status epilepticus. Philadelphia: FA Davis Company, 1989:256–80.
4. Aicardi J. Epilepsy in children. New York: Raven Press, 1986:240–59.
5. Dreifuss FE. Status epilepticus. In: Dreifuss FE, ed. *Pediatric epileptology*. Boston: John Wright/PSG, Inc., 1983:221–30.
6. Hauser WA. Status epilepticus: epidemiologic considerations. Neurology 1990; 40(Suppl 2):9–13.
7. Aicardi J, Chevrie JJ. Convulsive status epilepticus in infants and children. A study of 239 cases. Epilepsia 1970; 11:187–97.

7a. Hauser WA, Kurland LT. The epidemiology of epilepsy in Rochester, Minnesota, 1935 through 1967. Epilepsia 1975; 16:1–66.

8. Wilder BJ, Ramgel RJ. In: Levey R, Mattson R, Medrum B, Penry JK, Dreifuss FE, eds. Phenytoin, clinical use in antiepileptic drugs. New York: Raven Press, 1989.
9. Leppik JE. Status epilepticus: the next decade. Neurology 1990; 40(Suppl 2):4–9.
10. Leppik IE. Status epilepticus. Neurol Clin 1986; 4(3): 633–43.
11. Hauser WA. Status epilepticus: frequency, etiology, and neurological sequelae. In: Delgado-Escueta AV, Wasterlain CG, Treiman DM, Porter RJ, eds. Advances in neurology: Vol. 34. status epilepticus. New York: Raven Press, 1983:3–14.
12. Bittencourt PRM, Richens A. Anticonvulsant induced status epilepticus in Lennox–Gastaut syndrome. Epilepsia 1981; 22:129–34.
13. Porter RJ, Penry JK. Petit mal status. In: Delgado-Escueto AV, Wasterlain CG, Treiman DM, Porter RJ, eds. Advances in Neurology. Vol. 34. Status epilepticus. New York: Raven Press, 1983: pp. 61–67.
14. Pritchard PB III, O'Neal DB. Nonconvulsive status epilepticus following metrizamide myelography. Ann Neurol 1984; 16:252–54.
15. Rumpl E, Hinterhuber H. Unusual "spike wave stupor" in a patient with manic depressive psychosis treated with amitriptyline. J Neurol 1981; 226:131–35.
16. Niedermeyer E, Fineyre T, Riley T. Absence status (petit mal status with focal characteristics. Arch Neurol 1979; 38:417–21.
17. Aguilar NJ, Rasmussen T. Role of encephalitis in pathogenesis of epilepsy. Arch Neurol 1960; 2:663.
18. Rasmussen T, McCann W. Clinical studies of patients with focal epilepsy due to "chronic encephalitis." Trans Am Neurol Assoc. 1968; 93:89.
19. Aminoff MJ, Simon RP. Status epilepticus: causes, clinical features and consequences in 98 patients. Am J Med 1980; 69:657–66.
20. Stark LG, Chuang RY, Joy RM. (1987). Biochemical markers of exposure to proconvulsant and anticonvulsant chlorinated hydrocarbons (abstr). Epilepsia 1987; 28:584.
21. Meldrum BS, Horton RW. Physiology of status epilepticus in primates. Arch Neurol 1973; 28:1–9.
22. White PT, Grant P, Mosier J, Craig A. Changes in cerebral dynamics associated with seizures. Neurology (Minneap) 1961; 11:354–61.
23. Meldrum BS, Vigouroux RA, Brierley JB. Systemic factors and epileptic brain damage: prolonged seizures in paralyzed artificially ventilated baboon. Arch Neurol 1973; 29:82–87.
24. Wasterlain CG, Duffy TE. Status epilepticus in immature rats: protective effects of glucose on survival and brain development. Arch Neurol 1976; 33:821–27.
25. Tassinari CA, Daniele O, Michelucci R, Bureau M, Dravet C, Roger J. Benzodiazepines. Efficacy in status epilepticus. In: Delgado-Esueto AV, Wasterlain CG, Treiman DM, Porter RJ, eds. Advances in neurology. Vol. 34. Status epilepticus. New York: Raven Press, 1983:465–75.
26. Meldrum BS, Horton RW, Bloom SR, Butler J, Kennan J. Endocrine factors and glucose metabolism during prolonged seizures in baboons. Epilepsia 1979; 20:527–34.
27. Meldrum BS. Neuropathology and pathophysiology. In: Ladilaw J, and Richens A, eds. A textbook of epilepsy. Edinburgh: Churchill Livingstone, 1976:314–54.

28. Meldrum BS, Brierley JB. Prolonged epileptic seizures in primates. Ischemic cell changes and its relation to ictal physiological events. Arch Neurol 1973; 28:10–17.
29. Maytal J, Shinnar S, Moshé SL, Alvarez CA. Low morbidity and mortality of status epilepticus in children. Pediatrics 1989; 83:323–31.
30. Blennow G, Brierley JB, Meldrum BS, Siesjo BK. Epileptic brain damage. The role of systemic factors that modify cerebral energy metabolism. Brain 1978; 101:687–700.
31. Chapman AG, Meldrum BS, Siesjo BK. Cerebral metabolic changes during prolonged epileptic seizures in rats. J Neurochem 1977; 28:1025–35.
32. Menini C, Meldrum BS, Riche D, Silva-Comte C, Stutzmann JF. Sustained limbic seizures induced by intra-amyglyoid kainic acid in the baboon: symptomatology and neuropathological consequences. Ann Neurol 1980; 8:501–9.
33. Brown WJ, Babb TL. Effects of repeated seizures on hippocampal neurons in the cat. In: Fahn S, Marsden CD, Van Woert MH, eds. *Advances in Neurology*. Vol. 43. Myoclonus. New York: Raven Press, 1983:161–68.
34. Siesjo BK, Inguar M, Folbergrova J, Chapman AG. (1983). Local cerebral circulation and metabolism in bicuculin-induced status epilepticus: relevance for development of cell change. In: Delgado-Escueta AV, Wasterlain CG, Treiman DM, Porter RJ, eds. Advances in Neurology. Status epilepticus: Vol. 34. New York: Raven Press, 1983:217–30.
35. Meldrum BS. Metabolic factors during prolonged seizures and their relation to nerve cell death. In: Delgado-Escueta AV, Wasterlain CG, Treiman DM, Porter RJ, eds. Advances in neurology. Vol. 34, Status epilepticus. New York: Raven Press, 1983:261–76.
36. Trauner DA. Barbiturate therapy in acute brain injury. J. Pediatr 1986; vol 109:742–46.
37. Aicardi J, Chevrie JJ, (1983). Consequences of status epilepticus in infants and children. In: Delgado-Escueta AV, Wasterlain CG, Treiman DM, Porter RJ, eds. Advances in neurology. Vol. 34, Status epilepticus. New York: Raven Press, 1983: 115–25.
38. Goddard GV, McIntyre DC, Leech CK. A permanent change in brain function resulting from daily electrical stimulation. Exp Neurol 1969; 25:295–330.
39. McNamara JO, Byrne MC, Dasheiff RM, Fitz JG. The kindling model for epilepsy. A review. Prog Neurobiol 1980; 15:139–59.
40. Moshé SL, Alba BJ, Ackerman RF, Engel J Jr. Increased seizure susceptibility of the immature brain. Dev Brain Res 1983; 7:81–85.
41. Chevrie JJ, Aicardi J. Convulsive disorder in the first five years of life: neurological and mental outcome and mortality. Epilepsia 1978; 19:67–74.
42. Dunn DW. Status epilepticus in children; etiology, clinical features and outcome. *J Child Neurol* 1988; 3:167–73.
43. Aicardi J, Chevrie JJ. Status epilepticus. *Pediatrics* 1989; 84(5):939.
44. Engel J Jr, Troupin AS, Crandall PH, Sterman MB, Wasterlain CG. Recent developments in the diagnosis and therapy of epilepsy. Ann Intern Med 1982; 97:584–98.
45. Treiman DM. (1983). General principles of treatment. Responsive and intractable status epilepticus in adults. In: Delgado-Escueto AV, Wasterlain CG, Treiman DM,

Porter RJ, eds. Advances in neurology. Vol. 34. Status epilepticus. New York: Raven Press, 1983:377–89.

45a. Agurell S, Berlin A, Ferngran H, Hellstrom B. (1975). Plasma levels of diazepam after parenteral and rectal administrations in children. Epilepsia 1975; 16:277–83.

46. Browne TR, Penry JK. Benzodiazepines in the treatment of epilepsy. A review. Epilepsia 1973; 14:277–310.

47. Skerritt JH, Werz MA, McLean MJ, Macdonald RL. Diazepam and its anomalous P-chloro-derivatives RO5-4864. Comparative effects on mouse neurons in cell cultures. Brain Res 1974; 310:99–105.

48. Skerritt JH, Macdonald RL. Benzodiazepine receptors ligand actions on GABA responses: Benzodiazepines CL 218-872, Zopiclone. Eur J Pharmacol 1984; 101:127–34.

49. Delgado-Escueta AV et al. Management of status epilepticus. N Engl J Med 1983; 306:1337–40.

50. Franzoni E, Carboni C, Lambertini A. Rectal diazepam: a clinical and EEG study after a single dose in children. Epilepsia 1981; 24:35.

51. Knudsen FU. Rectal administration of diazepam in solution in the acute treatment of convulsions in infants and children. Arch Dis Child 1988; 54:855–57.

52. Louis S, Kutt H, McDowell F. The cardiocirculatory changes caused by intravenous Dilantin and its solvent. Am Heart J 1967; 74:523–29.

53. Hoppu K, Santavuori P. Diazepam rectal solution for home treatment of acute seizures in children. Acta Paediatr Scand 1981; 70:369–72.

54. Camfield CS, Camfield PR, Smith E, Dooley JM. Home use of rectal diazepam to prevent status epilepticus in children with convulsive disorders. J Child Neurol 1989; 4:125–26.

55. Treiman DM, Delgado-Escueta AV. Status epilepticus. In: Thompson RA, Green JR, eds. Critical care of neurologic and neurosurgical emergencies. New York: Raven Press, 1980.

56. Bell DS. Dangers of treatment of status epilepticus with diazepam. Br Med J 1969; 1:159–61.

57. Milligan N, Dhillon S, Richens A, Oxley J. Rectal diazepam in the treatment of absence status: a pharmacodynamic study. J Neurol Neurosurg Psychiatry 1981; 44:914–17.

58. Leppik IE, Derivan AT, Homan RW, et al. Double blind study of lorazepam and diazepam in status epilepticus. JAMA 1983; 249:1452–54.

59. Treiman DM, DeGiorgio CM, Ben-Menachem E, et al. Lorazepam vs. phenytoin in the treatment of generalized convulsive status epilepticus: report of an ongoing study (abstr). Neurology 1985; 35(Suppl 1):284.

60. Browne T. The pharmacokinetics of agents used in the treatment of status epilepticus. Neurology 1990; 40(Suppl 2):28–32.

61. Walker JE, Homan RW, Wasko MR, Growford IL, Bell RD, Tasker WD. Lorazepam in status epilepticus. Ann Neurol 1979; 6:207–13.

62. Graves NM, Kriel RL. Rectal administration of antiepileptic drugs in children. Pediatr Neurol 1987; 3:321–26.

63. Lockman LA. Treatment of status epilepticus in children. Neurology 1990; 40(Suppl 2):43–46.

64. Dreifuss FE. Treatment of status epilepticus. In: Swaiman K, Wright F,eds. Neurology in Childhood. St. Louis, Mo: CV Mosby Company, 1982.
65. Albani M. Phenytoin in infancy and childhood. In: Delgado-Escueta AV, Wasterlain CG, Treiman DM, Porter RJ, eds. Advances in neurology. Vol. 34. Status epilepticus. New York: Raven Press, 1983:457–464.
66. Cloyd JC, Bosch DE, Sawchuk RJ. Concentration profile of phenytoin after admixture with small volumes of intravenous fluids. Am J Hospital Pharm 1978; 34:313–18.
67. Wilensky AD, Lowden JA. Inadequate serum levels after intramuscular administration of diphenylhydantoin. Neurology 1973; 23:318.
68. Browne TR. Status epilepticus. Diagnosis and management. In: Brown TR, and Feldman RG, eds. Epilepsy. Boston: Little, Brown and Company, 1983:341–56.
69. Wilder BJ, Ramsay RE, Willmore LJ, et al. Efficacy of intravenous phenytoin in the treatment of status epilepticus. Kinetics of central nervous system penetrations. Ann Neurol 1977; 1:511–518.
70. Wilder BJ, Bruni J. Seizure disorders: pharmacological approach to treatment. New York: Raven Press, 1981.
71. Pellock JM, Low NL. Seizure disorders. In: Kelley VC, ed. Practice of pediatrics. Hagerstown, MD: Harper & Row, Publishers, Inc., 1980.
72. Shaner DM, McCurdy SA, Herring MO, Gabor AJ. Treatment of status epilepticus: a prospective comparison of diazepam and phenytoin versus phenobarbital and optional phenytoin. Neurology 1988; 38:202–7.
73. Browne TR. Paraldehyde, chlormethiazole and lidocaine. In: Delgado-Escueta AV, Porter RJ, Wasterlain CG, eds. Advances in Neurology, Vol. 34. Status epilepticus. New York: Raven Press, 1983:509–17.
74. Koren G, Butt W, Rajchgot P, et al. Intravenous paraldehyde for seizure control in newborn infants. Neurology 1986; 36:108.
75. Bastrom B. Paraldehyde toxicity during treatment of status epilepticus. Am J Dis Child 1982; 136:414–15.
76. Curless RG, Holzman BH, Ramsay RE. Paraldehyde therapy in childhood status epilepticus. Arch Neurol 1983; 40(8):477–80.
77. Congdon P, Forsythe W. Intravenous clonazepam in treatment of status epilepticus in children. Epilepsia 1980; 22:489–501.
78. Pinder RM, Brogden RN, Speight TM, Avery GS. Clonazepam: a review of its pharmacological properties and therapeutic efficacy in epilepsy. Drugs 1976; 5:321–61.
79. Tassinari CA, Daniele O, Michelucci R, Bureau M, Dravet C, Roger J. Benzodiazepines: efficacy in status epilepticus. In: Delgado-Escueto AV, Wasterlain CG, Treiman DM, Porter RJ, eds. *Advances in Neurology*. Vol. 34. Status epilepticus. New York: Raven Press, 1983:465–475.
80. Thorpy MJ. Rectal valproate syrup and status epilepticus. Neurology 1980; 30:1113–14.
81. Orlowski JP, Erenberg G, Luders H, et al. Hypothermia and barbiturate coma for refractory status epilepticus. *Crit Care Med* 1984; 12:367–71.
82. Simon RP. Management of status epilepticus. In: Pedley TA, Meldrum BS, eds. Recent advances in epilepsy. Vol. 2. New York: Churchill Livingstone, 1985: 137–60.

83. Sager DP, Bomar SK, Barbaccia JG. Intravenous medications. Philadelphia: JB Lippincott Company, 1980; 179.
84. Corkill G, Silvalingam S, Reitan JA, Gilory B, Helphrey M. Dose dependency of the post-insult protective effect of phenobarbital in the canine experimental stroke model. Stroke 1978; 9:10.
85. Gortein KJ, Mussafi H, Melamed E. Treatment of status epilepticus with thiopentone sodium anesthesia in a child. Eur J Pediatr 1983; 140:133–35.
86. Hoff JT, Smith AL, Hankinson HL, Nielsen SL. Barbiturate protection from cerebral infraction in primates. Stroke 1975; 6(1):28–33.
87. Goldberg MA, McIntyre HB. Barbiturates in the treatment of status epilepticus. In: Delgado-Escueta AV, Wasterlain CG, Treiman DM, Porter RJ, eds. Advances in Neurology. Vol. 34. Status epilepticus: mechanisms of brain damage and treatment. New York: Raven Press, 1983.
88. Crawford TO, Mitchell WG, Fishman LS, Snodgrass SR. Very high dose phenobarbital for refractory status epilepticus in children. Neurology 1988; 38:1035–40.
89. Prior PF, McLain GN, Scott DF, Laurance BM. Tonic status epilepticus precipitated by intravenous diazepam in a child with petit mal status. Epilepsia 1972; 13:467–72.
90. Levy RJ, Krall RL. Treatment of status epilepticus with lorazepam. Arch Neurol 1984; 41:605–11.

8

Febrile Seizures

JEROME V. MURPHY
*University of Missouri
and Children's Mercy Hospital
Kansas City, Missouri*

I. DEFINITION

A febrile seizure is a seizure accompanying a fever in a child several months to 5 years of age in the absence of an intracranial infection or toxin [1]. Excluded are children with prior afebrile seizures. Included are children with prior evidence of neurologic abnormalities (e.g., patients with cerebral palsy can have febrile convulsions). Febrile seizures are usually generalized tonic–clonic seizures [1]. Febrile seizures per se are not a symptom of epilepsy, as the seizure is provoked by fever and epilepsy is defined as an unprovoked seizure.

Febrile seizures are divided into simple and complex febrile seizures. Complex febrile seizures have at least one of three unusual features: (1) repeated episodes within 24 h, (2) long duration, and (3) focal seizures. Simple febrile seizures lack any of these features. The differentiation is important, as the child with a complex febrile seizure has an increased risk for unprovoked seizures or epilepsy [2].

Febrile seizures are the most common seizure disorder in childhood. In most nations the total incidence varies between 2.2 and 3.5% [3,4]. The highest reported incidence is about 14% in the children of the Mariana islands in the western Pacific [5]. As the whole family lives in the same room, the identification of febrile seizures might be more complete in this society. Allegedly, the incidence in China is the lowest in the world, and this relates to the reduced exposure to contagious febrile illnesses in the politically popular single-child families.

Febrile seizures occur more frequently in males than in females, and the reason is not known [4]. Fifty percent of children with febrile seizures experience their first event before the age of 2, and 90% before their third birthday. They are rare as a first event in the first 6 months of life, and it is also uncommon to have a first febrile seizure after the age of 3 years [6].

Most febrile seizures are brief (less than 15 min) [7]. Ten percent may last longer than 15 min, and 4% longer than 30 min [8]. Less than 10% of febrile seizures have focal features [2].

The most frequent complication of a febrile seizure is a recurrence of the event. About 30% of children with one febrile seizure will have a recurrence [3]. The risk is higher if the first febrile seizure occurs before the age of 18 months [4]. One report has correlated the risk of recurrence with a lower fever at the time of the first febrile convulsion [9]. Unfortunately, this study was not clearly prospective, excluded children with preexisting neurologic abnormalities, and included children with *Shigella* infections, in which a seizure may relate to the bacterial toxin [10].

Seven percent of children with a febrile convulsion will have an unprovoked seizure, a fivefold risk over children without a febrile convulsion. If the seizure is a simple febrile seizure, the risk for a spontaneous seizure is 2 to 4%. If a single complex feature is present, the risk increases to 6 to 8%. If the child's seizure has two of the complex features described above, the risk increases to 17 to 22%, and if all three features are present, the risk is 49% [2]. A positive family history of unprovoked seizures is also associated with the later appearance of an unprovoked generalized seizure [2]. Prophylaxis with an AED has not been demonstrated to change this risk [11].

Just as a child with previously diagnosed epilepsy can have another seizure concurrent with a fever, the opposite occurs. A child with a predisposition to epilepsy, either from a genetic epilepsy or from acquired disease, may have his or her initial seizure provoked by a fever (i.e., the first symptom of an epilepsy is brought forward by the fever and the unprovoked seizures occur later). Surveys of genetic epilepsies have demonstrated a higher-than-expected occurrence of prior febrile seizures (see Chapters 3 and 4). Nevertheless, all first febrile seizures are included in studies of febrile seizures, whether or not there is subsequent evidence of epilepsy [1].

As the temperature in a child with fever is not continually monitored, the proven concurrence of a fever and the convulsion is rare. The febrile convulsion generally occurs in a child either known to have a febrile illness or in a child found to have a fever immediately after a convulsion. In adults, the convulsion itself can produce a fever [12]. The production of a fever by a convulsion has not been reported in children.

Considering that fever is a very frequent sequela to immunization with the DPT vaccine in a very young child [13], it is hardly surprising that 1 in 1750 children will have a convulsion in the 24 h following immunization with DPT vaccine [14]. In one report a change in the scheduling of pertussis immunization was associated with a significant ($p = 0.004$) change in the time of febrile seizures between two cohorts of children [15]. If a child has a DPT immunization followed by a febrile convulsion, and if such a child has subsequent evidence of neurologic impairment, a component of the vaccine may be considered as etiologic in the neurologic impairment [16].

II. ETIOLOGY

Why a several-degree increase in the temperature of a young child's brain produces a seizure is unknown. Postulates concerning the etiology of febrile seizures include genetic factors, prenatal toxic exposures, rate of temperature change, the presence of bacteremia or viremia, and abnormal brain concentrations of an amino acid.

Given the frequently positive family history for this condition in children with febrile seizures, there may be a familial, or genetic, factor. If one parent has a febrile convulsion, about 20% of the offspring will have a febrile seizure; if both parents have febrile convulsions, this number rises to 55% [17]. In monozygotic twins the concordance rate for febrile seizures is 56%, and in dizygotic twins this falls to 14% [18]. These observations favor a genetic etiology for febrile seizures.

Considering that only 6% of children with febrile seizures have a positive family history for this illness, there must be alternative explanations [19]. An association between the later development of febrile seizures and prenatal maternal cigarette smoking and alcohol intake exists [19,20]. However, the presently popular elimination of these exposures during pregnancy will probably not have a great impact on the number of children with febrile seizures, as the statistically significant association occurs in only a small number of mothers of children with febrile convulsions.

Whether febrile convulsions relate to a rapid change in temperature or to a sustained elevation of temperature in the developing brain has been debated [21]. During prolonged EEG recordings in nine children after a febrile seizure, three had epileptic activity on the EEG with high-grade ($>$103°C) and sustained fever. One child with a strong genetic background for febrile seizures had such changes with only a low-grade fever [22]. These observations would suggest that the height of the fever is important in nonfamilial febrile seizures rather than the change in temperature.

The presence of bacteremia does not seem to relate to the presence or absence of a convulsion in a child with a febrile illness. In one study the number of children with bacteremia after a febrile convulsion (5.4%) was the same as the number of children evaluated for fever who had not had a febrile convulsion [23].

Viruses have been suspected to play a role in febrile seizures [24]. In one report where this was studied, 9 of 144 children (6%) with febrile convulsions had a virus isolated from their otherwise normal cerebrospinal fluid (CSF). These nine children had no unusual feature to their febrile convulsion [25]. Unfortunately, the authors did not include a control population of children with fever who had not had a febrile convulsion. Based on another publication, this number of viral-infested CSF specimens may not be unusual in children with febrile illnesses [26].

Amino acid concentrations in brain may have a role in causing seizures in some patients, as certain amino acids can serve as putative neurotransmitters in brain. One report analyzed amino acid concentrations in the CSF of children with a recent febrile convulsion and compared them with the concentration in CSF from age-matched controls. Although differences were discovered, they could have been secondary to the seizure rather than primary [27].

III. DIFFERENTIAL DIAGNOSIS

If one keeps in mind the definition of a febrile seizure, the differential diagnosis is limited. The person caring for the child with a fever and a convulsion must be satisfied that there is no evident central nervous system infection (i.e., meningitis, encephalitis, or brain abscess) or evidence of a toxin producing the clinical symptoms. Examples of toxins are a *Shigella* enteritis with fever and a convulsion [10]. The latter is secondary to a *Shigella* toxin. Lead toxicity could produce fever and a convulsion. Another example of a toxin that could have this effect would be an overdose of some drugs (e.g., tricyclic antidepressants, chlorpromazine, atropine, and aspirin) [28].

If a child with a fever and a convulsion has had a prior seizure without evident fever, that child has epilepsy and not febrile seizures. If the child with treated epilepsy has a fever and a convulsion, the treatment might not be adequate, and changes in the antiepileptic drug (AED) or the dose of the AED need to be considered.

IV. MANAGEMENT

A. Immediate

As most convulsions are very frightening events to observers, most patients with febrile convulsions are brought to emergency medical attention. Considering that they are brief, most have resolved by the time the patients reach emergency medical attention, and the diagnosis is based on the description of an observer. The medical management is then twofold (i.e., temperature control and evaluation for the cause of the fever).

As febrile seizures do not per se indicate the presence of an unusual febrile illness, the evaluation should be the same as that for a child with a similar fever and without the convulsion. If parental or medical concern necessitates hospitalization, the length of stay is generally brief [29].

If a child has evidence of a chronic infection or congenital heart disease, a brain abscess must be considered in the differential diagnosis. If papilledema is present, a neuroimaging procedure is mandatory before the performance of a lumbar puncture (LP). Fortunately, most children with brain abscesses tolerate an LP without major untoward response [30].

A prolonged febrile convulsion should be managed as it would be in any child with a prolonged afebrile convulsion. Generally, the seizure will stop concurrent with the administration of either diazepam or lorazepam. Immediate recurrences may warrant the temporary administration of longer-acting AEDs, such as phenytoin or phenobarbital.

Accurate rules for performing an LP are not available. The medically responsible person must be certain that the child does not have meningitis. An LP is a benign procedure that may be necessary to rule out that possibility. In general, the younger physician will more frequently perform an LP than will the experienced pediatrician [31]. This procedure will be performed more often in the infant below the age of 18 months in whom nuchal rigidity can be absent in the face of meningitis. If a child returns to the emergency room with a second febrile convulsion shortly after the first one, meningitis needs to be considered even if the original CSF was normal. Patients have been described in whom the CSF demonstrated signs of meningitis only in the second LP after the second convulsion [32].

No other study has been demonstrated to be of routine benefit in the child with a febrile convulsion [33]. EEGs are frequently performed after a febrile seizure but have never been demonstrated to have a therapeutic or predictive value. Eighty-eight percent of patients will have generalized slowing on the day after a febrile convulsions, and 33% will demonstrate this change 3 to 7 days later. Focal slowing may suggest a focal brain lesion and must be correlated with other clinical features. Epileptic changes are rare and not helpful [34].

There may be an investigational role for the performance of EEGs on children who have had a febrile seizure. This will help as a screen for the identification of children with genetic epilepsies, but it will not help in therapeutic decisions [34].

B. Long term

1. Continuous Prophylaxis

The long-term medical management of the patient with febrile convulsions has recently undergone a reappraisal. Continuous as opposed to intermittent prophylaxis with phenobarbital or valproic acid has been reported to reduce the risk of a recurrence of a febrile seizure from about 33% to 10% [35–37]. Whatever management is proposed, continuous prophylaxis, intermittent prophylaxis, or no prophylaxis, the family of the child with one febrile convulsion must be instructed in the reduction and control of fever using antipyretic agents [38].

Reported series describing prophylaxis with either phenobarbital or valproic acid have used randomization to therapy or placebo, but patients who were unable to comply with the continuous administration of an AED were eliminated from the study results (i.e., selection of patients for treatment results went beyond the randomization process, so comparison to the patients randomized to no treatment may be invalid) [39].

If one compares all patients randomized to valproic acid or to phenobarbital for the prophylaxis of febrile seizures to untreated control patients and does not eliminate from the results the patients unable to comply with the drug to which they have been randomized, these AEDs do not alter the recurrence risk as compared to controls [39]. In other words, just the assignment of a patient to either valproic acid or to phenobarbital for the prophylaxis of febrile seizures is not effective in reducing the number of subsequent febrile convulsions. Seemingly, the risk of recurrence can be lowered with either AED only if that AED is taken continuously at an appropriate dose.

Data have been presented demonstrating that the continuous prophylaxis of febrile seizures with phenobarbital for 2 years results in a significant reduction of IQ in the treated group as compared to a control population receiving placebo [40]. Unfortunately, only two-thirds of the phenobarbital-treated group in this study were still taking the drug at the end of the 2-year trial, and it is not clear if the children still on treatment with phenobarbital had an even lower IQ than the patients in the treatment group who did not comply with the phenobarbital protocol [40].

There is remote risk of a fatal hepatotoxicity in infants and young children treated with valproic acid [41]. Therefore, the risk from side effects of either phenobarbital or valproic acid may not warrant their chronic use of what is essentially a benign seizure disorder.

2. Intermittent Prophylaxis

An alternative and apparently effective method for the controlling recurrent febrile seizures is the administration of the intravenous formulation of diazepam, about 0.3 mg/kg body weight, rectally or orally every 12 h as long as the child has a temperature above 38.5 °C. Although diazepam may produce lethargy, this approach has the advantage that the patient is treated only at the time of the fever, and long-term adversity does not occur [42].

The intermittent use of diazepam may work only in children at high risk for recurrent febrile seizures [43]. In this study by Knudsen five high risk for recurrence factors were identified; less than 15 months of age at the first febrile seizures, epilepsy or febrile convulsions in first-degree relatives, a first complex febrile convulsion, and day nursery care. Children with $\geq$ 2 risk factors benefitted from intermittent diazepam, and children with $\leq$ 1 risk factor did not benefit.

Another study compared such intermittent use of diazepam with the use of valproic acid suppositories, which are not commercially available in this country. Both were given only at the time of fever, and both were equally effective in reducing the number of febrile seizures below a theoretical control number. Unfortunately, a control, unmedicated population was not included in this study [44].

Some doubt has been cast on this approach in a recently published double-blind, placebo-controlled trial of intermittent diazepam for the control of recurrent febrile seizures [45]. No difference was observed in febrile seizure recurrences between the children randomized to diazepam and those randomized to placebo. Fifteen of 93 patients assigned to intermittent diazepam prophylaxis recurred, and 18 of 92 children assigned to placebo recurred. However, careful scrutiny of the data demonstrated that of the 15 recurrences in the diazepam group, 14 never received diazepam! In other words, there were a total of 33 recurrences in 185 children. Thirty-two recurrences of febrile seizures were in children who had not received diazepam, and only one occurred in a child who had received diazepam. From this perspective diazepam should be an effective prophylaxis for the reduction recurrent febrile seizures [45].

There are two disadvantages to intermittent diazepam treatment of the child with a first febrile convulsion. Logically, the parent(s) may not be aware that a seizure is present until a convulsion has occurred, in which case the opportunity to administer an AED prophylactically has been lost. The second disadvantage is the frequency of noncompliance with intermittent management, described in all articles on intermittent therapy cited above [42–45].

In our clinic nurses have developed a 20- to 30-min protocol for the instruction of parents in the administration of diazepam intermittently during a febrile illness. This is followed by a video presentation of the technique. Studies on the efficacy of this approach are pending.

3. No Prophylaxis

Another approach to the long-term management of febrile seizures is no prophylactic therapy. In the best community-based studies febrile seizures carried too few sequelae to warrant chronic prophylaxis with an AED [7,46]. IQs of children with three or more febrile seizures were the same as those of control children when they later attended school [46]. Even febrile status epilepticus does not seem to have significant sequelae [8]. In the long run febrile seizures are not injurious to the brain, so their prophylaxis may be unnecessary. This approach assumes a moderate parental tolerance to the sight of a febrile convulsion

Table 1 Possible Managements Plans for Children with One Febrile Seizure

Drug	Method	Disadvantages
Chronic therapy		
Phenobarbital	Daily therapy with adequate amounts to maintain therapeutic levels	Small reduction in IQ with long-term use [40]
Valproic acid	Daily therapy with adequate amounts to maintain therapeutic levels	Remote risk of a fatal hepatotoxicity [41]
Intermittent therapy		
Diazepam	0.3 mg/kg every 12 h, temperature ≥ 38.5°C	Poor compliance [45], fever may not be recognized until the convulsion
Valproate suppository	150–300 mg	Poor compliance [44]
No therapy	Fever control without other AED[a]	Family distress when a convulsion is observed

[a]All proposed management plans have to utilize fever control with antipyretic agents.

in their child. It may be wise in this situation to instruct the parents on the use of rectally administered diazepam to stop a prolonged febrile seizure (see Chapter 5).

A summary of these approaches and their disadvantages is presented in Table 1. If a child has a febrile seizure, the physician must (1) instruct the family on the use of effective antipyretic agents, and (2) decide either to use intermittent prophylaxis with oral or rectal diazepam, or not to prophylax against recurrences, once the parents are instructed on the essentially benign nature of a febrile seizure. The decision on which path to chose will be a mutual decision involving physician and family.

V. PROGNOSIS

Two contrasting follow-up studies have appeared on the intellectual prognosis of children who had febrile seizures. One from England demonstrated that children with febrile seizures had a lower IQ than controls, and the degree of lowering varied with the number of febrile convulsions [47]. Contrariwise follow-up of children with febrile seizures who were in the Perinatal Collaborative Project indicated later IQs that were the same as the control population, even in the children with at least three febrile convulsions [46]. The difference in these two conclusions was reconciled by the differences in study populations. The English study was hospital-based, and therefore, one assumes, may have attracted the unusual febrile convulsion [47], whereas the study demonstrating no intellectual sequelae was derived from a community-based population [46].

The observation that children with febrile convulsions are as normal as control populations when they later enter school is extremely important. Since there is no long-term sequela from febrile convulsions, their prophylaxis may be unnecessary, and research into their prevention becomes less important.

Initial animal experiments studying febrile seizures demonstrated that animals with induced febrile seizures had long-term behavioral deficits [48]. More recent experiments using microwave hyperthermia have not demonstrated any behavioral changes in animals with febrile seizures. Therefore, one has to conclude that the method of provoking the febrile seizures in the earlier experiments damaged the brain rather than the febrile seizure itself [49].

As discussed in Chapter 5, retrospective studies of patients with mesial temporal sclerosis related to intractable complex partial seizures reveal a preponderance of patients with a history of a prolonged febrile seizure [50]. In such studies the conclusion is that prolonged febrile seizures are therefore not benign, as specific hippocampal neurones may be destroyed by the prolonged febrile seizures, secondarily establishing excitatory networks that predispose the patient to intractable complex partial seizures.

Prospective studies have not supported this theory [2,7,8,11]. Even if a relationship were to exist between prolonged febrile seizures and mesial temporal sclerosis, the compulsive treatment of children who have febrile seizures with AEDs would probably not be warranted. As only 4% of patients with febrile seizures have prolonged ictuses [8], and as not all febrile seizures can be prevented by such treatment, more than 96% of patients with febrile seizures would be treated unnecessarily to prevent the development of mesial temporal sclerosis if this were a reason for prophylactic treatment.

Another reason for the treatment of febrile seizures is to prevent the development of epilepsy. As this develops in only 3% of the population with simple febrile seizures, a large number of patients with febrile seizures would be treated for the protection of a few [2]. Also, there is no proof that such therapeutic intervention is effective in prevention of epilepsy, and there is proof that certain previously recommended therapies have significant adversities [11].

REFERENCES

1. Consensus statement on febrile seizures. In: Nelson KB, Ellenberg JH, eds. Febrile seizures. New York: Raven Press, 1981:301.
2. Annegers JF, Hauser WA, Shirts SB, Kurland LT. Factors prognostic of unprovoked seizures after febrile convulsions. N Engl J Med 1987; 316:493–98.
3. Hauser WA. The natural history of febrile seizures. In: Nelson KB, Ellenberg JH, eds. Febrile seizures. New York: Raven Press, 1981:5–17.

4. Forsgren L, Sidenvall R, Blomquist HK:son and Heijbel J. A prospective incidence of febrile convulsions. Acta Paediatr Scand 1990; 79:550–57.
5. Mathia KV, Dunn OP, Kurland LT, Reeder FA. Convulsive disorders in the Mariana Islands. Epilepsia 1968; 9:77–85.
6. Knudsen FU. Febrile convulsions. In: Dam M, Gram L, eds. Comprehensive epileptology. New York: Raven Press, 1991:133–44.
7. Nelson KB, Ellenberg JH. Prognosis in children with febrile seizures. Pediatrics 1978; 15:720–27.
8. Maytal J, Shinnar S. Febrile status eplepticus. Pediatrics 1990; 86:611–16.
9. el-Radhi, Banajeh S. Effect of fever on recurrence rate of febrile convulsions. Arch Dis Child 1989; 64:869–70.
10. Zvulunov A, Lerman M, Ashkenazi S, Weitz R, Nitzan M, Dinari G. The prognosis of convulsions during childhood shigellosis. Eur J Pediatr 1990; 149:293–94.
11. Wolf SM, Forsythe A. Epilepsy and mental retardation following febrile seizures in childhood. Acta Paediatr Scand 1989; 78:291–95.
12. Wachtel TJ, Steele GH, Day JA. Natural history of fever following seizure. Arch Intern Med 1987; 147:1153–55.
13. Rawson D, Petersen SA, Wailoo MP. Rectal temperature of normal babies the night after diphtheria, pertussis, and tetanus immunization. Arch Dis Child 1990; 65:1305–7.
14. Cody CL, Baraff LJ, Cherry JD, Marcy SM, Manclark CR. Nature and rates of adverse reactions associated with DTP and DT immunizations in infants and children. Pediatrics 1981; 68:650–60.
15. Jacobson V, Nielsen C, Buch D, Shields WD, Christenson P, Zachau-Christiansen B, Cherry JD. Relationship of pertussis immunization to the onset of epilepsy, febrile convulsions and central nervous system infections: a retrospective epidemiologic study. Tokai J Exp Clin Med 1988; 13(Suppl):137–42.
16. Golden GS. Pertussis vaccine and injury to the brain. J Pediatr 1990; 116:854–61.
17. Hauser WA, Annegers JF, Anderson VE, Kurland KT. The risk of seizure disorders among relatives of children with febrile convulsions. Neurology 1985; 35:1268–73.
18. Tsuboi T. Genetic analysis of febrile convulsions: twin and family studies. Hum Genet 1987; 75:7–14.
19. Nelson KB, Ellenberg JH. Prenatal and perinatal antecedents of febrile seizures. Ann Neurol 1990; 27:127–31.
20. Cassano PA, Koespell TD, Farwell JR. Risk of febrile seizures in childhood in relation to prenatal maternal cigarette smoking and alcohol intake. Am J Epidemiol 1990; 132:462–73.
21. Ouellette EM. The child who convulses with fever. Pediatr Clin North Am 1974; 21:467–81.
22. Minchom PE, Wallace SJ. Febrile convulsions: electroencephalographic changes related to rectal temperature. Arch Dis Child 1984; 59:372–73.
23. Chamberlain JM, Gorman RL. Occult bacteremia in children with simple febrile convulsions. Am J Dis Child 1988; 142:1073–76.
24. Lewis HM, Parry JV, Parry RP, Davies HA, Sanderson PJ, Tyrrell DAJ, Valman HB. Role of viruses in febrile convulsions. Arch Dis Child 1979; 54:869–76.

25. Rantala H, Uhari M, Tuokko H. Viral infections and recurrences of febrile convulsions. J Pediatr 1990; 116:195–99.
26. Wenner HA, Abel D, Olson LC, Burry VF. A mixed epidemic associated with echovirus types 6 and 11. Am J Epidemiol 1981; 114:369–78.
27. Cremades A, Penafiel R, Monserrat F, Ceron I, Perez-Flores D. Free amino acids in the cerebrospinal fluid of children with febrile seizures. Neuropediatrics 1989; 20:129–31.
28. Olson KR, Pentel PR, Kelley MT. Physical assessment and differential diagnosis of the poisoned child. Med Toxicol 1987; 2:52–81.
29. Green AL, MacFaul R. Duration of admission for febrile convulsions? Arch Dis Child 1985; 60:1182–84.
30. Johnson DL, Markle BM, Wiedermann BL, Hanahan L. Treatment of intracranial abscesses associated with sinusitis in children and adolescents. J Pediatr 1988; 113:15–23.
31. Lorber J, Sunderland R. Lumbar punctures in children with convulsions associated with fever. Lancet 1980; 1:785–86.
32. Rutter N, Smales ORC. Role of routine investigations in children presenting with their first febrile convulsion. Arch Dis Child 1977; 52:188–91.
33. Aicardi J. Epilepsy in children. New York: Raven Press, 1986:219–20.
34. Doose H, Ritter K, Volzke E. EEG longitudinal studies in febrile convulsions. Neuropediatrics 1983; 14:81–87.
35. Ngwane E, Bower B. Continuous sodium valproate or phenobarbitone in the prevention of simple febrile convulsions. Arch Dis Child 1980; 55:171–74.
36. Wallace SJ, Smith JA. Successful prophylaxis against febrile convulsions with valproic acid or phenobarbitone. Br Med J 1980; 280:353–60.
37. Wallace SJ. Prevention of recurrent febrile seizures using continuous prophylaxis: sodium valproate compared with phenobarbital. In: Nelson KB, Ellenberg JH, eds. Febrile seizures. New York: Raven Press, 1981:135–42.
38. Ipp MM, Gold R, Greenberg S, Goldbach M, Kupfert BB, Lloyd DD, Maresky DC, Saunders N, Wise SA. Acetaminophen prophylaxis of adverse reactions following vaccination of infants with diphtheria–pertussis–tetanus–polio vaccine. Pediatr Infect Dis J 1987; 6:721–25.
39. Newton RW. Randomised controlled trials of phenobarbitone and valproate in febrile convulsions. Arch Dis Child 1988; 64:1189–91.
40. Farwell JR, Lee YJ, Hirtz DG, Sulzbacher SI, Ellenberg JH, Nelson KB. Phenobarbital for febrile seizures: effects on intelligence and on seizure recurrence. N Engl J Med 1990; 322:364–69.
41. Dreifuss FE, Langer DH, Moline KA, Maxwell JE. Valproic acid hepatic fatalities. II. US experience since 1984. Neurology 1989; 39:201–7.
42. Knudsen FU. Effective short-term diazepam prophylaxis in febrile convulsions. J Pediatr 1985; 106:487–90.
43. Knudsen FU. Recurrence risk after febrile seizure and effect of short-term diazepam prophylaxis. Arch Dis Child 1985; 60:1045–49.
44. Daugbjerg P, Brems M, Mai J, Ankerhus J, Knudsen FU. Intermittent prophyllaxis in febrile convulsions: diazepam or valproic acid? Acta Neurol Scand 1990; 82:17–20.

45. Autret E, Billard C, Bertrand P, Motte J, Pouplard F, Jonville AP. Double-blind, randomized trial of diazepam versus placebo for prevention of recurrence of febrile seizures. J Pediatr 1990; 117:490–94.
46. Ellenberg JH, Nelson KB. Febrile seizures and later intellectual performance. Arch Neurol 1978; 35:17–21.
47. Smith JA, Wallace SJ. Febrile convulsions: intellectual progress in relation to anticonvulsant therapy and to recurrence of fits. Arch Dis Child 1982; 57:104–7.
48. Vanucci RC. Metabolic and pathological consequences of experimental febrile seizures and status epilepticus. In: Nelson KB, Ellenberg JH, eds. Febrile seizures. New York: Raven Press, 1981:43–57.
49. Hjeresen DL, Diaz J. Ontogeny of susceptibility to experimental febrile seizures in rats. Dev Psychobiol 1988; 21:261–75.
50. Sagar HJ, Oxbury JM. Hippocampal neuron loss in temporal lobe epilepsy: correlation with early childhood convulsions. Ann Neurol 1987; 23:334–40.

9

Myoclonic Epilepsy

FEREYDOUN DEHKHARGHANI
University of Missouri
and Children's Mercy Hospital
Kansas City, Missouri

I. INTRODUCTION

The myoclonic epilepsies of childhood and adolescence are difficult to classify and there is a divergence of opinion over nomenclature. The term *myoclonus* is an abbreviated form of *paramyoclonus multiplex*, which was initially used by Friedreich to describe the involuntary movements [1].

Myoclonus is a complex disorder with varied etiologies and widespread sites of origin in the central nervous system. Upon physiological grounds, myoclonus has been classified as cortical, reticular, or spinal origin. This chapter is limited to myoclonus, whose site of origin is cortical or presumed to be cortical and falls in the category of *myoclonic seizures seen in myoclonic epilepsies*.

II. DEFINITION

Myoclonus is a sudden, brief, shocklike involuntary muscle contraction. Myoclonus can occur singly or repetitively; it may be focal, segmental, generalized, unilateral, bilateral, symmetrical, or asymmetrical. Myoclonic jerks should be differentiated from tics, chorea, dystonia, and tremor. *Nocturnal myoclonus* is a movement disorder seen during sleep and should be differentiated from nocturnal epilepsy.

In *action myoclonus*, muscular jerking is initiated by movement, attempt of movement, or even intention to move. This type of myoclonus is not an epileptic phenomena. However, it is seen in some forms of epilepsy, such as Unverricht–Landborg disease, a form of progressive myoclonic epilepsy, and Lafora body disease. The same phenomenon is observed as a sequel to hypoxic encephalopathy.

In nonepileptic myoclonus, the muscular contractions are usually irregular and precipitated or aggravated by sensory stimuli such as light, noise, or tapping. Postural changes may aggravate the intensity or frequency of spasms. Like many other movement disorders, nonepileptic myoclonic jerks disappear during sleep [2].

III. SPECTRUM OF MYOCLONIC SEIZURES AND MYOCLONIC EPILEPSY

Myoclonic seizures with associated electroencephalogram (EEG) spikes are seen in a wide variety of neurological diseases and syndromes. They may be progressive or static. Myoclonic epilepsy may complicate an underlying neurological disorder as seen in progressive myoclonic epilepsy, cerebral lipidosis, infantile hemiplegia, viral encephalitis, and anoxic encephalopathy.

Myoclonic attacks are seen in many types of epilepsies in different age groups and may be the only or the predominant type of seizure. They are frequently associated with other types of seizures [3]. Tonic and atonic seizures, when they are very brief, can be mistaken by myoclonic seizures. A combination of tonic or atonic seizures with myoclonic seizures is not infrequent, such as massive myoclonia, followed by loss of postural tone. Polygraphic investigation can help to differentiate these features by showing suppression of motor activity on the electromyogram (EMG) of atonic seizure, presence of prolonged bursts of motor activities in tonic seizures, and burst of synchronized activity on the EMG of true myoclonic seizures [4]. In epileptic myoclonus, muscle jerks are preceded by EEG spike, but due to a very short time lag, the EEG representation of seizure (spikes) may be difficult to differentiate from movement artifact without the use of specific techniques [5].

Although most myoclonic jerks are associated with spike discharges on the EEG, the association does not necessarily imply that the cortex is the initial site of a lesion. Subcortical levels, including the brainstem, cerebellum, even the extrapyramidal region, may be the prime site of a pathological abnormality [6].

Action myoclonus is seen in different types of cerebral storage diseases, which may become complicated by progressive epileptic encephalopathy. Association of cerebellar and basal ganglia disorder with action myoclonus and epilepsy has been known for many years [7]. The presence of myoclonus in childhood or adolescence in conjunction with cerebellar or other neurological disorders should raise the possibility of progressive myoclonic epilepsy [8].

Table 1 Classification of the Myoclonic Epilepsies of Childhood

Progressive myoclonic encephalopathies
1. With demonstrated or probable metabolic disturbances
2. Genetic syndromes without known metabolic basis
3. Subacute sclerosing panencephalitis

Nonprogressive myoclonic epilepsies
1. With mainly pseudomyoclonic seizures (with tonic type seizure)
   a. Infantile spasms
   b. Lennox–Gastaut syndrome
2. With mainly true myoclonic seizures
   a. Several types of cryptogenic myoclonic epilepsies
   b. Myoclonus associated with petit mal absences
   c. Myoclonic absences
   d. Eyelid myoclonia with absences
   e. Myoclonic epilepsy of adolescence

Source: Modified from Ref. 4.

IV. COMMON MYOCLONIC EPILEPSY OF CHILDHOOD

Marsden et al. divide myoclonus into four major etiologic categories: physiologic, essential, epileptic, and symptomatic [4,8a]. Major categories of the myoclonic epilepsies of childhood are presented in Table 1. The following epileptic disorders, which are manifested by myoclonic seizures, are discussed in this chapter: (1) West syndrome (infantile spasms), (2) Lennox–Gastaut syndrome, (3) benign myoclonic epilepsy in infancy, (4) severe myoclonic epilepsy in infancy, (5) early myoclonic encephalopathy, (6) juvenile myoclonic epilepsy (impulsive petit mal), (7) early infantile epileptic encephalopathy, (8) epilepsy with myoclonic absences, (9) epilepsy with myoclonic astatic seizures, and (10) progressive myoclonic epilepsies. For the place of these epileptic disorders in the international classification of epilepsy and epileptic syndromes, see Chapter 3.

A. Infantile Spasms

Infantile spasms (West syndrome) are an age-specific convulsive disorder of infancy and early childhood. Infantile spasms were first reported by W.J. West in his own child [9]. He described clinical features of this affliction with characteristic spasms and developmental retardation. This unique form of epilepsy is presently recognized by the triad of myoclonic spasm, psychomotor retardation, and a characteristic EEG pattern.

1. Epidemiology

Incidence of infantile spasms is 1 in 4000 to 6000 live births [10–12] due to multifactorial susceptibility and the significant role of environmental precipitating factors; it is difficult to calculate the recurrence rate of infantile spasms [13]. It constitutes 7.5 to 15% of childhood seizure disorders [14].

2. Age of Onset

Eighty-five percent of cases of infantile spasms began at under 1 year of age with the peak incidence of 2 to 7 months. Onset of infantile spasms before the age of 3 months is uncommon. Boys are more often affected as seen in 60% of cases collected by Lacy and Penry [12]. A family history of infantile spasms is not common, but a family history of epileptic seizures of any type is found in 6 to 17% of cases [13,15]. West syndrome results from acquired brain disorders in 15 to 67% of cases [12].

3. Clinical Features

The most common clinical presentation of infantile spasms consists of brief episodes of muscle contraction manifested by sudden extension or flexion of extremities (i.e., myoclonic seizures). Infantile spasms may be associated with tonic or atonic components. Respiratory irregularities, crying at the end of a cluster, flushing, abnormal eye movement, smiling, or grimacing are seen in 30 to 50% of cases [16]. Laughter has occasionally been noted during or following myoclonic jerks. Seizures are rare during sleep but are more frequent during drowsiness and especially upon awakening. Repetitive spasms are rare after the age of 3 years. The most common clinical presentation of myoclonic seizures are mixed flexor–extensor spasms. Spasms may involve the muscles of the neck, trunk, and extremities simultaneously. Child may have predominant flexor or extensor spasms. Myoclonic jerks are usually followed by a brief episode of motor arrest and attenuation of responsiveness. Frequently, autonomic disturbances such as irregular respiration, color changes, and rarely tachycardia are seen during the spasm. Spasms may be preceded by a cry or nonspecific vocalization.

Flexor spasms have been described as "jackknife" when flexor is very prominent and legs are drawn up. In *salaam spasms*, sudden postural changes resemble the Moro reflex. *Cheerleader spasms* and *lightning spasms* are other descriptive terms for myoclonic jerks in this disorder when spasms occur in clusters. Seizures are much more frequent during wakefulness. They occur in clusters, frequently after arousal from sleep. At times, initial episodes are mistaken for colic or simple startles. There is no consensus of opinion as to whether there is any disturbance of consciousness [17]. Mental retardation or psychomotor regression is seen in about 95% of the cases.

4. Atypical Infantile Spasms

There are three types of atypical infantile spasms: (1) when hypsarrhythmia on the EEG is not associated with clinical evidence of myoclonic seizures, (2) when the onset of West syndrome is before the age of 3 months or after the age of 1 year, and (3) when infantile spasms are associated with other types of seizures.

5. Differential Diagnosis

Infantile spasms should be differentiated from a *benign myoclonus of early infancy*. Benign myoclonus of early infancy is recognized by (1) earlier age of onset (3 to $8\frac{1}{2}$ months), (2) a normal neurological examination and developmental maturation, (3) a normal EEG, (4) resolution of spasms by the age of 2 years, and (5) myoclonia with more cephalic involvement than extremities. Clinically, these infants exhibit episodes of tonic or myoclonic activities during wake and sleep or as a cluster similar to infantile spasms [18–20].

Benign neonatal sleep myoclonus (benign infantile nocturnal myoclonus) is a condition that consists of repeated episodes of rapid brief flexor contraction of the upper extremities. The following features are helpful for differentiation: (1) occurrence during sleep, (2) a normal EEG, (3) normal neurological examination, (4) age of onset in the first week of life, and (5) improvement within a few months. They may be repetitious and mimic myoclonic epilepsy. These are sudden involuntary brief lightning-like movements of one or more extremity. It may happen singly or four or five in a series. Etiology of this condition is not known. No treatment is needed and this should be differentiated from benign myoclonus of early infancy. In benign myoclonus of early infancy, the age of onset is after 3 months and myoclonus is not limited to sleep time [21].

Infantile spasms should also be differentiated from benign myoclonic epilepsy, myoclonic–astatic epilepsy, and early myoclonic encephalopathy. In atypical form, when the age of onset is after the age of 1 year, infantile spasms should be differentiated from Lennox–Gastaut syndrome.

According to Jeavons, the absence of psychomotor retardation or atypical age of onset does not exclude the diagnosis of West syndrome. However, if at least two EEGs are normal, including a sleep recording, an infant in whom the onset of spasm was later than 3 months, West syndrome is excluded [17]. The absence of hypsarrhythmia is not an exclusion criterion, as it is not always present in West syndrome in routine EEGs. Spasms may not be present initially, but their occurrence is sometimes essential.

6. EEG of Infantile Spasms

The electroencephalographic pattern of hypsarrhythmia was first described by Gibbs and Gibbs [22]. The electroencephalogram consists of a chaotic pattern of diffuse high-voltage slow activities intermixed with multifocal spike discharges. In typical cases, there is a significant interhemispheric asynchrony. Hypsarrhythmia is usually seen in the earlier stages of the disease. This EEG finding becomes very prominent during quiet sleep [non-rapid eye movement (REM) sleep]. During the myoclonic seizures, the EEG consists of high-voltage, slow-wave transients followed by attenuation (sudden depression of amplitude) of background rhythm.

Occasionally, ictal patterns are associated with sudden attenuation of background rhythm on the EEG. Clinically, spasms may precede the appearance of hypsarrhythmia, or hypsarrhythmia may precede infantile spasms [16].

A hypsarrhythmic pattern is seen in 66% of infants with West syndrome. In some cases, the EEG pattern of hypsarrhythmia may be seen only during sleep. Some patients may show suppression and burst activity on their EEG before the age of 4 months. Another common pattern is high-voltage irregular slow rhythms, with or without spikes, followed by a period of flattening of activity for several seconds. The EEG during an attack may also show high-amplitude spikes and slow waves with or without attenuation of background rhythm. A similar pattern is seen during sleep without clinical seizures. Disturbance of the sleep organization in patients with infantile spasms has been documented by prolonged overnight recordings. Reduction of REM stage sleep and reduction of total sleep time has been reported. Dysfunction of the brainstem has been postulated as the cause for sleep disturbance in patients with infantile spasms [23]. There is no increase in total sleep time in those who received hormone therapy, whether or not it was successful. However, an increase in the REM time is seen during therapy. A hypsarrhythmia pattern may disappear at times, particularly during REM sleep.

7. Etiology

Infantile spasms occur in a wide variety of disorders, some of which are genetically determined [17]. Two main groups, idiopathic (cryptogenic) and symptomatic (secondary to another disease process), are recognized. Earlier studies indicated 40% of cases as being cryptogenic. Recent studies suggest that only 9 to 14% of cases are cryptogenic [24,25]. Sixty percent of cases are considered to be symptomatic. The inciting events of infantile spasms may date back to prenatal, perinatal, and postnatal events.

Twenty-six percent of the symptomatic group are secondary to a prenatal disorder. Examples are: intrauterine infection (e.g., toxoplasmosis, herpes, syphilis, and cytomegalovirus) [12,26,27], chromosomal abnormalities, and genetic disorders. Among chromosome abnormalities are Down syndrome, and of genetic disorders, tuberous sclerosis, phenylketonuria (PKU), vitamin B_6 dependency, and urea cycle disorders have been reported with infantile spasms [12,28–31].

The most common reported perinatal factors are trauma during delivery, intrapartum asphyxia, prematurity with intraventricular hemorrhage, and sepsis. Of postnatally occurring diseases, infections are considered the most important causes of infantile spasms [12]. Every attempt should be made to identify the etiology. It may help to treat the underlying causes, make the prognosis clear, and help in providing genetic counseling.

The relationship of *pertussis immunization* to the onset of infantile spasms is controversial [32,33] and has generated the most concern. Several investigators believe that the relationship is a time coincidence between the age at which immunizations are given and the age that infantile spasms occur [34–36]. Due to the remote possibility that there is an unproven relationship, it is recommended that pertussis immunization be deferred in children with a history of convulsions and progressive central nervous system dysfunction [37]. In one study when the age of vaccination was changed, the distribution of infantile spasms remained unchanged [38,39]. In another study that compared two groups of children, one that received Diphtheria-Pertussis-Tetanus (DPT) and the other that received Diphtheria-Tetanus (DT), no differences in the occurrence of infantile spasms was noted. Bellman believes that pertussis immunization is not a risk factor for development of infantile spasms in normal children, but the presence of a pre-existing neurological disorder may be an important risk factor for precipitation of infantile spasms after immunization [40].

The British National Childhood Encephalopathy study has not revealed a significant association between infantile spasms and pertussis immunization [40]. The present evidence indicates that the relationship between infantile spasms and DPT immunization is coincidental [39].

Infantile spasms are associated with a diverse range of pathological findings affecting the cortical and brainstem regions. Present neuroimaging techniques [magnetic resonance imaging (MRI), computerized tomography (CT), sonography, etc.] are not always sensitive enough to detect developmental anomalies of the cortical region, minor gyral malformation, or defective cortical migration [12,41]. The most common abnormalities are cerebral atrophy and congenital malformation [42,43]. Seventy percent of children with infantile spasms have an abnormal CT scan, including cerebral atrophy, hydrocephalus, or other focal or generalized abnormalities [12,42–44].

Sleep alterations and EEG changes in children with infantile spasms are believed to be secondary to a brainstem dysfunction. It is postulated that both disorders are caused by dysfunction of a neurotransmitter system. This disorder may be secondary to failure, delayed formation, or later destruction of a neurotransmitter system [45]. An immunologic defect has also been considered as a possible underlying pathophysiology [46].

In general, treatment of infantile spasms is difficult. Only the benzodiazepines, valproic acid, adrenocorticotrophic hormone (ACTH), and corticosteriods have been found efficacious [12,47].

8. Conventional Anticonvulsant Therapy

a. Benzodiazepines. Three major benzodiazepines used in treatment of infantile spasms are (1) clonazepam, (2) nitrazepam, and (3) diazepam. Varying degrees of effectiveness is reported [16,48–51]. The dose for clonazepam is 0.2 mg/kg per day in three divided doses. Clonazepam has been used with good response in approximately 20% of the patients [49]. The diazepam dose is 0.3 mg/kg per day in two doses. The nitrazepam* dose is 0.5 to 1 mg/kg per day in two to three divided doses. Nitrazepam has resulted in a 50% satisfactory response rate [53]. Benzodiazepines are, in general, less effective than steroids [47]. In Hrachovy's study, patients who failed to respond to both ACTH and prednisone remained refractory to clonazepam.

b. Valproic Acid. The recommended dose of valproic acid is 15 to 20 mg/kg per day at the onset of treatment that could be increased gradually to 60 mg/kg per day. In a double blind, randomized, controlled, crossover study, a beneficial effect was noted when valproic acid was given to infants with infantile spasms who failed to respond to ACTH and/or prednisone. Another study has shown a high degree of efficacy of valproic acid alone or in combination with ACTH [54,55]. The possibility of hepatic toxicity, particularly in infants, has to be taken into consideration. Valproic acid has been effective in 40 to 66% of cases [54,56,57]. There is no evidence that the combination of benzodiazepines or valproic acid increases the effectiveness of either treatment [16].

Pyridoxine has been used in the treatment of infantile spasms, but no conclusion can be drawn from the literature [39].

c. Hormonal Therapy. In the late 1950s, Sorel and Dusaucy-Bauloye reported the effectiveness of low-dose, short-duration ACTH therapy in infantile spasms. Later, oral corticosteriod treatment was also found to be effective [58]. The duration and dosage are varied by different investigators; long-acting ACTH as low as 10 IU/day and as high as 180 units has been used [59,60]. Duration of therapy as short as 3 weeks or as long as 10 months have been recommended [16]. Several studies concluded that steroids are as effective as ACTH, but many investigators suggest starting treatment with ACTH and using steroids in case of a relapse, ineffectiveness of ACTH, or when daily injection is not practical.

The mode of action of ACTH in controlling infantile spasms is not known. A direct stimulating effect on the adrenal glands and function as a neurotransmitter with a direct effect on the central nervous system has been hypothesized [41,61].

Present information suggests that the most effective therapy is hormonal therapy and that patients who are going to respond do so within the first 2 weeks of this treatment. Clinical response is usually seen within 1 week. If spasms continue to be observed after 2 weeks and the EEG continues to show a hypsarrhythmic pattern, it is recommended the duration of treatment be extended to a full 6-week course [58]. If the patient fails to respond to the 6-week therapy,

---

*Nitrazepam is not approved by the Food and Drug Administration for use in the United States, despite one study demonstrating its efficacy [52].Nitrazepam can be obtained through Hoffmann–LaRoche Co., but its use requires an investigational new drug (IND) number from the Food and Drug Administration (FDA).

treatment could be changed from ACTH to prednisone. Numerous studies have shown the effectiveness of ACTH and corticosteriods in cessation or amelioration of infantile spasms. Sixty to 70% of cases of infantile spasms are controlled, and 20% will show improvement. Cryptogenic spasms are more often improved with ACTH therapy than are symptomatic ones. The relapse rate is about 30% [41]. A British study has shown that infants whose spasms have stopped within 1 month after therapy had a better prognosis than those with spasms continuing for longer periods [16].

Optimal dose, duration of therapy, and the relationship of response to lag time between the appearance of the spasms and initiation of treatment has been the subject of different studies with varying conclusions. Some investigators believe that the response to hormonal therapy is all or none: complete control or no control [47,62–64]. Hrachovy et al. [62,65] have shown the same degree of effectiveness when ACTH gel 20 units/day was compared with prednisone 2 mg/kg per day. They did not find major differences in the effectiveness of ACTH and prednisone in improving the EEG findings. The overall response of the patients to either ACTH or prednisone was 67%. There were patients who failed to respond to ACTH but responded to prednisone during a crossover, and vice versa. In this study, 31% of the patients who responded to either drug relapsed between 12 and 33 months, but 80% of the relapsed group responded to the second course of therapy. Delayed initiation of treatment had no effect in response to treatment.

A recent report by Snead et al. reveals that a treatment regimen with a high dose of ACTH 150 IU/m^2 of body surface area daily for 1 week was enough to control the spasms in 14 of 15 children (93%) and normalize their EEGs. They showed that plasma cortisol rose rapidly within 1 h of ACTH administration and continued at a slower rise for 12 to 24 h. They concluded that a sustained plateau of cortisol may be more effective in controlling infantile spasms than the pulse effect expected with oral steroid or lower doses of ACTH. Seizure control was achieved in 93% of patients, and one-third of the controlled patients relapsed [62]. They recommend the following regimen: (1) ACTH gel 150 IU/m^2 per day, divided into two doses, for the first week; (2) 75 IU/m^2 per day as a single daily dose for the second week; (3) 75 IU/m^2 per day every other day for 2 more weeks. After the fourth week of therapy, ACTH is tapered and discontinued over a period of 8 weeks.

We, however, recommend the low dose reported by Hrachovy [62]. Both regimens are outlined in Table 2. It is not clear if ACTH is more effective than corticosteriods [32,58]. Corticosteriod therapy is recommended for patients in whom IM injection of ACTH is not practical. The recommended dose for prednisone is 2 to 3 mg/kg per day. Duration of therapy is similar to ACTH. Response to treatment is generally a complete cessation of spasm and improvement in the EEG.

Table 2 Two Different Treatment Regimens with ACTH for Infantile Spasms

(A) First week	150 units/m^2 per day IM in two divided doses
Second week	75 units/m^2 per day IM once daily
Third and fourth weeks	75 units/m^2 per day IM every other day
Final 8 weeks	Taper
(B) First and second weeks	20 units ACTH gel/day IM
	If patient responds to treatment, the dosage is tapered and the drug is discontinued over a 1-week period
	If no response to therapy, increase ACTH gel to 30 units/day IM
Additional 4 weeks	ACTH gel 30 units IM/day
Seventh and eighth weeks	Taper and discontinue ACTH

Source: (A) Modified from Ref. 63; (B) modified from Ref. 62.

Side effects of hormonal therapy: The side effects of corticotropin and steroids are frequent, occurring in 37% of patients [66]. Arterial hypertension is reported in one-third of patients [47]. Episodic irritability, crying spells, electrolyte imbalance, suppression of the immune system, excessive weight gain, GI bleeding, intracranial hemorrhage, and cataracts are among the potential side effects of hormonal therapy [67,68]. Hypokalemia has been reported in 12% of patients [60]. Cushingoid appearance, hirsutism, irritability, and sleep disturbance are transient and disappear after discontinuation of therapy. Cerebral shrinkage, manifested by dilatation of the ventricles and large subarachnoid space, is seen on the CT scan of infants treated with ACTH or corticosteriods [69,70]. Hypertrophic cardiomyopathy is a potentially fatal complication of ACTH therapy [71]. With prolonged ACTH therapy, suppression of function in the hypothalamic–pituitary–adrenal axis has been reported [72]. ACTH should not be stopped abruptly; the patient should be provided with appropriate cortisol substitution and/or [73] ACTH should be tapered slowly [74].

9. Prognosis

Approximately half of the children with infantile spasms will have cessation of clinical spasms and disappearance of hypsarrhythmia on their EEG by the age of 3 years [12]. However, 65% experience other types of seizures [58]. Eighty-five percent of children with infantile spasms show some degree of mental and developmental retardation. Prognosis for future psychointellectual development is poor in the symptomatic group and is probably related to the underlying disease. One study reports 10% of the symptomatic group and 44% of the cryptogenic group are normal at a 6-year follow-up. Two reports suggest that the earlier the onset of treatment, the better the outcome, but these studies are retrospective and poorly controlled [25,75]. Hrachovy et al. have shown in their patients that delayed initiation of treatment had no effect on response [62].

It seems that the determining factor for patients' future neurointellectual development is in the underlying pathological process. Mental retardation is observed in 71 to 85% of all patients, and 55 to 60% of patients will develop other types of seizures. Thirty to 50% of children demonstrate clinical signs of cerebral palsy [16]. Some investigators have found a similar outcome in both treated and untreated patients [39]. Hrachovy reports the overall prognosis is poor, with only 5% of the total population having normal outcomes. Response to hormonal therapy does not affect the long-term outcome, and delayed treatment also has had no effect. Thirty-eight percent of the cryptogenic group were normal, in contrast to 5% of the symptomatic patients.

Mortality of infantile spasms in recent years has been reduced from 20% (16) to 5% due to the availability of better general medical care [76]. Factors influencing a good prognosis include (1) idiopathic etiology, (2) normal development prior to spasms, (3) good response to ACTH therapy, (4) short interval from the beginning of the spasm to the onset of therapy, and (5) idiopathic group.

B. Lennox–Gastaut Syndrome

Lennox–Gastaut syndrome (LGS) is a seizure disorder of extreme severity with poorly understood pathogenesis. In the International Classification of Epilepsies and Epileptic Syndromes (ICE) 1989, the Lennox–Gastaut syndrome (LGS) is in the category of the generalized cryptogenic and/or symptomatic epilepsies. Karbowski [77] has reviewed historical aspects of this syndrome and given convincing evidence that Tissot, a famous Swiss physician, in his description of symptomatic epilepsies in 1770, has referred to a disorder resembling what presently is known under the eponym of Lennox–Gastaut syndrome. Several monographs in the nineteenth century refer to intractable childhood seizures with mental retardation and myoclonic jerks. In 1939, Gibbs discovered an electroencephalographic pattern of slow spikes and waves but considered it a variant of petit mal [78]. William Lennox, in 1950, gave an accurate description of this syndrome and its EEG correlate. Later, Gastaut reviewed a large number of patients with this condition and characterized different aspects of this intractable form of epilepsy and proposed the name *Lennox syndrome* [79]. Gastaut described the triad of frequent tonic seizures and absences with pronounced mental retardation and an interictal EEG of slow spike–wave discharges. This triad has remained the core diagnostic feature of this syndrome and will be discussed in detail. The various clinical manifestations have been termed akinetic seizures, astatic seizures, astatic–myoclonic petit mal, and myokinetic epilepsy with drop attacks [80]. Gastaut believes that the myoclonic component represents the least frequent phenomenon in this syndrome [81].

The Lennox–Gastaut syndrome is reported in adulthood [82], with similar clinical features except for the age of onset. Bauer [82] found 72 cases out of 1251 patients with epilepsy. This adult group of Lennox–Gastaut syndrome is divided into those who have had the onset of their seizures below the age of 6 years but continued to have typical Lennox–Gastaut syndrome after the age of 18 years. The second group had started their seizures after 6 years of age but continued with typical features of the Lennox–Gastaut syndrome. In the third group, patients who had started with generalized primary epilepsy with absence and tonic–clonic seizures deteriorated to Lennox–Gastaut syndrome.

Lennox–Gastaut syndrome has a prevalence of 6.2% of all epilepsies and 10.3% of epilepsies in children [81]. In general, the age of onset is after the age of 1 or 2 years and before that of 7 years. Giovanari Rossi, in a study of epileptic children from 3 months to 18 years, found that 13.7% had myoclonic epilepsy and reports that 6.5% of all their epileptic patients had Lennox–Gastaut syndrome [80]. In this study, 21% of the cases, the most frequent type, were epilepsy with myoclonic absences. Cryptogenic intermediate myoclonic epilepsy of childhood constitutes 16.2% of cases. In Rossi's study, 12.9% of the cases were unclassified.

1. Clinical Presentation of Lennox–Gastaut Syndrome

Tonic seizures that consist of sustained contraction of muscle group and atypical absences are the most common type of seizure in this syndrome. However, tonic–clonic, clonic, unilateral, and partial seizures may also occur. A fall often occurs with the seizure. Patients may have a massive myoclonus. There is disagreement as to the homogenicity or heterogenicity of the syndrome and as to the exact limits of the syndrome. At times, myoclonic seizures become the most prominent feature of Lennox–Gastaut syndrome (LGS); some investigators believe that this should be distinguished as a subgroup of Lennox–Gastaut syndrome which may carry a better prognosis. This syndrome is not well delineated, and the development of both clinical and electroencephalographic criteria is needed. There may be a continuum of cases as described by Aicardi in 1986 [83]. In Aicardi's series of 40 cases of Lennox–Gastaut syndrome as defined by Gastaut's triad, 100% of them had tonic seizures, 50% atonic, 27.5% myoclonic, and 60% of atypical absence seizures [84]. Chevrie and Aicardi (1972) report 9 to 15% of the myoclonic epilepsies of childhood are considered to be a variant of Lennox–Gastaut syndrome [85,86]. Tonic seizures of Lennox–Gastaut syndrome are frequently nocturnal. Many other types of attacks are observed in a smaller number of patients.

Status epilepticus is observed in 72.4% of patients with Lennox–Gastaut syndrome when they are followed for several years. Beaumanoir et al. [87] distinguished five types of status epilepticus in patients with Lennox–Gastaut syndrome. Confusional or subconfusional state is present in all five types. Clinically, seizures may be myoclonic, tonic, atonic, or a combination of each of these types of seizures. Duration of different types of seizures were extremely variable. In 33% of their patients, the first status epilepticus constituted the first epileptic sign. Fifty percent of this group have had a previous history of infantile spasms. Nocturnal sleep studies in patients with Lennox–Gastaut syndrome by Baldy-Moulinier [88] have shown that the majority of patients with Lennox–Gastaut syndrome have a tonic seizure during their sleep.

The violent falls often cause head and facial injuries. Due to the brief duration of seizures, loss of consciousness may go undetected. Atonic attacks lead to drop attacks. A fall can be caused by myoclonic jerks preceding the tonic seizure or atonic attacks [89,90]. Ikeno [91] believes that purely atonic types are rare in contrast to tonic types as a cause of drop attacks.

Drop attacks are also seen in other types of epilepsies, such as primary generalized myoclonic–astatic epilepsy, atypical benign partial epilepsy of childhood, and myoclonic epilepsy of childhood. Violent falls are also caused by myoclonic jerks or atonia. Focal EEG abnormality, slowing of the background rhythm, mental retardation, developmental delay, and age of onset of seizures are helpful to differentiate these conditions. Other disorders associated with drop attacks should also be considered: narcolepsy–cataplexy syndrome, breath-holding spells, syncope, pallid syncope, orthostatic collapse, prolonged QT syndrome, arterioventricular block, sick-sinus syndrome, progressive familial left bundle branch block, congenital aortic stenosis, obstructive cardiomyopathy, and congenitally corrected transposition of the great vessels [92]. Nonepileptic drop attacks can usually be distinguished from epileptic falls by a careful history taking and simultaneous EEG-video recording with special electrode placement.

The boundaries between Lennox–Gastaut syndrome and West syndrome are vague. Thirty percent of symptomatic cases of infantile spasms turn into Lennnox-Gastaut syndrome. On the other hand, 20% of patients with Lennox–Gastaut syndrome evolve from infantile spasms [93].

Some intermediate and unclassified epileptic syndromes are recognized which could be considered subsets of Lennox–Gastaut syndrome. *Myoclonic variant* LGS is characterized by an onset around 4 years of age and frequent myoclonic seizures. According to Aicardi, this subtype has a better prognosis and mental retardation is less frequent. The majority of cases are cryptogenic. A variant of *intermediate petit mal* is considered an intermediate category between absence epilepsy (petit mal) and Lennox–Gastaut syndrome. This form fulfilled all clinical and electroencephalographic properties of Lennox–Gastaut syndrome in addition to frequent absences with 3 Hz, often irregular spike slow wave, and sensitivity to hyperventilation. It does not carry a specific prognosis. *Epilepsy with myoclonic-astatic seizures* was initially presented and discussed by Doose in 1964. These children have a positive family history for epilepsy and may be associated with absences. The age of onset is also between 6 months and

6 years. Several authors believe that this syndrome includes different forms of infantile myoclonic epilepsy [80].

2. EEG Findings in Lennox–Gastaut Syndrome

Clinically, tonic seizures last from 5 to 20 s and are associated with clouding of consciousness. Typically, the EEG starts with a slow wave or slow spike followed by a very brief desynchronization of the background recording and the presence of low-voltage fast (18 to 25 Hz) activity or spikes and slow waves. This episode usually terminates with high-voltage slow activities [94]. Respiratory changes, apnea, or irregular noisy respiration are frequently seen during tonic seizures, representing autonomic alteration.

Abundance of spike and slow waves on the EEG has no correlation with mental retardation or prognostic value for seizure control. Hyperventilation usually does not activate these discharges. During a deeper stage of sleep, spike discharges may change to polyspikes, at times interrupted with a burst of 10- to 20-Hz fast frequency. The ictal EEG may manifest with sudden attenuation of background rhythm and the appearance of fast rhythmic activities in the beta range. Myoclonic seizures are associated with high-voltage spike or polyspikes and wave activity. Atonic seizures may present with brief bisynchronous frontal fast activities. Atypical absences are manifested by continuous slow spike–wave discharges.

There is experimental evidence which suggests that spikes and slow waves in Lennox–Gastaut syndrome are caused by an abnormal interaction of thalmocortical afferent volleys to the injured cortex [95,96]. Tonic seizures, myoclonic attacks, and their EEG findings may represent cortical dysfunction activated by the brainstem reticular formation. The fact that tonic seizures are exacerbated during sleep, and occasionally by benzodiazepines, both influencing reticular formation function, support this view. At times, it is difficult to differentiate the sleep EEG of these patients from electrical status epilepticus [97]. But electrical status epilepticus of sleep does not have a slow-wave component or, at least, it is not as alternating as is seen in Lennox–Gastaut syndrome.

Whether the EEG of Lennox–Gastaut syndrome represents a primary generalized or rapid secondary bilateral synchrony from a frontal focus has remained unresolved. It has been shown that in addition to a symptomatic partial lesion, a constitutional epileptic predisposition also plays a role in secondary bilateral synchrony. Thirty-seven percent of patients with Lennox–Gastaut syndrome have a family history of seizures [98]. Gastaut specifies that simple transcallosal propagation to homologous contralateral hemisphere is not adequate to explain generalization in Lennox–Gastaut syndrome. Practical importance of this finding is in the surgical treatment of this condition with corpus callosotomy for intractable drop attacks. The slow spike–wave complexes may not be present on all tracings [99]. The paroxysmal EEG activity is generally increased during sleep.

3. Etiology

LGS has multiple etiologies; cryptogenetic and symptomatic forms exist. Most secondary cases are related to encephalopathies. Tuberous sclerosis is relatively common.

In a study of 127 subjects with Lennox–Gastaut syndrome, Ohtahara et al. [100] found that 22% were idiopathic with no underlying disorders, no neuroradiological abnormality, and normal psychomotor development prior to the onset of LGS. They found 67.9% of the idiopathic develop mental retardation over a 3-year follow-up. Another study of Lennox–Gastaut syndrome found that 67.5% of children were purely symptomatic. Of those, 20% were pre- and postnatal asphyxia or birth injury, 15% had a history of central nervous system (CNS) inflammatory disease, and 20% had a brain malformation or a neurometabolic disorder. In the symptomatic group, the epilepsy preceded typical EEG changes in 74% of patients. The onset of seizures prior to slow spike waves was mostly during infancy. They also found that the earlier the onset of slow spike–waves and clinical seizures, the worse the prognosis [101]. Fifty percent of the patients with Lennox–Gastaut syndrome have an abnormal CT scan of the head [84].

4. Differential Diagnoses

Lennox–Gastaut syndrome should be differentiated from the following: 1. Atypical benign partial epilepsy of childhood, lack of tonic seizures, and presence of focal seizures are helpful.

2. Continuous spike–wave activity during sleep (known as electrical status epilepticus of slow sleep). This EEG abnormality is not associated with seizures, particularly if there is no tonic seizure.

3. Traumatic partial epilepsy with bilateral slow spike–wave complexes. In this condition the seizures are usually partial complex in type.

4. Atypical absence epilepsy. The age of onset of LGS is lower than typical absence seizures. Abnormality of background of EEG, preexisting history of a brain dysfunction, and severe mental retardation are helpful in the differential diagnosis.

5. Epilepsy with myoclonic absences has an age of onset of 4 to 9 years, with positive family history, an abnormal EEG of 3-Hz spikes and slow waves, a mild degree of mental retardation, and behavior problems common.

6. Severe myoclonic epilepsies in infancy. History of febrile and nonfebrile convulsions is frequent and a high percentage have a family history of epilepsy. Tonic seizures are rare and they have photosensitivity on their EEGs.

7. Progressive degenerative brain disorders, associated clinical features of each disorder, and clinical course are helpful [84].

True myoclonic epilepsies generally are not associated with a tonic seizure, but they may have atonic attack. The Lennox–Gastaut syndrome has been seen in patients with well-defined focal lesions, suggesting secondary generalized epilepsy. History of complex partial seizures before the onset of Lennox–Gastaut syndrome and partial attacks following a prolonged period of typical Lennox–Gastaut syndrome are helpful [102, 103].

5. Treatment

The treatment of Lennox–Gastaut syndrome is frequently difficult, and seizures often become intractable. Benzodiazepines have been used in treatment of LGS with some success. Some patients show an initial response, but they may have a breakthrough in their seizure control. This phenomenon is thought to be secondary to a decrease in benzodiazepine receptors. Sometimes patients refractory to one benzodiazepine may respond to another. Alternate-day therapy with benzodiazepam has also been recommended [104]. Three commonly used benzodiazepines are the following:

1. *Clonazepam* has a recommended dose of 0.1 to 0.2 mg/kg per day. It should be started in a low dose and gradually increased over a period of 5 days to its final dose. Sedation is a limiting factor, especially at the onset of treatment.
2. *Nitrazepam* has been found to be effective in patients who have not responded to clonazepam. Recommended initial dose is 0.5 mg/kg per day, gradually increased to 1 mg/kg per day in two to three divided doses. Excessive sedation, drooling, and increased bronchial secretion are troublesome, especially in children with severe mental retardation and preexisting dysfunction of the upper airway. This drug is not approved for use by the Food and Drug Administration. Its use therefore requires an investigational new drug (IND) number. Hoffman–LaRoche Co. will supply this drug under those circumstances.
3. *Diazepam* with a dose of 0.3 mg/kg per day in two divided doses can also be used.

Antiepileptic drugs with a sedative effect should be avoided, as a number of seizures are increased in inactive and drowsy patients. Status epilepticus in patients with Lennox–Gastaut following IV diazepam has been reported [105,106].

Sodium valproate is probably the most effective antiepileptic drug for the treatment of Lennox–Gastaut syndrome. The effectiveness of valproate has been shown in many studies in patients with this and other generalized epilepsies. At times, it is used in combination with benzodiazepine. Effective dose of valproate is between 20 and 50 mg/kg per day. Treatment should start with 15 to 20 mg/kg per day in two divided doses. Measurement of trough drug level is indicated when the patient develops side effects or when doses much higher than the recommended therapeutic range are used. Blood levels should also be followed when the patient is on polytherapy.

Other anticonvulsant drugs have been found less effective and they may even increase the number of seizures. *Primidon*, *ethosuximide*, and *carbamazepine* have been used *in conjunction* with other anticonvulsants, especially when tonic–clonic seizures or complex partial seizures are complicating clinical features of this syndrome.

ACTH and steroids have been used in patients with Lennox–Gastaut syndrome on the same theoretical basis as their efficacy in infantile spasms. Yamatogi [107] reports that 50% of patients responded to treatment but that 50% of those patients relapsed within 6 months. Acetazolamide, in conjunction with other drugs, can sometimes be helpful. Limited information is available on effectiveness of investigational antiepileptic drugs with gabamimetic properties.

Ketogenic diets have been used successfully in some centers. The principle of this diet is to produce ketosis by a proportionately high intake of fat compared to both carbohydrates and proteins. Huttenlocher [108] introduced a modification of this diet by using medium-chain triglycerides (MCT) with higher ketogenic potential. MCT oil is more ketogenic than the standard ketogenic diet. As a result, only 50 to 70% of the total calories need to be supplied by this preparation. To ensure that the patient remains ketotic, urine needs to be tested for the presence of ketones. On this diet, 60% of the total caloric intake is provided by a MCT, and 30% of the caloric requirement is provided by protein and carbohydrates and the remaining 10% by unsaturated fatty acids. Patients need to be hospitalized for the early phase of treatment, as it requires starvation and frequent determination of blood glucose. The most common side effects are nausea, vomiting, abdominal cramps, and diarrhea. Drowsiness or insomnia has also been reported and the child needs careful monitoring during intercurrent infection and febrile illness. This diet should not be used simultaneously with acetazolamide or valproate.

Numerous reports have described the clinical efficacy of the ketogenic diet. Thirty to 54% of patients successfully respond to the ketogenic diet. Higher success rates are achieved in young children [109–111]. Myoclonic and astatic seizures respond better than partial seizures. The precise mechanism of action of the ketogenic diet is not known. It is postulated that ketone bodies have intrinsic anticonvulsant properties [112].

In the past, unpalatability of the diet and supplying most of the daily calories in the form of fats has limited use of this dietary regimen [13]. The introduction of MCT has improved tolerance of this diet. The effectiveness of this treatment is unpredictable [109]. Schwartz reported 25% improvement in children with drop attacks [114]. A ketogenic diet may change the level of anticonvulsant medication, causing side effects [113]. The plasma levels of β-hydroxybutyrate (BHB) and acetoacetate show a significant correlation with the anticonvulsant effect of the diet [108]. Cerebral capacity of neonates and infants to oxidize ketone bodies is five to four times higher than that of adults. It is believed that the effectiveness of the diet in younger patients is due to a higher ability of their brain to metabolize ketone bodies.

Unconventional drugs, such as thyrotrophin-releasing hormone (TRH) and ACTH, have been used. Immunoglobulin, tryptophan, and amantadine have been tried with varying degrees of success by some investigators [115–117]. Immunological therapy has been used based on a report of significant association between certain HLA subtypes and epilepsy. Lennox–Gastaut syndrome has been attributed to the HLA-A7 phenotype [118,119] The possible clinical benefit of immunoglobulins might be due to their immunosuppressive effect assuming an underlying autoimmune pathogenesis in the idiopathic Lennox–Gastaut syndrome. Oligoantigenic diet has not been effective [120].

6. Surgical Approach

Corpus callosotomy has been used in the treatment of patients with focal or lateralized epileptic abnormality with secondary generalization. There is usually cessation or significant reduction in severe drop attacks. Result of transection of corpus callosum in patients with Lennox–Gastaut syndrome is comparable with those of patients with secondary bilateral synchrony. The best outcome is seen in patients with hemispheric lesions and secondary bilateral synchrony in EEG.

7. Prognosis

The disability of the epileptic condition decreases in adulthood with the reduction of seizures. Some patients continue with the same, and others will develop a partial and complex partial type of seizure. The mild form may show some global improvement in psychosocial function. Anticonvulsant medication is needed to continue as their reduction may cause a recurrence and exacerbation of seizures. The electroencephalogram is not a reliable guide for termination of therapy.

Oller-Daurella and Oller [93] report on 368 cases of LGS, of which 163 have been followed for more than 5 years. In this study 26.4% of idiopathic and 15.4% of symptomatic Lennox–Gastaut syndrome achieved a symptom-free period of more than 5 years. They report that 17% of their patients had intellectual recovery, and most of these suffered from the idiopathic form of Lennox–Gastaut syndrome.

C. Benign Myoclonic Epilepsy in Infancy

Benign myoclonic epilepsy in infancy is characterized by bursts of generalized myoclonus occurring several times a day and starting between 6 months to 2 years of life. Limb movements are associated with an upward–outward movement of the upper extremities. Consciousness is not lost. A family history of convulsive disorder is frequent. The patient may develop a mild delay in intellectual development.

Some authors believe that this type of epilepsy may be the earliest expression of primary generalized epilepsy [121]. The EEG shows bursts of generalized spike–wave activities during the early stages of the disease. This electrographic abnormality may persist for several years.

This condition was described in 1981 by Dravet and is considered to be a rare form of epilepsy, comprising 2% of epilepsies in children less than 1 year of life [121,122]. At times, the clinical presentation is manifested by head nodding and later shows drop attacks; eye rolling is frequent. Occasional rhythmic jerking movements are seen lasting less than 10 s. The EEG shows spike waves or polyspike waves with a rate of 3 Hz. A history of simple febrile seizures is not unusual. Discharges are less frequent during deeper levels of sleep. The clinical examination is normal.

A condition similar to this syndrome has occasionally been reported in the literature under the name of infantile myoclonic epilepsy. Benign myoclonic epilepsy of infancy should be differentiated from (1) benign, nonepileptic myoclonus of infancy, which is associated with normal EEG and spontaneous recovery [18,121]; (2) infantile spasms by the EEG, lack of psychomotor regression, and later age of onset; (3) Lennox–Gastaut syndrome, differentiated by lack of tonic seizures and typical slow spike–wave discharges on their EEG; and (4) severe myoclonic epilepsy in infants, which as its name implies is manifested by myoclonic seizures preceded by severe repeated convulsive seizures and development is seriously disturbed after the child's second year.

Sodium valproate is the drug of choice. It causes normalization of the EEG and improvement in the clinical condition. Without treatment, the child will continue to have myoclonic seizures. Phenobarbital or benzodiazepines may aggravate both clinical and EEG disturbances [86,121]. Without treatment, the epilepsy may be accompanied by a relative slowing down of intellectual development. Benign myoclonic epilepsy is the only type of myoclonic epilepsy that starts early in life and has a benign prognosis. This is a rare type of myoclonic epilepsy.

D. Severe Myoclonic Epilepsy in Infants

The incidence of severe myoclonic epilepsy in infants is unknown. A high percentage have a family history of epilepsy or convulsions. Seizures begin during the first year of life. The average age of onset is 5 months, ranging from 2 to 10 months. There is no disturbance in consciousness unless seizures occur at very close intervals of a few seconds.

Initially, EEG recordings are normal. During the second year, paroxysmal abnormalities appear in the form of rapid, generalized spike–waves or polyspike–waves. Photosensitivity appears very early during the first year of life. Localized paroxysmal abnormalities are also seen. Seizures are extremely resistant to any kind of treatment. Epilepsy remains active, at times, up to the age of 11 or 12 years, then tends to occur at less frequent intervals. The myoclonic jerks may change into atypical absences. Intellectual retardation and severe language dysfunction are frequent.

The onset of seizures is associated with slight rise of temperature and interpreted as febrile convulsions. History of prolonged or unilateral seizures associated with fever and status epilepticus is frequently preset in those patients. Clinically, by the time that myoclonic seizures occur, the EEG shows spike/slow-wave activities. This condition should also be differentiated from benign myoclonic epilepsy and Lennox–Gastaut syndrome [123].

E. Early Myoclonic Encephalopathy

Early myoclonic encephalopathy was described by Aicardi [124,125] in infants with severe encephalopathy and burst suppression on the EEG. These infants do not have gross developmental or structural anomalies of the brain before the onset of seizures. This severe form of epilepsy consists of myoclonic jerks, partial motor seizures, and tonic spasms. The syndrome starts in neonatal life in children with severe neurological impairment, and there is a high mortality before the age of 6 months [26]. Undetermined metabolic defects are frequently suspected in these children. This condition is seen in nonketotic hyperglycinemia [126]. Children with this syndrome should have a complete metabolic workup. Organic acidemia or a severe structural brain defect may be found. The relationship of neonatal myoclonic encephalopathy with early infantile epileptic encephalopathy is not entirely clear.

F. Early Infantile Epileptic Encephalopathy

Early infantile epileptic encephalopathy was reported by Ohtahara et al. [127] as characterized by tonic spasms and a burst-suppression pattern on the EEG. Age of onset is in the neonatal period. This syndrome frequently evolves into infantile spasms at about 4 to 6 months of age [16]. Several workers do not consider early infantile epileptic encephalopathy as a separate entity from early myoclonic encephalopathy. Characteristics of early infantile epileptic encephalopathy are onset at early infancy, tonic spasms, burst suppression in EEG, severe psychomotor retardation, intractable seizures, poor prognosis, polyetiology, and evolution into the West syndrome [127]. In a study of 14 cases of early infantile epileptic encephalopathy by Ohtahara et al., three were idiopathic [100] Table 3.

G. Juvenile Myoclonic Epilepsy

Juvenile myoclonic epilepsy is also known as impulsive petit mal of Janz. This is a form of primary generalized epilepsy with age-related onset manifested by

Table 3 Underlying Pathologies in Patients with Three Types[a] of Age-Dependent Epileptic Encephalopathies Associated with Myoclonic Seizures

Category	EIEE	WS	LGS	
Cryptogenic	3	46	56	
Cryptogenic with mental defect		3	12	
Pathological mental defect		12	32	
Cerebral palsy with mental defect		60	66	
Cerebral palsy		4	8	
Post encephalitis		9	33	
Sequelae of the West syndrome			21	
Hydrocephalus		7	5	
Multiple anomalies		6	2	
Microcephaly or brain atrophy	6	5	3	
Others	5	29	27	
Total	14	181	265	cases

Source: Modified from Ref. 100.
[a]EIEE, Early-infantile epileptic encephalopathy with suppression burst; WS, west syndrome (infantile spasms); LGS, Lennox–Gastaut syndrome.

bilateral, singular, or repetitive myoclonic jerks involving predominantly the upper extremity, frequently with associated drop attacks. It is a well-defined epileptic syndrome with a frequency of 2.8 to 4.3% of all epileptic patients [3,128,129]. The upper extremities are more affected than are the lower extremities. When lower extremities are involved, myoclonic attacks are associated with a fall. At times, myoclonic jerks are frequent and consecutive and become myoclonic status epilepticus. Consciousness usually remains intact during the myoclonic seizures. Frequently, a family history of seizures is present. The patient may also have generalized tonic–clonic seizures. Myoclonic jerks occur, typically, shortly after awakening or at the end of the day [3, 128]. Sleep deprivation precipitates the attacks. Generalized tonic–clonic seizures occur in 85% of patients with this condition [6,130]. Myoclonic jerks precede generalized tonic–clonic seizures by months or years. Ten percent of patients have associated absence attacks.

The interictal EEG shows rapid generalized irregular spike–wave discharges. The ictal EEG shows generalized 18- to 20-Hz spikes followed by slow waves. The background rhythm of the EEG is normal and without focal abnormalities. Approximately 30 to 40% of patients have photoconvulsive response during photic stimulation [131].

The neurological and intellectual functions remain normal. The age of onset is between 12 and 18 years [3]. The terms *myoclonic epilepsy of adolescence, benign myoclonic juvenile epilepsy*, and *impulsive petit mal* have been used by different authors to describe this condition. There is no history of a progressive CNS disorder. Spontaneous recovery is rare, and seizures may recur several days after discontinuation of medication.

The neurodiagnostic workup is unrevealing. Genetic factors play a significant role. Various types of seizures are seen in 27.3% of relatives of patients with juvenile myoclonic epilepsy. Of them, 15% of affected relatives have myoclonic attacks, 17% awakening grand mal, and 14% absence seizures. Juvenile myoclonic epilepsy is considered in the category of primary generalized epilepsy of adolescence [3]. This syndrome represents 4% of persons with epilepsy (131).

Juvenile myoclonic epilepsy can be differentiated from epilepsy with generalized tonic–clonic seizures upon awakening by the presence of early morning myoclonic jerks in impulsive petit mal. Juvenile absence epilepsy may be associated with myoclonic seizures, but absence remains the predominant feature and myoclonic are very infrequent. However, they both may represent two variations of the same disorder. Juvenile myoclonic epilepsy should be differentiated from Lennox–Gastaut syndrome with myoclonic astatic seizures and myoclonic absence seizures by their age of onset and normal mental functions in juvenile myoclonic epilepsy. It should also be differentiated from nonepileptic progressive myoclonus, which is usually associated with dementia or cerebellar dysfunction and have poor prognosis. Their EEG findings are also different.

Sodium valproate remains the drug of choice for treatment of juvenile myoclonic epilepsy; it controls both myoclonic and tonic–clonic seizures in 75 to 85% of cases. Control of myoclonic jerks may be improved by regular sleep and reducing stress [132,133]. Prognosis is good with appropriate treatment.

Juvenile myoclonic epilepsy may become worse with the use of barbiturates and benzodiazepine.

H. Epilepsy with Myoclonic Absences

The onset of this epilepsy is around the age of 7 years, with male preponderance. The exact nosological place of this type of epilepsy is not known [3,134]. It may be a variant of absence seizures. Some believe that it is a distinct syndrome [135]. The outlook is less favorable than that of typical absence epilepsy but better than that for patients with myoclonias without absence [3]. Twenty percent of patients have associated tonic seizures and sometimes tonic–clonic convulsions. The ictal and interictal EEG resembles typical absence pattern. Prognosis is poor because of resistance to treatment and mental deterioration in some cases [136]. Valproate, ethosuximide, and benzodiazepines such as clonazepam are the recommended antiepileptic drugs.

I. Epilepsy with Myoclonic–Astatic Seizures

This type of epilepsy starts during the first 5 years in 94% of patients and in 24% during the first year of life [137], mostly 2 to 5 years. Boys are affected twice as much as girls. Myoclonic seizures consist of symmetrical violent jerks of the arms and shoulders. Astatic seizures are associated with abrupt loss of muscle tonus. Mild astatic attacks may appear as brief head nodding or slight knee bending. Myoclonic astatic seizures are a combination of myoclonic jerks and atonic attacks. Development of the child is usually normal.

Interictal EEG shows monomorphic theta rhythms with partial attenuation. The EEG is usually normal at the onset of this epilepsy. Theta rhythms may be preceded or followed by spike–wave paroxysmal discharges. During a seizure, the EEG shows continuous 2- to 3-Hz spikes and waves. During sleep, spikes and waves are regularly activated.

Sudden loss of tone is preceded by symmetrical myoclonia of the arms. Brief loss of consciousness is seen during absence attacks. Slurring of speech and drooling is frequent. Febrile and afebrile grand mal attacks are seen in two-thirds of the patients. Tonic seizures and focal seizures are not infrequent.

The course of this epilepsy is variable and the patient's seizures later become predominantly absence type. A small group of patients continue with myoclonic and/or astatic seizures and occasional major motor convulsions. Fifty percent of patients will have developmental and intellectual retardation.

It is also called the *centrencephalic myoclonic–astatic epilepsy of early childhood* with a high incidence of possible family history for epilepsy. Some authorities believe that this is a variant of Lennox–Gastaut syndrome. This form of epilepsy was initially described by Doose in 1964. It has several features of Lennox–Gastaut syndrome. Age of onset is similar between 6 months and 6 years. Myoclonic–astatic epilepsy is differentiated from Lennox–Gastaut syndrome by (1) genetic predisposition, (2) normal development before the onset of seizures, (3) relatively good prognosis, and (4) absence of neurological deficit and generalized discharges manifested by irregular spike waves, theta rhythm, and photosensitivity without focal abnormality on EEG. Doose has discussed the great variability of the clinical and EEG manifestation of this disease [137].

Valproate with or without ethosuximide may completely control seizures. This condition should be differentiated from infantile spasms and Lennox–Gastaut syndrome [138].

J. Progressive Myoclonic Epilepsies

Progressive myoclonus epilepsies must be differentiated from the primary type of myoclonic epilepsy: The diagnosis rests on the presence of mental deterioration, the occurrence of other types of myoclonus, particularly erratic and intension myoclonus, the EEG findings, and clinical presentation [139]. The most common types of progressive myoclonic epilepsies include Lafora disease, Unverricht–Landborg disease, sialidosis, neuronal ceroid-lipofuscinosis, and mitochondrial encephalopathy. Myoclonus may occur as part of generalized diseases of the cerebral gray matter, which include lipid storage disease, subacute sclerosing panencephalitis (SSPE), Creutzfelt–Jakob disease, and progressive poliodystrophy (Alper disease).

1. *Lafora disease* is an autosomal recessive disorder that manifests between the age of 11 and 18 years, with a multiple type of seizure, myoclonus and rapid development of dementia, periodic agitation, and loss of language. The clinical picture of deterioration is completed within 2 years. The diagnosis can be made by examination of a skin biopsy. Lafora bodies can be seen by light microscopic in the eccrine sweat gland duct cells [140]. Lafora bodies are seen in substantia nigra, dentate nucleus, superior olive, pontine, and thalamic nuclei. Cerebellar and cerebral cortex are also involved [141]. The electroencephalogram shows diffuse slowing and disorganization of the background rhythm. Bilaterally symmetric spikes and polyspikes or spikes and slow waves are also seen on the EEG.

2. *Unverricht–Landborg disease* is an autosomal recessive disease resembling Baltic myoclonus. The age of onset is between 8 and 13 years and it is manifested by prominent myoclonic jerks and tonic–clonic seizures. Ataxia and mental retardation is frequently seen at the beginning of illness and gradually becomes worse. It can be differentiated from Lafora type of PME by the absence of inclusion bodies on skin biopsy. In Unverricht–Landborg disease the patient has stimulus sensitive myoclonic jerks and grand mal seizures. The patient's early developmental maturation is normal; then clumsiness, drop attacks, and myoclonic jerks complicate the clinical picture. Neuroimaging studies are normal. Phenobarbital can suppress myoclonic jerks; sodium valproate and clonazepam both in high doses have been recommended for treatment of seizures in this condition. There is a very slow decline in intellectual functions and emotional stability. The electroencephalogram shows generalized spike–wave activities with gradual disorganization of background rhythm over a period of years. Photoparoxysmal response and photoconvulsion are noted following prolonged photic stimulation.

3. *Sialidosis* is a lysosomal storage disorder: Two clinically recognizable types are reported. Type I has its onset in adolescence with myoclonus and gradual visual loss. Tonic–clonic seizures, ataxia, and cataract and peripheral neuropathy are major clinical symptoms. Type II is associated with myoclonus, tonic–clonic seizures, coarse facies, and dysostosis multiplex. Hearing loss and mental impairment are evident from early life. The diagnosis rests on biochemical studies and enzyme assay in fresh fibroblasts or other tissues.

4. *Ceroid-lipofuscinosis (Batten disease)* is characterized by retinal degeneration, dementia, seizure, and myoclonus. The condition is inherited as an autosomal recessive disease. Infantile, late infantile, juvenile, and adult forms are reported; all are associated with varying degrees of seizure frequencies. The infantile form is thought to present during the age of 8 and 18 months with regression of motor milestones, hypotonia, ataxia, dementia, and impaired vision.

Diagnosis rests on the clinical presentation, retinal changes, and demonstration of inclusions on skin biopsy by electron microscope.

5. *Mitochondrial myopathy*, with "ragged red" muscle fibers, is associated with intellectual retardation, generalized motor seizures, progressive ataxia, and myoclonus. The diagnosis rests on the demonstration of typical histological changes in muscles.

Treatment

Valproic acid, and benzodiazepines such as clonazepam, are effective for the symptomatic treatment of the myoclonus seen in these conditions. The use of antiepileptic drugs that can produce ataxia should be avoided [140]. In progressive myoclonic epilepsy, myoclonus is a part of a progressive neurological disease and not a part of the primary epileptic symptomatology. There is no medication that satisfactorily inhibits the progression of these disorders. Valproic acid is effective in ameliorating seizures and also has antimyoclonic action. The myoclonic seizures are well controlled by valproate, which elevates the cortical level of inhibitory neurotransmitter γ-aminobutyric acid (GABA). However, the anticonvulsant effect of valproate is not absolutely dependent on cerebral GABA elevation. Benzodiazepines and barbiturates also interact with GABA-receptor complex and augment the inhibitory action of GABA [142].

REFERENCES

1. Hallett M. Early history of myoclonus. In: Advances in neurology. Vol. 43. Myoclonus. Fahn S, Marsden CD, Van Woert MH, eds. New York: Raven Press, 1986.
2. Menkes JH. Paroxysmal disorders. In: Menkes JH, ed. Textbook of neurology. Philadelphia: Lea & Febiger, 1985:608–76.
3. Aicardi J. Myoclonic epilepsies of late childhood and adolescence. In: Aicardi J, ed. Epilepsy in childhood. New York: Raven Press, 1986:66–72.
4. Aicardi J. Myoclonic epilepsies of infancy and childhood. In: Fahn S, Marsden CD, Van Woert MH, eds. Advances in Neurology. Vol. 43. Myoclonus. New York: Raven Press, 1986:11–31.
5. Shibasaki H, Yamashita Y, Tobimatus S, Neshige R. Electroencephalographic correlates of myoclonus. In: Fahn S, Marsden CD, Van Woert MH, eds. Advances in neurology. Vol. 43. Myoclonus. New York: Raven Press, 1986 357–72.
6. Dreifuss FE. Myoclonic seizures. In: Dreifuss, FE, ed. Pediatric epileptology. Boston: John Wright/PSG, Inc., 1983:109–19.
7. Naito H, Oyanagi S. Familial myoclonus epilepsy and choreoathetosis: hereditary dentatorubral–pallidoluysian atrophy. Neurology 1982; 32:798–807.
8. Lance J. Action myoclonus, Ramsay–Hunt syndrome, and other cerebellar myoclonic syndromes. In: Fahn S, Marsden CD, Van Woert MH, eds. Advances in neurology. Vol. 43. Myoclonus. New York: Raven Press, 1982:33–56.

8a. Marsden CD, Hallett M, and Fahn S. The nosology and pathophysiology of myoclonus. In: Marsden CD, Fahn S, eds. Movement disorders. London: Butterworth Scientific, 1982:196–248.
9. West WJ. On a peculiar form of infantile convulsions. Lancet 1841; 1:724.
10. Nelson K. Discussion in Alter. The epidemiology of epilepsy: a workshop. National Institute of Neurological Disorders and Stroke monograph. Vol. 14. Washington, DC: US Government Printing Office, 1972.
11. Riikonen R, Donner M. Incidence and aetiology of infantile spasms from 1960 to 1976. A population study in Finland. Dev Med Child Neurol 1979; 21:333–43.
12. Lacy JR, Penry JK Infantile spasms. New York: Raven Press, 1976.
13. Fleiszar KA, Daniel WL, Imrey PB. Genetic study of infantile spasms with hypsarrhythmia. Epilepsia 1977; 18:55–62.
14. Dreifuss FE. Infantile spasms. In: Dreifuss FE, ed. Pediatric epileptology. Boston: John Wright/PSG, Inc., 1983:97–108.
15. Millichap JG, Bickford RG, Miller RH, Backus RE. Infantile spasms, hypsarrhythmia and mental retardation: a study of etiologic factors in 61 patients. Epilepsia 1962; 3:188–97.
16. Aicardi J. Infantile spasms and related syndromes. In: Aicardi J, ed. Epilepsy in childhood. New York: Raven Press, 1986:17–38.
17. Jeavons PM. West syndrome: infantile spasms. In: Dravet C, Bureau M, Dreifuss FE, Wolf P, Roger J, eds. John Libbey Eurotext Ltd., 1985:42–50.
18. Lombroso CT, Fejerman N. Benign myoclonus of early infancy. Ann Neurol 1977; 1:138–43.
19. Coulter DL, Allen RJ. Benign neonatal sleep myoclonus. Arch Neurol 1982; 39:191.
20. Dooley JM, Killam IW. Myoclonus in children. Arch Neurol 1984; 41:138.
21. Blennow G. Benign infantile myoclonus. Acta Paediatr Scand 1985; 74:505–7.
22. Gibbs FA, Gibbs EL. Atlas of electroencephalography. Epilepsy. Vol. 2. Reading, MA: Addison-Wesley Publishing Co., Inc., 1952.
23. Hrachovy RA, Frost JD Jr, Kellaway P. Sleep characteristics in infantile spasms. Neurology 1981; 31:688–94.
24. Riikonen RA. A long-term follow-up study of 214 children with the syndrome of infantile spasms. Neuropediatrie 1982; 13:14–23.
25. Matsumoto A, Watanabe K, Negoto T, et al. Long-term prognosis after infantile spasms: statistical study of prognostic factors in 200 cases. Dev Med Child Neurol 1981; 23:51–65.
26. Crichton JV. Infantile spasms in children of low birth weight. Dev Med Child Neurol 1979; 10:36.
27. Feldman RA, Schwartz JF. Possible association between cytomegalovirus infection and infantile spasms. Lancet 1968; 1:180.
28. Roth JC, Epstein CJ. Infantile spasms and hypopigmented macules: early manifestations of tuberous sclerosis. Arch Neurol 1971; 25:547.
29. Shih VE, Efron ML, Moser HW. Hyperornithinemia, hyperammonemia, and homocitrullinuria: a new disorder of amino-acid metabolism associated with myoclonic seizures and mental retardation. Am J Dis Child 1969; 117:83.

30. Duffner PK, Cohen ME. Infantile spasms associated with histidinemia. Neurology 1975; 25:195.
31. Low NL, Bosma JF, Armstrong MD, et al. Infantile spasms with mental retardation. Clinical observation and dietary experiments. Pediatrics 1958; 22:1153.
32. Jeavons PM, Bower BD. Infantile spasms: a review of the literature and a study of 112 cases. In: Jeavons PM, Bower BD, Clinics in developmental medicine. no. 15. London: William Heinemann Medical Books Ltd., 1964:1–82.
33. Kulenkampft M, Schawartzman JS, Wilson J. Neurological complications of pertussis inoculation. Arch Dis Child 1974; 49:46.
34. Melchior JC. Infantile spasms and early immunization against whooping cough. Danish survey from 1970 to 1975. Arch Dis Child 1977; 52:134.
35. Fukuyama Y, Tomori N, and Sugitate M. Critical evaluation of the role of immunization as an etiological factor of infantile spasms. Neuropediatrie 1977; 8:224.
36. Tsuchiya S, Kagawa K, Fu Kuyama Y. Critical evaluation of the role of immunization as an etiological factor in infantile spasms (second report). Brain Dev 1978; 3:171.
37. Committee on Infectious Diseases 1983–1984 of the American Academy of Pediatrics. Pertussis vaccine. Pediatrics 1984; 74:303.
38. Melchior JC. Infantile spasms and immunization in the first year of life. Neuropediatrie 1971; 3:3.
39. Hrachovy RA, Frost JD Jr. Infantile spasms. Pediatr Clin North Am 1989; 36(2):311–29.
40. Bellman MH, Ross EM, Miller DL. Infantile spasms and pertussis immunization. Lancet 1983; 1:1031.
41. Riikonen R. Infantile spasms: some new theoretical aspects. Epilepsia 1983; 24:159–68.
42. Gastaut H, Gastaut JL, Regis H, Bernard R, Pinsard N, et al. Computerized tomography in the study of West's syndrome. Dev Med Child Neurol 1978; 20:21–27.
43. Singer WD, Haller JS, Sullivan LR, Wolpert S, Mills C, and Rabe EF. The value of neuroradiology in infantile spasms. J Pediatr 1982; 100:47–50.
44. Kellaway P, Frost JD Jr, et al. Precise characterization and quantification of infantile spasms. Ann Neurol 1979; 6:214.
45. Silverstein F, Johnston MV. Cerebrospinal fluid monoamine metabolites in patients with infantile spasms. Neurology 1984; 34:102.
46. Hrachovy RA, Frost JD Jr, Pollack M, et al. Serologic HLA typing in infantile spasms. Epilepsia, 1987; 28:613.
47. Kellaway P, Frost JD Jr, Hrachovy RA. Infantile spasms. In: Morselli PL, Pippenger CE, and Penry JK, Antiepileptic drug therapy in pediatrics. New York: Raven Press, 1983: 115–136.
48. Dumermuth G, Kovacs E. The effect of clonazepam (R05-4023) in the syndrome of infantile spasms and hypsarrhythmia and in petit mal variant or Lennox syndrome. ACTA Neurol Scand (Suppl 53) 1973; 49:25.
49. Vassella F, Pavlincova E, Schneider HI, et al. Treatment of infantile spasms and Lennox–Gastaut syndrome with clonazepam (Rivotril). Epilepsia 1973; 14:165–75.

50. Geller M, Christoff N. Diazepam in the treatment of childhood epilepsy. JAMA 1971; 215:2087.
51. Weinber WA, Harwell JL. Diazepam (Valium) in myoclonic seizures: a favorable response during infancy and childhood. Am J Dis Child 1965; 109:123.
52. Dreifuss F, Farwell J, Holmes G, et al. Infantile spasms. A comparative trial of nitrazepam and corticotropin. Arch Neurol 1986; 43:1107–10.
53. Hrachovy RA, Frost JD, Kellaway P, et al. A controlled study of prednisone therapy in infantile spasms. In: Wada JA, Penry JK, eds. Advances in epileptology. New York: Raven Press, 1980.
54. Bachman DS. Use of valproic acid in treatment of infantile spasms. Arch Neurol 1982; 39:49–52.
55. Dyken PR, Durant RH, Minden DB, et al. Short term effects of valproate on infantile spasms. Pediatr Neurol 1985; 1:34–37.
56. Pavone L, Incorpora G, LaRosa M, Livolti S, Mollica F. Treatment of infantile spasms with sodium dipropylacetic acid. Dev Med Child Neurol 1981; 23:454–61.
57. Simon D, Penry JK. Sodium di-*n*-propylacetate in the treatment of epilepsy. A review. Epilepsia 1975; 16:549–73.
58. Glaze GD, Zion TE. Infantile spasms. Chicago: Year Book Medical Publishers, Inc., 1985: 25–27.
59. Sato S, Takeshi E, Hara H, Fu Kuyama Y. Brain shrinkage and subdural effusion associated with ACTH administration. Brain Dev 1982; 4:13–20.
60. Lombroso CT. A prospective study of infantile spasms. Clinical and therapeutic correlations. Epilepsia 1983; 24:135–58.
61. Willig RP, Lagenstein I. Use of ACTH fragments in children with infantile spasms. Neuropediatrics 1982; 13:55–58.
62. Hrachovy RA, Frost JD, Kellaway P, Zion TE. Double blind study of ACTH vs. prednisone therapy in infantile spasms. J Pediatr 1983; 103:641–45.
63. Snead OC, Benton JW Jr, Hosey LC, Swann JW, et al. Treatment of infantile spasms with high dose ACTH: efficacy and plasma levels of ACTH and cortisol. Neurology 1989; 39:1027–31.
64. Hrachovy RA, Frost JD Jr, Kellaway P, et al. A controlled study of ACTH therapy in infantile spasms. Epilepsia 1980; 21:631.
65. Hrachovy RA, Frost JD, Kellaway P, Zion T. A controlled study of prednisone therapy in infantile spasms. Epilepsia 1979; 20:403–7.
66. Riikonen R, Donner M. ACTH therapy in infantile spasms: side effects. Arch Dis Child 1980; 55:664–72.
67. Fitzhardinnge PM, Eisen A, Lejtenyl C. Sequelae of early steroid administration to the newborn infant. Pediatrics 1974; 53:877.
68. Johnson DE, Munson DP, Thompson TR. Effect of antenatal administration of betamethasone on hospital cost and survival of premature infants. Pediatrics 1981; 68:633.
69. Langenstein L, Willig RP, Kuhne D. Cranial computed tomography (CCT) findings in children treated with ACTH and dexamethasone: first results. Neuropediatrics 1979; 10:370–84.
70. Carollo C, Marin G, Scanarini M, et al. CT and ACTH treatment in infantile spasms. Childs Brain 1982; 9:347–353.

71. Young RSK, Fripp RR, Stern DR. Cardiac hypertrophy associated with ACTH therapy for childhood seizure disorder. J Child Neurol 1987; 2:311–12.
72. Rao JK, Willis J. Hypothalamo-pituitary-adrenal function in infantile spasms: effects of ACTH therapy. J Child Neurol 1987; 2:220–23.
73. Perheentupa J, Riikonen R, Dunkel L, Simell O. Adrenal hyporesponsiveness after treatment with ACTH of infantile spasms. Arch Dis Child 1986; 61:750–53.
74. Ross D. Suppressed pituitary ACTH. Response after ACTH treatment of infantile spasms. J Child Neurol 1986; 1:34–37.
75. Lerman P, Kivity S. The efficacy of corticotropin in primary infantile spasms. J Pediatr 1982; 101:294.
76. Glaze DG, Hrachovy RA, Frost JD Jr, et al. Prospective study of outcome of infants with infantile spasms treated during controlled studies of ACTH and prednisone. J Pediatr 1988; 112:389–96.
77. Karbowski K. (1988). Developments in epileptology in the 18th and 19th centuries prior to the delineation of the Lennox–Gastaut syndrome. In: Niedermeyer E, Degen R, eds. The Lennox–Gastaut syndrome. New York: Alan R Liss, Inc., 1988:1–8.
78. Gibbs FA, GIbbs EL, Lennox WG. The influence of the blood sugar level on the wave and spike formation in petit mal epilepsy. Arch Neurol Psychiatr 1939; 41:111–16.
79. Gastaut H, Rogers J, Soulayrol R, Tassinari C, Regis H, et al. Childhood epileptic encephalopathy with diffuse slow spike waves (otherwise known as "petit mal variant") or Lennox syndrome. Epilepsia 1966; 7:139–79.
80. Giovanari Rossi G, Gobbi G, Melideo G, Parmeggiani A. Myoclonic manifestations in the Lennox–Gastaut syndrome and other childhood epilepsies. In: Niedermeyer E, Degen R, eds. The Lennox–Gastaut syndrome. New York, Alan R Liss, Inc., 1988:137–58.
81. Gastaut H. The Lennox–Gastaut syndrome: comments on the syndrome's terminology and nosological position amongst the secondary generalized epilepsies of childhood. In: Broughton RJ, ed. Henry Gastaut and Marseille School's contribution to the neurosciences. Amsterdam: Elsevier Biomedical Press (EEG Suppl 35), 1982:71–84.
82. Bauer G., Benke, T., and Bohr, K. The Lennox–Gastaut syndrome in adulthood. In: Niedermeyer E, Degen R, eds., The Lennox–Gastaut syndrome. New York: Alan R Liss, Inc., 1988:317–27.
83. Aicardi J. (1986). Lennox–Gastaut syndrome and myoclonic epilepsies of infancy and early childhood. In: Aicardi J, ed. Epilepsy in children. New York: Raven Press, 1986:39–65.
84. Aicardi J, Gomes AL. The Lennox–Gastaut syndrome. Clinical and electroencephalographic features. In: Niedermeyer E, and Degen R, eds. The Lennox–Gastaut syndrome. New York: Alan R Liss, Inc., 1988:25–46.
85. Aicardi J. Childhood epilepsies with brief myoclonic, atonic or tonic seizures. In: Laidlaw J, Richens A, eds. A textbook of epilepsy. Edinburgh, Churchill Livingstone, 1982:88–96.
86. Dravet C, Roger J, Bureau M, Dalla Bernardina B. Myoclonic epilepsies in childhood. In: Akimoto H, Kazamatsuri H, Seino M, Ward A, eds. Advances in

epileptology. 13th Epilepsy international symposium. New York: Raven Press, 1982:135–140.
87. Beaumanoir A, Foletti G, Magistris M, Volanchi D. Status epilepticus in the Lennox–Gastaut syndrome. In: Niedermeyer E, Degen R, eds. The Lennox–Gastaut syndrome. New York: Alan R Liss, Inc., 1988:283–99.
88. Baldy-Moulinier M, Touchon J, Billiard M, Carriere A, Besset A. Nocturnal sleep studies in the Lennox–Gastaut syndrome. In: Niedermeyer E, Degen R, eds. The Lennox–Gastaut syndrome. New York: Alan R Liss, Inc., 1988:243–60.
89. Gastaut H, Regis H. On the subject of Lennox's "akinetic" petit mal. Epilepsia 1961; 2:198–305.
90. Egli M, Mothersill I, O'Kane M, O'Kane F. The axial spasm. The predominant type of drop seizures in patients with secondary generalized epilepsy. Epilepsia 1985; 26:401–15.
91. Ikeno T, Shigematsu H, Migakoshi M, Ohba A, Yagi K, Seino M. An analytic study of epileptic falls. Epilepsia 1985; 26:612–21.
92. Nolte R, Wolf M, Krageloh-Mann I. The atonic (astatic) drop attacks and their differential diagnosis. In: Niedermeyer E, Degen R, eds. The Lennox–Gastaut syndrome. New York: Alan R Liss, Inc., 1988:95–108.
93. Oller-Daurella L, Oller F-V L. The Lennox–Gastaut syndrome: synopsis. In: Niedermeyer E, Degen R, eds. The Lennox–Gastaut syndrome. New York: Alan R Liss, Inc., 1988:387–97.
94. Tassinari CA, Ambrosetto G. Tonic seizures in the Lennox–Gastaut syndrome: semiology and differential diagnosis. In: Niedermeyer E, Degen R, eds. The Lennox–Gastaut syndrome. New York: Alan R Liss, Inc., 1988:109–24.
95. Avoli M, Gloor P. Role of the thalamus in generalized penicillin epilepsy: observations on decorticated cats. Exp Neurol 1982; 77:386–402.
96. Pellegrini A, Musgrave J, Gloor P. Role of afferent input of subcortical origin in the genesis of bilaterally synchronous epileptic discharges of feline generalized penicillin epilepsy. Exp Neurol 1979; 64:155–73.
97. Patry G, Lyagoubi S, Tassinari CA. Subclinical "electrical status epilepticus" induced by sleep in children. Arch Neurol (Chicago) 1971; 24:242–52.
98. Gastaut H, Zifkin BG. Secondary bilateral synchrony and Lennox–Gastaut syndrome. In: Niedermeyer E, Degen R, eds. The Lennox–Gastaut syndrome. New York: Alan R Liss, Inc., 1988:221–42.
99. Niedermeyer E. The generalized epilepsies. Springfield, IL: Charles C Thomas, 1972:74–86.
100. Ohtahara S, Ohtsuka Y, Yoshinaga H, Iyoda K, et al. Lennox–Gastaut syndrome: etiological considerations. In: Niedermeyer E, Degen R, eds. The Lennox–Gastaut syndrome. New York: Alan R Liss, Inc., 1988:47–63.
101. Weiermann G, Jacobi G. An analysis of clinical and electroencephalographic data in 120 patients with Lennox–Gastaut syndrome. In: Niedermeyer E, Degen R, eds. The Lennox–Gastaut syndrome. New York: Alan R Liss, Inc., 1988:399–408.
102. Pazzaglia P, D'Alessandro R, Ambrosetto G, Lugaresi E. Drop attacks: an ominous change in the evolution of partial epilepsy. Neurology 1985; 35:1725–30.
103. Angelini L, Broggi G, Riva D, Solero CL. A case of Lennox–Gastaut syndrome successfully treated by removal of parieto-temporal astrocytoma. Epilepsia 1979; 20:665–69.

104. Sher PK. Alternate day clonazepam treatment of intractable seizures. Arch Neurol 1985; 42:787–88.
105. Papini M, Pasquinelli A, Orlandi D, et al. Alertness and incidence of seizures in patients with Lennox–Gastaut syndrome. Epilepsia 1984; 25:161–67.
106. Bittencourt PRM, Richens A. Anticonvulsant-induced status epilepticus in Lennox–Gastaut syndrome. Epilepsia 1981; 22:129–34.
107. Yamatogi Y, Ohtsuka Y, Ishida T, et al. Treatment of the Lennox–Gastaut syndrome with ACTH: a clinical and electroencephalographic study. Brain Dev 1979; 4:267–76.
108. Huttenlocher PR. (1976). Ketonemia and seizures: metabolic and anticonvulsant effects of two ketogenic diets in childhood epilepsy. Pediatr Res 1976; 10:530–40.
109. O'Donohoe NV. Epilepsies of childhood. 2d ed. London: Butterworth & Company (Publishers) Ltd., 1985.
110. Helmholz HF. The treatment of epilepsy in childhood. JAMA 1927; 88:2028–32.
111. Livingston S. Ketogenic diet in the treatment of childhood epilepsy. Dev Med Child Neurol 1977; 19:833–34.
112. Withrow CD. The ketogenic diet: mechanism of anticonvulsant action. In: Glasser GH, Penry JK, Woodbury DM, eds. Antiepileptic drugs: mechanisms of action. New York: Raven Press, 1980:635–42.
113. Brett M. The Lennox–Gastaut syndrome: therapeutic aspects. In: Niedermeyer E, Degen R, eds. The Lennox–Gastaut syndrome. New York: Alan R Liss, Inc., 1988:329–39.
114. Schwartz RH, Eaton J, Aynsley-Green A, Bower BD. Ketogenic diet in the management of childhood epilepsy. In: Rose FC, ed. Research progress in epilepsy. London: Pitman Books Ltd., 1983:326–32.
115. Matsumoto M, Kumagi T, Takeuchi T, Miyazaki S, et al. Clinical effects of thyrotropin-releasing hormone for severe epilepsy in childhood: a comparative study with ACTH therapy. Epilepsia 1987; 28(1):49–55.
116. Sandstedt P, Kostulas V, Larsson LE. Intravenous gammaglobulin for post-encephalitis epilepsy. Lancet 1984; 2:1154–55.
117. Shields WD, Saslow E. Myoclonic, atonic and absence seizures following institution of carbamazepine therapy in children. Neurology (Cleve) 1983; 33:1487–89.
118. Smeraldi E, Smeraldi RS, Cazullo CL, Cazullo AG, et al. Immunogenetics of the Lennox–Gastaut syndrome: frequency of HLA antigens and haptotype in patients and first-degree relatives. Epilepsia 1975; 16:699–703.
119. Gilhus NE, Aarli JA, Thorsby E. HLA antigens in epileptic patients with drug-induced immunodeficiency. Int J Immuno pharmacol 1982; 4:517–20.
120. Muller K, Lenard HG. The Lennox–Gastaut syndrome: therapeutic aspects including dietary measures and general management. In: Niedermeyer E, Degen R, eds. The Lennox–Gastaut syndrome. New York: Alan R Liss, Inc., 1988:341–55.
121. Dravet C, Bureau M, Roger J. Benign myoclonic epilepsy in infants. In: Roger J, Dravet C, Bureau M, Dreifuss FE, Wolf P, eds. Epileptic syndromes in infancy, childhood and adolescence. London: John Libbey Eurotext Ltd., 1985:51–57.
122. Dalla Bernardina B, Colamaria V, Capovilla G, Bondavalli S. Nosological classification of epilepsies in the first three years of life. In: Nistico G, Di Perri R, Meinardi H, eds. Epilepsy: an update on research and therapy. New York: Alan R Liss, Inc., 1983:165–83.

123. Dravet C, Bureau M, Roger J. Severe myoclonic epilepsy in infants. In: Roger J, Dravet C, Bureau M, Dreifuss FE, Wolf P, eds. Epileptic syndromes in infancy, childhood and adolescence. London: John Libbey Eurotext Ltd., 1985:58–67.
124. Dalla Bernardina B, Dulac O, Fejerman N, et al. Early myoclonic epileptic encephalopathy. Eur J Pediatr 1983; 140:248–52.
125. Aicardi J, Goutieres F. Encéphalopathie myoclonique néonatale. Rev EEG Neurophysiol 1978; 8:99–101.
126. Dalla Bernardina B, Aicardi J, Goutieres F, Plouin P. Glycine encephalopathy. Neuropediatrics 1979; 10:209–25.
127. Ohtahara S, Ohtsuka Y, Yamatogi Y, Oka E. The early-infantile epileptic encephalopathy with suppression-burst. Developmental aspects. Brain Dev 1987; 9(4):371–76.
128. Asconape J, Penry JK. Some clinical and EEG aspects of benign juvenile myoclonic epilepsy. Epilepsia 1984; 25: 108–14.
129. Jeavons PM. Nosological problems of myoclonic epilepsies in childhood and adolescence. Dev Med Child Neurol 1977; 19:3–8.
130. Janz D. The natural history of primary generalized epilepsies with sporadic myoclonias of the ''impulsive petit mal'' type. In: Lugaresi E, Pazzaglia P, Tassinari CA, eds. Evolution and prognosis of epilepsies. Bologna, Italy: Aulo Gaggi, 1973:55–61.
131. Wolf P. Juvenile myoclonic epilepsy. In: Rogers J, Dravet C, Bureau M, Dreifuss FE, Wolf P, eds. Epileptic syndromes in infancy, childhood and adolescence. London: John Libbey Eurotext Ltd., 1985: 247–58.
132. Janz D. Epilepsy with impulsive petit mal (juvenile myoclonic epilepsy). Acta Neurol Scand 1985; 72:449–59.
133. Engel J Jr. Epileptic syndromes. In: Engel J Jr, ed. Seizures and epilepsy. Philadelphia: FA Davis Company, 1989:179–220.
134. Tassinari CA, Burea M. Epilepsy with myoclonic absences. In: Roger J, Dravet C, Bureau M, Dreifuss FE, Wolf P, eds. Epileptic syndromes in infancy, childhood and adolescence. London, John Libbey Eurotext Ltd., 1985:194–204.
135. Lugaresi E, Pazzaglia P, Franck L, Roger J, and Bureau-Paillas M, et al. Evolution and prognosis of primary generalized epilepsies of the petit mal absence type. In: Lugaresi E, Pazzaglia P, Tassinari CA, eds. Evolution and prognosis of epilepsies. Bologna, Italy: Aulo Gaggi, 1973:3–22.
136. Tassinari CA. (1985). Epilepsy with myoclonic absences. In: Roger J, Dravet C, Bureau M, Dreifuss FE, Wolf P, eds. Epileptic syndromes in infancy, childhood and adolescence. John Libbey Eurotext Ltd., 1985:321.
137. Doose H. Myoclonic astatic epilepsy of early childhood. In: Roger J, Dravet C, Bureau M, Dreifuss FE, Wolf P, eds. Epileptic syndromes in infancy, childhood and adolescence. John Libbey Eurotext Ltd., 1985:78–88.
138. Doose H. Myoclonic astatic epilepsy [cortico-reticular epilepsy with minor seizure (and grand mal) of early childhood]. In: Roger J, Dravet C, Bureau M, Dreifuss FE, Wolf P, eds. Epileptic syndromes in infancy, childhood and adolescence. John Libbey Eurotext Ltd., 1985:319.
139. Aicardi J. Myoclonic epilepsies associated with progressive degenerative disorders of the central nervous system: progressive myoclonic epilepsies, myoclonus-

epilepsy. In Aicardi J, ed. Epilepsy in children. New York: Raven Press, 1986:73–78.

140. Andermann F, Berkovic S, Andermann E. The progressive myoclonus epilepsies. In: Merritt Putnam quarterly. Green Brook, NJ: Park Davis, Division of Warner-Lambert Company, 1989.

141. Koskiniemi ML. Baltic myoclonus. In: Fahn S, Marsden CD, Van Woert MH, eds. Advances in neurology. Vol. 43. Myoclonus. New York: Raven Press, 1986:57–64.

142. MacDonald RL, Barker JL. (1979). Enhancement of GABA-mediated post synoptic inhibition in mammalian spinal cord neurons: a common mode of anticonvulsant action. Brain Res 1979; 167(2):323–36.

10

Effects of Epilepsy on Behavior

STANLEY BERENT and BRUNO GIORDANI
University of Michigan
Ann Arbor, Michigan

I. INTRODUCTION

Behavior refers to the thoughts, feelings, and actions that are mediated by the nervous system and manifested in the person's continuing survival. Behavior is a general term that is used in lay as well as professional communications. It is a word that is easily misinterpreted because its use often varies from one instance to another. This is because behavior is not a unitary concept. It is multifactorial, and its component parts are both interactive (e.g., the effect of motivation on a child's school performance) and relatively independent (e.g., memory). For instance, it is necessary to determine the component part, or parts, of behavior that are adversely affected by an event (e.g., seizure or other occurrence) in order to understand how the person's behavior has been affected more generally.

Although a number of schemes are possible, one model separates behavior into areas, each with previously demonstrated, relative functional autonomy in comparison to the others [1]. These components include (1) *general intellect*, (2) *cognition* (i.e., the various aspects of learning, memory and language), (3) *sensory-perceptual* and *motor* function, (4) *affect* (e.g., anxiety and/or depression), and (5) *adjustment* strategies (including adjustment failures; psychopathology). Dividing behavior into these component parts is a necessary step toward objective assessment because it lays the foundation for operational definitions of each term. An *operational definition* is one that describes a concept in terms of events that are identifiable and repeatable. In scientific inquiry, operationalism contributes to the discovery of information that is generalizable from one situation to another. Analogously, the use of operational definitions in the clinical setting leads to clarity in communication, reducing the likelihood of misunderstandings between doctor and patient or between practitioners.

In this vein, "intelligence" has been a subject of careful study. It has come to be almost universally defined by formal psychometric criteria, that is, by performance on a given test (e.g., most often, the Wechsler Intelligence Scales [2,3]). As a result, we know a great deal about this important aspect of behavior and events that affect it. It is known, for example, that normal intellectual development is greatly influenced by education and other life experiences. Two-thirds (68%) of the general population will reflect a level of general intellect that falls within plus or minus 1 standard deviation (1 SD = 15 points on the Wechsler Scale) of the mean (a full scale IQ of 100) and approximately one-sixth (16%) reflect intelligence quotients of 116 or higher. Hopefully, in the majority of cases it does not, but epilepsy can interfere with normal intellect in a variety of ways. When the onset of epilepsy is before the age of 5 years, for example, normal intellectual development is more likely to be adversely affected in comparison to persons with epilepsy of later onset, after 10 years of age [4]. Similarly, children with epilepsy evidence, as a group, show less academic progress than would be expected on the basis of age and IQ [5]. These children are often found to be about one year behind age expectations in terms of reading ability, with 20% of such children reflecting severe and specific reading disability [6]. Specific cognitive impairment(s) may subserve these difficulties in schooling and intellectual development. Impairments in verbal-language abilities and attention concentration, for instance, appear to be particularly involved in poor academic progress [7].

Although many persons with epilepsy may evidence only minimal behavioral symptoms, abundant evidence exists that epilepsy is associated with a variety of behavioral problems. The specific nature of these problems and their underlying causes are yet to be identified in many instances. There is much that is understood, however, and the remainder of this chapter is devoted to a presentation and discussion of the way in which epilepsy-related phenomena can affect the various aspects of behavior. It is hoped that this information will help clinicians and the patients they treat to be aware of the signs and symptoms of epilepsy-related abnormal behaviors, to recognize the mechanisms contributing to the condition in a given case, and to intervene effectively and early to ameliorate the difficulty.

II. EPILEPSY AS A SYNDROME

According to Dreifuss [8], epilepsy is a syndrome with special implications for children. In addition to the seizure, the most easily observed phenomenon in epilepsy, the syndrome is defined by etiology, course, prognosis, and family history. To this, one could add the concept of "treatment." Whether pharmacologic, surgical, or psychological, treatment often becomes a chronic component of the child's life with its own consequences for behavior. Variables that are associated with any part of the syndrome can have consequences for the child's behavior. The seizure itself can interfere directly with behavior. The type of seizure determines the particular medication to be used. Medications and other treatment, in turn, have their own impact on behavior. Childhood epileptics have etiologies that are often different from those in adult life, and the specific nature of a given etiology contributes to behavioral complications. The course can determine the extensiveness of intervention and/or the need for continued treatment. Familial history, including both genetic and cultural contributions, are reflected in the nature of the syndrome and is an important determinant of the behavioral picture in a given case. Just as behavior is multifactorial, so may "cause" be multiple. Identification of the various contributions to observed behavior is a necessary step in effective clinical intervention.

III. SEIZURE AND BEHAVIOR IN EPILEPSY

In considering their effects on behavior, seizures have primarily been characterized in six ways: (1) type, (2) Age of onset, (3) Duration, (4) Frequency, (5) Severity, and (6) Phase (i.e., preictal, ictal, postictal, and interictal). With regard to seizure *type*, an elaborate and comprehensive description becomes a process of diagnosis. Historically speaking and from a world viewpoint, the field of epilepsy research has suffered from a lack of standardization in the clinical diagnosis of epilepsy and in the classification of epileptic seizures. Relatively recent international cooperation has attempted to rectify this situation (Commission on Classification and Terminology, International League Against Epilepsy, [9,10]). In clinical research, seizures are most often and most simply classified as being either partial or general. (For a fuller discussion of clinical diagnosis and classification, the reader is referred to Chapter 3 in the present volume. See also Dreifuss [8] and Roger et al. [11].) Briefly, a *partial seizure* is one that originates in a focal area of one cerebral hemisphere. The seizure may remain focal with no effect on the individual's consciousness (a simple partial seizure), or it may involve impairment of consciousness (a complex partial seizure). A simple seizure can evolve into a complex one. Either simple or complex partial seizures may progress to a secondary seizure, generalized to both cerebral hemispheres. A *generalized seizure* begins with involvement of both brain hemispheres.

The nature of seizure lends itself to *operational definition*. Such definitions may be based on instrumentation (e.g., an initial bilateral ictal electroencephalographic pattern for diagnosing a generalized seizure), procedure (e.g., a defined pattern of impairment on neuropsychological test results), observation (e.g., a convulsive movement limited to one side of the body for a partial seizure), or some combination of the three.

Studies on type of seizure and behavior have made it clear that this factor (i.e., seizure type), though interactive with the other variables to be discussed, has important implications in itself for the affected patient's behavior. It is important to keep in mind not only the interactions between factors, as just mentioned, but the concept of ''individual differences'' as well. Everyone is an individual, in other words, and for every rule there is an exception.

It has long been held that generalized motor seizures are associated with greater impairment of intellectual and cognitive abilities than are partial seizures [12]. Patients with either primary or secondarily generalized seizures have been found to evidence impairments on tasks that reflect attention, concentration, and visual-perceptual problem solving [13]. Partial seizures are more likely to result in deficits that are focal, reflecting the specific locus of underlying cerebral dysfunction. In one study [14] of 50 patients with epileptogenic foci localized to either the left or the right brain hemisphere; for example, individuals with a left-hemisphere seizure focus performed more poorly than did those with a right-hemisphere seizure focus on a verbal learning task. On a visual, nonverbal task, these left-hemisphere-affected patients did no more poorly than did their right-hemisphere counterparts. A number of studies have found that patients with temporal lobe electroencephalographic foci experience difficulties on tasks of general learning and memory [15–17]. The clearest findings of this sort have been with patients who have structural lesions [18–25]. A demonstrable structural lesion is not necessary, however, and focal, functional abnormalities can subserve modality specific cognitive impairment [26]. It has even been demonstrated that generalized epileptiform electroencephalogram (EEG) discharges that are unaccompanied by overt clinical changes may be associated with cognitive impairments that are transitory and either general or specific depending upon and consistent with type of seizure [27].

When *age of onset* is considered, the distinctions between generalized and partial seizure effects become less clear [28]. Regardless of seizure type, it appears that an early onset of seizure (i.e., before 5 years of age) is associated with poorer intellectual function than is a later onset (i.e., after age 10) [4,28,29]. In general, the earlier the onset, the greater the behavioral deterioration when measured at a later age [30]. Tasks as measured by routine intelligence tests appear to be most ''at risk'' for impairment by seizures of early onset [4,28,31,32]. Such tasks are greatly influenced by education, and as indicated earlier in this chapter, it may be that early onset of seizure interferes with schooling and the normal course of intellectual development. In the authors' own studies, for example, it was found that individuals with partial seizures who successfully completed high school showed no differences in cognitive and intellectual tasks from one another, regardless of age of onset [33].

The kind of behavior being considered is a factor as well. While early onset seizure has been associated with greater intellectual difficulties, an adolescent onset of either partial or generalized seizures has been associated with a higher risk for psychosocial problems (e.g., psychopathology) as measured by the Minnesota Mutiphasic Personality Inventory (MMPI) [34].

Duration is a complex variable. Depending on how one defines the term, duration can be confounded with onset and/or seizure frequency. In some studies it is unclear whether the authors have based their measure of duration on length of time of the ictus, the period the patient has experienced a seizure disorder, an aspect of the epileptic syndrome unrelated to seizure per se, or simply the time elapsed since the initial diagnosis of epilepsy [35]. Clear, operationally defined terms would allow for comparison of results between studies and determination of the generalizability of findings.

The results of most studies that have addressed duration as a variable lead to the general and perhaps common sensical conclusion that longer duration of seizure disorder is related to a progressive decline in neuropsychological test performance [36–38]. The relationship between duration and progressive decline is clearest in cases of generalized seizures of early onset [39].

There are those who hold that duration of seizure is of relatively little importance in its contribution to intellectual impairment in comparison to a factor such as age of onset [40]. Others argue that duration contributes to both intellectual and educational difficulties in the relative short term and that persistent, refractory seizures may very well eventuate in premature aging and deterioration of the brain over the life span of the patient [41]. Rodin [41] suggests longitudinal, interdisciplinary studies to address these questions.

As with many of the other seizure-related variables under consideration, other factors associated with the syndrome of epilepsy may interact with duration to produce an affect on behavior. Depending on the specific etiology, for example, underlying disease processes may lead to progressive worsening of the patient's condition. Brain degeneration may occur over the course of the illness and eventuate not only in progressive decline of behavioral efficiency but in a changing seizure symptom picture as well. A syndrome such a familial progressive myoclonic epilepsy, for example [1], leads to dementia as the disorder progresses. In the course of such progression (and correlated with duration, of course), the child might be expected to show decline in general intellect, increasing difficulty in school and social, interpersonal situations, with eventual and gross dysfunctions of learning, memory, and other aspects of basic cognition.

Rodin [41] would argue that even when one excludes epileptic syndromes and treatments that eventuate in overt cerebral disease, there are patients who show what appears to be premature behavioral decline that seems to be predictable solely on the basis of long duration of seizures.

Questions related to the influence of seizure on behavior are deserving of continued attention by both scientists and clinicians. The answers to these questions will guide the clinician's treatment interventions in terms of the kind(s) of treatment(s) to use. From a research point of view, the answers to these questions will enable us to direct resources to areas that are likely to advance our understanding of epilepsy and brain–behavior relationships more generally. Such advances in knowledge will, in turn, allow for the development of improved treatment strategies.

With regard to *seizure frequency*, the results of formal studies have been mixed [42]. While some investigations have concluded an adverse effect on behavior as a result of frequency of seizures [4,43,44], others have found conflicting evidence for such relationship [45,46]. The strongest evidence that frequency may be important in predicting behavioral impairment derives from studies that have employed test–retest designs to look at changes in behavior that occurred either as a result of fluctuations in symptoms over time or of successful treatment. Such studies have led to the general observation that good seizure control is associated with better neuropsychological functioning than in poor seizure control [42]. In one specific study [47], for instance, patients were monitored over time in their performance on the Wechsler Intelligence scales. The patients were retrospectively divided into two groups: seizure improved (SI) and seizure unimproved (SU). While patients from both groups showed improvement in scores from one test session to the next (a probable practice effect), only the SI group evidenced statistically significant improvement on overall IQ measures as well as on scores for all subtests of the Wechsler scales.

Treatment of epilepsy is a complex undertaking. It may involve the initiation of a new medication and very often includes a change from poly- to monopharmacy. Also, changes in the patient's motivation and/or attitude and thus in his or her compliance picture might result from improved rapport with the treating clinician or from direct counseling which may be a component of the treatment regimen. These and other treatment-related factors are often confounded with outcome variables (e.g., reduction of seizure frequency) and compete as explanations for observed changes in behavior. Giordani et al. [13,48] studied a group of 25 patients who were treated successfully in an impatient setting for seizures that had been previously refractory to conventional outpatient intervention. Patients were administered a comprehensive battery of neuropsychological tests at the time of their admission to the inpatient unit and again at their first clinic visit after discharge from the hospital. The results of these studies reflected improvement in neuropsychological function as a result of successful treatment intervention, but the analysis of variance design revealed that reduction in number of antiepileptic drugs and, especially, withdrawal of barbiturates were related to the improved test performance. Reduction in seizure frequency, itself, was unrelated to behavioral changes.

At first glance it would appear that *severity* of seizure would represent a good variable for scientific inquiry. This has not been the case in actuality. The reason for this is that no one has been able to establish a reliable and valid measure of severity. Nussbaum and O'Connor [49] proposed a method for assessing severity, but their approach rests on observation, is highly subjective in places, and does not lend well to the scientific requirement of operationalism.

Following what was said earlier about methods for operationalyzing epilepsy relevant variables, both observation, as employed by Nussbaum and O'Connor [49], and procedure (e.g., results on formal psychometrics) suffer from a common problem. They are both usually employed as dependent variables, allowing one to determine the effects of independent variables (e.g., onset). Confusion at times occurs when these variables are used as independent variables in the same study. The same caution applies to instrumentation (e.g., electroencephalography). Various aspects of EEG have been used, in fact, to study epilepsy. In combination with observation and procedure, the EEG has proven a valuable approach. Mirsky and Van Buren [50], to give but one example, demonstrated that spike–wave activity on the EEG was associated in some cases with impairment of sustained concentration and attention. One could argue that EEG manifestations such as these reflect "severity," but consensually and precedentially this use of EEG has not been established. Phenomena associated with EEG have either been viewed as representing the "type" of seizure or the more neutral type of EEG phenomenon per se.

In terms of *phase*, the disruption of behavior during an ictus is clinically obvious in many instances and often represents the basis on which the diagnosis of epilepsy is made [1]. Since seizures occur sporadically, the clinician often may not witness the attack directly. As in making the diagnosis of epilepsy itself, history, EEG, clinical neurologic examination, neuropsychological testing, and other procedures are used to determine the nature and extent of behavioral impairment that occurs during a seizure. There are some seizures (e.g., *absence*) that may occur frequently enough to be observed during the examination [1]. Usually, however, the examination reveals the patient's interictal state. This phase of the patient's disorder is hardly silent, and the EEG and other laboratory tests may reveal paroxysmal irregularities and/or other signs of neurologic abnormality [1]. Clinical observation, history, and psychological testing should be employed to provide clinical correlation to other laboratory findings, so the behavioral consequences of seizure to a given patient can be understood and treated appropriately.

The phase of a seizure disorder can be divided into four parts: immediate preictal, ictal, immediate postictal, and interictal. Behavioral disruption can accompany each phase in characteristic fashion for a given individual. One phase holds implication for behavior that may occur during another. Bonnie, for example, was a 20-year-old young woman who had been followed at our clinic since her early adolescence. She suffered from both simple and complex partial seizures that often secondarily generalized. Clinical neurologic examination of this patient was essentially normal even though her EEG reflected abnormalities in the left cerebral hemisphere. Formal neuropsychological testing clearly revealed cognitive impairments interictally that included lowered efficiency in verbal learning and memory in comparison to her nonverbal abilities. Despite these interictal impairments, Bonnie reflected an average general intellect and had completed high school successfully with a C average and a secretarial training program at a business college.

The psychological testing also showed a person with very low self-esteem and depression. A series of clinical interviews revealed a very timid and naive young lady, one who seemed more like 16 than 20. Interpersonally, she reported one boyfriend whom she had dated steadily since her adolescence. Recently, they had experienced difficulty in the relationship because of what she perceived as his demands for an increase in their sexual activities, which had theretofore been limited to kissing and light petting. The boyfriend had proposed marriage, but this apparently frightened her as much as the idea of sexual intercourse itself. As far as marriage was concerned, her family sided with the boyfriend, and this had led to difficulties between she and them as well.

Occupationally, Bonnie had been unable to hold a job for more than a few weeks. Despite her secretarial training, she seemed unable to perform in the actual work setting. One job was lost when she experienced a "seizure" at work and it was discovered that she had neglected to tell them about her epilepsy on the employment application form. Bonnie had most recently been hired as a waitress but planned to quit because, she reported, the male employees were pressuring her to "go out with them."

It is clear from these brief descriptions that Bonnie's interictal behavior is complainable, that is, adversely affecting her everyday life. Every area of behavior as described earlier in the chapter is affected. Although this young person had been able to complete formal course work in the benign environment of school, it is very likely that cognitive and intellectual impairments interfere with on-the-job performance. Her ability to cope with what may be the usual stresses of life, interpersonal and occupational, and some less usual stresses associated with her epilepsy may be reduced as well. Consequently, she is manifesting depression and other abnormal behaviors that without appropriate intervention may worsen over time.

Periodic seizures are a part of this person's experience. In her descriptions of these attacks, it becomes clear that they hold both immediate consequences for her behavior as well as implications in terms of anxiety and other interictal reactions. These attacks, directly observed by the clinician during interview on two occasions, often begin with interruption of ongoing behavior followed by lip smacking, drooling, and garbled speech. The immediate preictal state, she says, may at times involve automatisms where she may tug at her clothing or buttons. This progresses to mild "shaking" of one or both sides of the body and then a period of seeming quiescence. There is a postictal confusion, and the patient reports that she may be amnesic for periods ranging from minutes to hours following a seizure.

Bonnie reflects great concern about her seizures and their effects. She was most alarmed when late one night she "found" herself confused, some distance from home, in a secluded spot, and her clothes in disarray. She has no memory of any specific violation that occurred, but her concerns are quite understandable. She worries about the stigma of such behavior and lives in fear of recurrences.

From the viewpoint of the syndrome of epilepsy as earlier presented, it is clear that the clinician needs to recognize and treat not only Bonnie's seizures but the behavioral consequences of those seizures as well. In this particular case, these behaviors may include pseudo- as well as electrographic seizures. It is well established that patients who manifest pseudoseizures are very likely to suffer from electrographic seizures as well, and the presence of one of these types of seizures should never be taken to rule out the other [51]. By recognizing the consequences of the various phases of seizure to the patient's everyday life, the clinician will be in a position to intervene effectively either directly or through appropriate referral. At the least, such intervention will include brief counseling and provision of information, but it may include involvement in support groups and/or formal psychotherapy as well.

As with other medical disorders, the person with epilepsy may experience thoughts and feelings that in themselves interfere with normal behavioral efficiency. A first experience with a seizure, for example, is very likely to be alarming to the patient and to their family, friends, and others who are close to them (e.g., classroom teachers). In some cases, there may be a lack of understanding as to the true nature of the event, and such ignorance can in itself stimulate anxiety or even panic. Fantasy may replace confusion with further misunderstanding. Specific thought content may vary from one person to another. While one person may worry about loss of control during an attack, another may become concerned about underlying disease and its eventual course. It is important that the clinician be aware of these "nonmedical" aspects of the patient's condition and correct ignorance whenever possible. This can be especially challenging because often such fears are left unstated or communicated only indirectly. In addition, stigmatization by others is an ever-present threat. Although societal views about epilepsy have perhaps improved in recent years, the clinician should help the patient deal with the fact that carrying a diagnosis of epilepsy may affect how others perceive and interact with the patient and how the patient views himself or herself as well.

IV. TREATMENT AND BEHAVIOR

Ideally, the treatment of epilepsy would be free of iatrogenesis. However, there are side effects associated with all clinical interventions. Interventions in epilepsy primarily include pharmacologic, surgical, and/or psychological treatment. To this list one might add inpatient hospitalization, family, and other environmental adjustments (e.g., changes in employment or school). Finally, the human factor must be considered. Individual differences in response to treatments at both a physical and psychological level influence the nature of symptoms and their control.

A. Drug Treatment

Although medication might not be necessary in every case of epilepsy [8], the use of an antiepileptic drug (AED) or drugs occupies a central position in the treatment of seizures. The choice of a specific drug to be used in a given case is usually determined by the patient's type of seizure, while the syndromal aspects of the case determine the need for medication and its continuance [8] in addition to other types of intervention. A partial list of some commonly used AEDs include carbamazepine, phenytoin, and/or phenobarbital for partial seizures; carbamazepine, phenytoin, and/or valproic acid for generalized seizures; ethosuximide, valproic acid, and/or clonazepam for absence seizures [1]. In addition, a large number of "new" and potential AEDs are currently proceeding through formal clinical trials, and these will presumably become available to patients in the coming years. These potential medications are largely derived from compounds that affect neuronal synapses or cell membranes as well as receptor sites and other aspects of inter- and/or intracellular transmission [52,53]. Many of these drugs are benzodiazepine-like agents or barbituric derivatives [52,53], and these compounds could conceivably affect normal learning and other cognitive and perceptual behaviors along with their inhibition of seizures. Formal neuropsychological assessment procedures have been used increasingly in clinical trials and should be required in addition to establishing clinical efficacy and other potential side effects in all new drug development. (The reader is referred to Chapter 2 for a comprehensive discussion of the clinical use of AEDs in epilepsy). Although all currently used drugs have established efficacy in terms of seizure control, they produce side effects as well. Many of these are undesirable effects on cognitive and other aspects of behavior. In children, such side effects can have unique consequences because, as emphasized by Dreifuss [8], they occur during a vulnerable time when the developing person is engaged in acquisition of knowledge and social and personal coping skills (p. 1).

Studies that have examined the effects of AEDs on behavior have usually attended to three primary aspects of drug treatment: the type of medication (e.g., phenytoin versus carbamazepine), the number of drugs (e.g., poly- versus monotherapy), and/or dosage (e.g., blood level of a given medication).

1. Drug Type

Regardless of type, it appears that all AEDs at dose levels sufficient to control seizures might also impair neuropsychological function to some extent.

In his review of the literature, Trimble [54] concluded that carbamazepine had little or no adverse effect on cognitive ability in comparison to phenobarbital, phenytoin, or sodium valproate. Dodrill [55], on the other hand, stated that *all* AEDs have "slight to mild adverse effects on abilities." While carbamazepine seemed to have the fewest cognitive side effects, Dodrill argued that methodological problems plague many studies in the area and prevent a final conclusion regarding which AED might have the least negative effect. In a recent paper [56], the authors conclude that phenobarbital has such adverse effects on cognitive performance that these outweigh the potential benefits of the drug in terms of seizure control.

2. Polypharmacy

While polypharmacy may be necessary in the treatment of some (intractable) epilepsy syndromes [57], there is apparent consensus that monotherapy may decrease side effects and even be of greater efficacy in terms of seizure control than is polypharmacy [48,57–62]. Monotherapy is often achieved in clinical practice by reducing the number of medications, and it has been shown that the cognitive and other benefits that result from such change may not be apparent for some months following treatment modification [61]. Cognitive effects of AEDs may persist differentially between changes in drug types, and this could be a factor in delayed changes in behavior. The effects of phenobarbital, for example, have been shown to outlast the administration of the drug by several months [56].

3. Drug Dose

Dose-related effects on behavior are demonstrable even in monotherapy [63]. When serum AED levels are within a toxic range, general neuropsychological impairments can be expected [64,65]. Such changes, related to plasma levels, in a child's usual behavior can be expected across drug types [66]. Changes can occur in one or more behavioral domains [67,68] and/or adversely affect intelligence in general [69]. Since dose-related behavioral responses can be independent of other "physical" side effects of a medication, occurring at levels that are "subtoxic" [70,71]; the clinician need be ever vigilant to their possible presence.

Individual differences in drug responses remain an important consideration for the clinician. Organismic variables that are seemingly removed from the direct mechanisms of action of a given AED can interact with drug type or dose to alter the level at which toxicity becomes a factor. These might include such events as hormonal changes during puberty [72], other pathologies [73], other drugs [74], or pregnancy [75], to give a few examples. Motivational factors associated with patient compliance must be included in this list. A 16-year-old young man, to provide a clinical example, confided that embarrassment and fear of becoming stigmatized by his peers led him to conceal his epilepsy. He avoided taking his medications in public and this led to sporadic dosing, with concomitant wide fluctuations in AED blood levels and toxic side effects. In a separate case, a young woman with predominantly nocturnal seizures developed a fear of sleep and avoided going to bed in a vain attempt to ward off another attack. Her consumption of large amounts of coffee and frequent all-night socializing in order to avoid sleep may have paradoxically contributed to the intractableness of her epilepsy and severity of adverse side effects through their adverse affects on her compliance with the medication regimen as well as directly affecting her metabolism. A combined intervention that included inpatient hospitalization to monitor and "correct" her medications along with brief psychological counseling helped produce a beneficial outcome in this particular case.

B. Surgical Treatments

The earliest surgical treatments for epilepsy were performed by Dr. Victor Horsely at "Queen Square" in London, England and were limited to patients with clear structural lesions [76]. These procedures were later more broadly applied by Drs. Penfield and Jasper in Montreal to include cases with focal abnormalities but often without associated structural abnormalities [76]. Today, surgery for epilepsy is employed fairly widely [77,78]. Modern surgical procedures primarily include focal resections, hemispherectomy, and corpus collosum sectioning [76]. Wyler [76] reflects what may be the growing popularity of surgical intervention in arguing that such treatment should be considered "at the earliest possible age when it has become evident that medical management will not be sufficient to control a patient's seizure disorder" (p. 173). He premises his argument for surgery by observing that continued seizures in an individual are associated with long-term, adverse effects on intelligence, psychosocial developmental, educational, and vocational aptitude, and increased potential for "sudden death" (p. 174).

Successful surgical treatment of epilepsy can lead to improved behavioral adjustment, presumably through reduction of seizure occurrences [79,80]. Cognitive impairment can result from surgery as well. The nature of impairment may be either highly specific or general, but it is likely to be consistent with the area of surgically lesioned tissue [79]. Focal resection of the left temporal cortex, for instance, could result in decreased verbal learning capacity in comparison to presurgical levels of performance, while leaving nonverbal learning ability generally unaffected.

In determining the advisability of surgery in a given case, the clinician must evaluate the patient's current condition against the potential benefits and costs that might result should surgery proceed. It has been established that the estimate of seizure reduction is only part of such prognostication and that attention must include the individual's neuropsychological functioning as well [81,82]. The inclusion of formal neuropsychological assessment, along with EEG, Wada testing, and other clinical and laboratory test, has become a routine part of both pre- and postsurgical monitoring.

V. CONCLUSION

Formal neuropsychological services are now, in fact, recommended at all specialized centers for the diagnosis and treatment of epilepsy [83]. These include tertiary referral centers, fourth-level medical centers, and fourth-level surgical centers. In the arena of independent practice, as well, accessibility to neuropsychological services is usually easily obtainable.

In systematically and objectively attending to the various aspects of behavior that were outlined earlier in the chapter, several objectives important to the patient's clinical management can be accomplished. These include a description of present signs that might subserve the patient's complains or symptoms, establishment of a baseline for future comparison, and determination of changes over time. These changes could be adverse, signaling side effects of intervention or worsening of underlying disease, but they could also be positive and reinforce the correctness of treatment strategies. Behavioral information can also be used to estimate changes from premorbid state and to provide a basis for prognostic statements. Or, such information can provide a basis for determination of type and extent of disability, providing guidance for educational and/or vocational interventions. Even when formal testing is not undertaken, the neuropsychological perspective, as emphasized here and elsewhere by the authors [1,84], represents an important component in the clinician's armamentarium in the fight against epilepsy.

REFERENCES

1. Berent S, Sackellares JC. Clinical monitoring of children with epilepsy: a neurologic and neuropsychologic perspective. In: Hermann B, Seidenberg M, eds. The childhood epilepsies: neuropsychological, psychosocial and intervention aspects. New York: John Wiley & Sons, Inc., 1989: 15–31.
2. Wechsler D. Manual for the Wechsler intelligence scale for children—revised. New York: Psychological Corporation, 1974.
3. Wechsler D. Manual for the Wechsler adult intelligence scale—revised. New York: Psychological Corporation, 1981.

4. Dikmen S, Matthews CG. Effect of major motor seizure frequency upon cognitive-intellectual functions in adults. Epilepsia 1977; 18:21–29.
5. Seidenberg M, Beck N, Geisser M, Giordani B, Sackellares JC, Berent S, Dreifuss FE, Ball TJ. Academic achievement of children with epilepsy. Epilepsia 1986; 27:753–59.
6. Yule W. Educational achievement. In: Kulig BM, Meinardi H, Stores G, eds. Epilepsy and behavior. Lisse, The Netherlands: Swets en Zeitlinger, 1980:162–68.
7. Seidenberg M, Beck N, Geisser M, O'Leary D, Giordani B, Berent S, Sackellares JC, Dreifuss FE, Boll TJ. Neuropsychological correlates of academic achievement of children with epilepsy. 1988; Epilepsy 1:23–29.
8. Dreifuss FE. Childhood epilepsies. In: Hermann BP, Seidenberg M, eds. Childhood epilepsies: neuropsychological, psychosocial and intervention aspects. New York: John Wiley & Sons, Inc., 1989:1–13.
9. Commission on Classification and Terminology, International League Against Epilepsy. Proposed revisions of clinical and electroencephalographic classification of epileptic seizures. Epilepsia 1981; 22:480–501.
10. Commission on Classification and Terminology, International League Against Epilepsy; Proposal for classification of epilepsies and epileptic syndromes. Epilepsia 1985; 26:268–78.
11. Roger J, Dravet C, Bureau M, Dreifuss FE, Wolf P. Epileptic syndromes in infancy, childhood and adolescence. London, John Libbey Eurotext Ltd., 1985.
12. Klove H, Matthews CG. Neuropsychological studies of patients with epilepsy. In: Reitan RM, Davison LA, eds. Clinical neuropsychology: current status and applications. New York: John Wiley & Sons, Inc., 1974.
13. Giordani B, Sackellares JC, Miller S, Berent S, Sutula T, Seidenberg M, Boll TJ, O'Leary D, Dreifuss FE. Improvement in neuropsychological performance in patients with refractory seizures following intensive diagnostic and therapeutic intervention. Neurology 1983; 33:489–93.
14. Berent S, Giordani B, Sackellares JC, O'Leary D, Boll TJ. Cerebrally lateralized and epileptogenic foci and performance on a verbal and visual-graphic learning task. Percept Mot Skills 1983; 56:991–1001.
15. Glowinski H. Cognitive deficits in temporal lobe epilepsy. 1973; 157:129–37.
16. Dennerll RD. Cognitive deficits and lateral brain dysfunction in temporal lobe epilepsy. Nerv Ment Dis 1973; 157:129–37.
17. Quadfasel AF, Pruyser PW. Cognitive deficits in patients with psychomotor epilepsy. Epilepsia 1955; 4:80–90.
18. Bender MB, Teuber HL. Spatial organization of visual perception following injury to the brain. AMA Arch Neurol Psychiatry 1947; 58:721–39.
19. Bender MB, Teuber HL. Spatial organization of visual perception following injury to the brain. AMA Arch Neurol Psychiatry 1948; 59:39–62.
20. Meyer V, Yates AJ. Intellectual changes following temporal lobectomy for psychomotor epilepsy: preliminary communication. Neurol Neurosurg Psychiatry 1955; 18:44–52.
21. Milner B. Psychological defects produced by temporal lobe excision. Res Nerv Ment Dis 1958; 36:224–57.

22. Milner B. Visually guided maze learning in man: effects of bilateral hippocampal, bilateral frontal, and unilateral cerebral lesions. Neuropsychologia 1965; 3:317–38.
23. Milner B. Visual recognition and recall after right temporal lobe excision in man. Neuropsychologia 1968; 6:191–209.
24. Milner B. Interhemispheric differences in the localization of psychological processes in man. Br Med J 1971; 27:272–77.
25. Reitan RM. Certain differential effects of left and right cerebral lesions in human adults. J Comp Physiol Psychol 1955; 48:474–77.
26. Berent S, Sackellares JC, Abou-Khalil B, Gilman S, Siegel G, Hichwa R, Hutchins G. PET studies of cerebral glucose metabolic activity in temporal lobe epilepsy: the functional implications of lateralized hypometabolism. Neurology 1986; 36:337.
27. Aarts JH, Binnie CD, Smit AM, Wilkins AJ. Selective cognitive impairment during focal and generalized epileptiform EEG activity. Brain 1984; 101:293–308.
28. O'Leary DS, Lovell MR, Sackellares JC, Berent S, Giordani B, Seidenberg M, Boll TJ. The effects of age of onset of partial and generalized seizures on neuropsychological performance in children. J Ner Ment Dis 1983; 171:624–29.
29. Dikmen S, Matthews CG, Harley JP. The effect of early versus late onset of major motor epilepsy upon cognitive-intellectual performance. Epilepsia 1975; 16:73–81.
30. Lennox WG. Brain injury drugs and environment as causes of mental decay in epileptics. Am J Psychiatry 1942; 99:174–80.
31. Collins AL. Epileptic intelligence. J Consult Psychol 1951; 15:392–99.
32. Keith HM, Ewert JC, Green MW, Gage RP. Mental status of children with convulsive disorders. Neurology 1955; 5:419–425.
33. Giordani B, Berent S, Sackellares JC, Rourke D, Seidenberg M, O'Leary DS, Dreifuss FE, Boll TJ. Intelligence test performance of patients with partial and generalized seizures. Epilepsia 1985; 26:37–42.
34. Hermann BP, Schwartz MS, Karnes WE, Vahdat P. Psychopathology in epilepsy: relationship of seizure type to age at onset. Epilepsia 1980; 21:15–23.
35. Besag FMC. Cognitive deterioration in children with epilepsy. In: Trimble MR, Reynolds EH, eds. Epilepsy, behavior, and cognitive function. Chichester, West Sussex, England: John Wiley & Sons Ltd., 1988:113–127.
36. Lennox WG, Lennox MA. Epilepsy and related diseases. Boston: Little, Brown and Company, 1960.
37. Delaney RC, Rosen AJ, Mattson RH, Novelly RA. Memory function in focal epilepsy. Cortex 1980; 16:103–17.
38. Ladavas E, Umilta C, Provincialli L. Hemisphere-dependent cognitive performances in epileptic patients. Epilepsia 1979; 20:493–502.
39. Dodrill CB. Neuropsychology of epilepsy. In: Filskov SB, Boll TJ, eds. Handbook of clinical neuropsychology. New York: John Wiley & Sons, Inc., 1981:336–95.
40. Hung TP. Intellectual impairment and behavior disorder in 500 epileptic patients. Pro Aust Assoc Neurol 1968; 5:163–70.
41. Rodin E. Prognosis of cognitive functions in children with epilepsy. In: Hermann BP, Seidenberg M, eds. Childhood epilepsies: neuropsychological, psychosocial and intervention aspects. New York: John Wiley & Sons, Inc., 1989:33–50.

42. Cull CA. Cognitive function and behavior in children. In: Trimble MR, Reynolds EH, eds. Epilepsy, behavior and cognitive function. Chichester, West Sussex, England: John Wiley & Sons, Ltd., 1988:97–111.
43. Mazurowa M. Psychological evaluation of children with post traumatic epilepsy (catamnestic examinations). In: Majkowski J, ed. Posttraumatic epilepsy and pharmacological prophylaxis. Warsaw: International League Against Epilepsy, 1977:69–73.
44. Niemann H, Boenick HE, Schmidt RC, and Ettlinger G. Cognitive development in epilepsy: the relative influence of epileptic activity and of brain damage. Eur Arch Psychiatry Neurol 1985; 234:399–403.
45. Rodin EA. The prognosis of patients with epilepsy. Springfield, IL: Charles C Thomas, 1968.
46. Raina I, Veres J. Life events and seizure frequency in epileptics: a follow-up study. Acta Med Hung 1989; 46:169–87.
47. Seidenberg M, O'Leary DS, Berent S, Boll TJ. Changes in seizure frequency and test–retest scores on the WAIS. Epilepsia 1981; 22:75–83.
48. Giordani B, Sackellares JC, Miller SM, Sutula TP, Boll TJ, Dreifuss FE, Berent S. Changes in neuropsychological test performance following improved seizure control and elimination of barbiturate antiepileptic drugs. Epilepsia 1982; 23:437.
49. Nussbaum K, O'Connor S. Impairment severity in seizure disorders: some suggestions for reliable assessment. J Occup Med 1977; 19:615–18.
50. Mirsky AF, Van Buren JM. On the nature of the "absence" in centren cephalic epilepsy: a study of some behavioral, electroencephalographic and autonomic factors. Electroencephalogr Clin Neurophysiol 1965; 18:334–48.
51. Sackellares JC, Giordani B, Berent S, Seidenberg M, Dreifuss FE, Vanderzant CW, Boll TJ. Patients with pseudoseizures: intellectual and cognitive performance. Neurology 1985; 35:116–19.
52. Porter RJ. Mechanisms of action of new antiepileptic drugs. Epilepsia 1989; 30(Suppl):29–34.
53. Porter RJ. New antiepileptic drugs. Cleve Clin J Med 1989; 56(Suppl):260.
54. Trimble MR. Anticonvulsant drugs and cognitive function: a review of the literature. Epilepsia 1987; 28(Suppl):37–45.
55. Dodrill CB. Effects of antiepileptic drugs on abilities. J Clin Psychiatry 1988; 49(Suppl):31–34.
56. Farwell JR, Lee YJ, Hirtz, DG, Sulzbacher SI, Ellenberg JH, Nelson KB. Phenobarbital for febrile seizures: effects on intelligence and on seizure recurrence. N Engl J Med 1990; 322:364–69.
57. Porter RJ, Schulman EA, Penry JK. Phenytoin monotherapy in intractable epilepsy. Pro 11th Epilepsy Int Symp 1979:126.
58. Trimble MR, Cull CA. Antiepileptic drugs, cognitive function, and behavior in children. Cleve Clin J Med 1989; 56(Suppl):140–46.
59. Vining EP. Cognitive dysfunction associated with antiepileptic drug therapy. Epilepsia 1987; 28(Suppl):18–22.
60. Richens A. Drug treatment of epilepsy. London: Henroy Kimpton, 1976.
61. Thompson PJ, Trimble MR. Anticonvulsant drugs and cognitive functions. Epilepsia 1982; 23:531–44.

62. Shorvon SD, Reynolds EH. Reduction in polypharmacy of epilepsy. Br Med J 1979; 2:1023–25.
63. Thompson PJ. Anticonvulsant drugs, cognitive function, and behavior. Epilepsia 1983; 24(Suppl):55–63.
64. Dekaban AS, Lehman EJB. Effects of different dosages of anticonvulsant drugs on mental performance in patients with chronic epilepsy. Acta Neurol Scand 1975; 52:319–30.
65. Matthews CG, Harley JP. Cognitive and motor sensory performance in toxic and non-toxic epileptic subjects. 1975; 25:184–88.
66. Trimble M, Corbett J. Anticonvulsant drugs and behaviour: preliminary report. Proc 11th Epilepsy Int Symp 1979:47–48.
67. Loiseau P, Strube E, Broustat D, Battellochi S, Gomeni C, Morselli PL. Learning impairment in epileptic patients. Epilepsia 1983; 24:183–92.
68. Oxley J, Richens A, Wadsworth J. Improvement in memory function in epileptic patients following a reduction in serum phenobarbitone levels. Pro 11th Epilepsy Int Symp 1979:52.
69. Bourgeois BFD, Prensky AL, Palkes HS, Talent BK, Busch SG. Intelligence in epilepsy: a prospective study in children. Ann Neurol 1983; 14:438–44.
70. Thompson P, Huppert FA, Trimble M. Phenytoin and cognitive function: effects on normal volunteers and implications for epilepsy. Br J Clin Psychol 1981; 20:155–62.
71. Berent S, Sackellares JC, Giordani B, Wagner JG, Donofrio PD, Abou-Khalil B. Zonisamide (1,2-benzisoxazole-3-methanesulfonamide [CI-912]) and cognition: results from preliminary study. Epilepsia 1987; 28:61–67.
72. Niijima S, Wallace SJ. Effects of puberty on seizure frequency. Dev Med Child Neurol 1989; 31:174–80.
73. Britten N, Wadsworth ME, Fenwick PB. Stigma in patients with early epilepsy: a national longitudinal study. J Epidemiol Community Health. 1984; 38:291–95.
74. Sackellares C, Dreifuss F, Sato S, Penry JK. The effects of other antiepileptic drugs on plasma valproate levels. Pro 11th Epilepsy Int Symp 1979:147.
75. Schmidt D, Canger R, Avanzini G, Battino D, Cusi C, Beck-Mannagetta G, Koch S, Rating D, Janz D. J Neurol Neurosurg Psychiatry 1983; 46:751–55.
76. Wyler AR. The surgical treatment of epilepsy. In: Hermann BP, Seidenberg M, eds. Childhood epilepsies: neuropsychological, psychosocial, and intervention aspects. New York: John Wiley & Sons, Inc. 1989:173–88.
77. Luders H, Wyllie E, Rothner DA, Bourgeois B, Kotagal P. Surgery of localization related epilepsies in children. Brain Dev 1989; 11:98–101.
78. Henriksen O. Surgical treatment of epilepsy: clinical aspects in children. Acta Neurol Scand 1988; 117(Suppl):47–51.
79. Rausch R, Crandall PH. Psychological status related to surgical control of temporal lobe seizures. Epilepsia 1982; 23:191–202.
80. Hermann BP, Wyler AR, Ackerman B, Rosenthal T. Short-term psychological outcome of anterior temporal lobectomy. 1989; 71:327–34.
81. Crandall PH. Postoperative management and criteria for evaluation. In: Purpura DP, Penry JK, Walter RD, eds. Advances in neurology. New York: Raven Press, 1975:265–79.

82. Wannamaker BB, Matthews CG. Prognostic implications of neuropsychological test performance for surgical treatment of epilepsy. J Nerv Ment Dis 1976; 163:29–34.
83. National Association of Epilepsy Centers. Recommended guidelines for diagnosis and treatment in specialized epilepsy centers. Epilepsia 1990; 31(Suppl):1–12.
84. Berent S. Modern approaches to neuropsychological testing. In: Smith D, Treiman D, Trimble M, eds. Advances in neurology. New York: Raven Press, 1991:423–37.

11

Adverse Effects of Antiepileptic Drugs

KEVIN FARRELL
University of British Columbia
Vancouver, British Columbia, Canada

I. INTRODUCTION

The objective of antiepileptic drug therapy is to prevent seizures without causing side effects. Consequently, the decision to use medication should be based on an assessment of the risk of having another seizure, the risks associated with a seizure, and the possible side effects of drug therapy. To do this, the potential side effects associated with each antiepileptic drug should be appreciated. In this chapter we review briefly some of the principles behind drug toxicity and describe both the serious and the common side effects associated with the antiepileptic drugs used most often.

II. GENERAL PRINCIPLES

A. Idiosyncratic Adverse Effects

Idiosyncratic side effects occur very infrequently, are not related to the dose of the drug, and are often serious. Idiosyncratic reactions are associated with a significant risk of severe morbidity or even death. Consequently, the medication should be discontinued promptly in such patients unless there are definite reasons to continue that treatment. The problem is complicated further in patients who develop an idiosyncratic reaction to phenobarbital, phenytoin, or carbamazepine, in that these patients are at a much higher risk of a similar reaction to one of the other two drugs [1].

Fever, skin rash, jaundice, and lymphadenopathy are the most common clinical manifestations of an idiosyncratic drug reaction [1]. Erythema multiforme, the Stevens–Johnson syndrome, and toxic epidermal necrolysis are classical manifestations of an idiosyncratic drug reaction. These conditions may be life-threatening and drug should be stopped immediately if they occur. Scarlatiniform or maculopapular rashes occur more commonly and are often difficult to distinguish from the exanthem associated with certain viral infections. The occurrence of a similar rash in siblings or close contacts would suggest that the rash related to a viral infection. In contrast, the presence of eosinophilia, raised liver enzyme activity, raised antinuclear antibodies, or an abnormal urinalysis would favor the diagnosis of a drug reaction. The decision whether to stop a drug in the presence of a scarlatiniform or maculopapular rash depends on several factors. These include the likelihood of the rash being related to the drug and also the degree of difficulty with which seizure control was acheived in that child. The physician must always bear in mind, however, that a scarlatiniform or maculopapular rash may be the initial manifestation of a life-threatening drug reaction. Consequently, if a decision is made to continue drug treatment, the parents should be made aware of the risks and the child should be monitored closely.

The pathophysiology of idiosyncratic side effects is not understood fully but may involve a genetically determined abnormality in drug metabolism. When lymphocytes from patients who have had a serious drug reaction to phenobarbital, phenytoin, or carbamazepine are incubated with the involved drug, they exhibit a much higher cell death than that of lymphocytes from patients who do not develop a reaction to that drug [1]. Furthermore, lymphocytes from the parents of such patients demonstrate an intermediate degree of toxicity [2]. The abnormal lymphocyte toxicity is observed only when a microsomal system is added to the incubation process. This suggests that a microsomal metabolite of the drug may be involved in the toxicity.

B. Concentration-Dependent Adverse Effects

Although gastrointestinal side effects may be the result of a direct local effect, most common side effects are related to the concentration of the drug in the blood. Such side effects become more obvious as the dose is increased and diminish as the dose is decreased. The blood level of a drug reflects the concentration of the drug in the body and is determined for the most part by a few basic principles. An understanding of these basic principles can help to prevent side effects caused by inappropriate dosage changes, and is important in the interpretation and proper use of antiepileptic blood levels.

The absorption of certain drugs, such as carbamazepine and valproic acid, may be rapid and result in a marked variation in the blood levels throughout the

Table 1 Pharmacokinetic Parameters of Antiepileptic Drugs

Drug	Half-life (hours)	Time to steady state (days)	Protein binding (%)	Therapeutic range (μg/mL)
Phenobarbital	60–100	12–21	45–55	10–40
Phenytoin	See text	5–21[a]	80–95	10–20
Ethosuxmide	15–68	3–14	<10	30–100
Carbamazepine	15–24	3–5	65–80	4–12
Valproic acid	10–18	2–4	80–90	30–100
Clonazepam	20–30	4–6	80–90	Not established

[a]The time to reach steady state at higher phenytoin concentrations is at the uppper end of the range (see the text).

day. Transient side effects may occur when the blood level reaches a peak. When a side effect occurs at a particular time of the day, the possibility that it relates to a high "peak level" should be considered and the blood level measured at that time of day. Absorption is determined partly by the formulation of the drug. Formulations of certain drugs, including valproic acid, have been developed which result in a slower rate of absorption and less fluctuation in blood levels throughout the day. When a sustained-release formulation is not available, the side effects may resolve if the same amount of drug is administered as smaller doses given more frequently.

The blood level of a drug rises progressively after treatment is begun until a steady state is reached. The time taken to reach steady state is determined by the rate at which the body metabolizes the drug and is approximately five times the drug's half-life—the time it takes for the blood level of the drug to fall by half. Antiepileptic drugs are metabolized at different rates and the approximate times taken to reach steady state for these drugs are listed in Table 1. Adjusting the drug dosage after the drug level has reached a steady state will reduce the risk of blood levels within the toxic range. The elimination of phenytoin is more complex than that of most drugs. At higher phenytoin blood levels, the drug is cleared more slowly and the time taken to reach steady state may be much longer. For this reason, dosage increases of phenytoin should be limited to 25 mg when the blood level is within the therapeutic range and 50 mg when the level is below the therapeutic range.

The aim of antiepileptic drug treatment is to control seizures without side effects, not to achieve a blood level within the therapeutic range. There is considerable variation between patients in both the blood level required to control seizures and that at which side effects occur. Thus seizures are controlled in many patients at drug levels below the therapeutic range. Similarly, patients often experience no side effects at drug levels above the therapeutic range. In con trast, dose-dependent side effects may occur in some patients at blood levels within the therapeutic range. For these reasons, the adjustment of drug dosage should be based mainly on clinical assessment and the measurement of blood levels should be used to answer specific clinical concerns. The side effects of certain drugs, particularly phenobarbital and phenytoin, may be insidious and difficult to detect, especially in the handicapped child. In that situation, monitoring of blood levels may alert one to the possibility of drug toxicity.

Many antiepileptic drugs are bound to plasma proteins (Table 1), and only the unbound portion is pharmacologically active. The blood level measured in most laboratories is the total drug level, which includes both the bound and unbound fractions of the drug. Because the protein binding of drugs does not usually vary significantly in the majority of patients, the total drug level is a reasonable reflection of the unbound drug level. On the other hand, protein binding may be decreased by hepatic dysfunction, renal failure, pregnancy, disorders causing hypoproteinemia, and by other medications. If the protein binding is altered in highly bound drugs such as phenytoin or valproic acid, the total blood level is not a true reflection of the unbound level. In that situation, side effects may occur at total levels within the therapeutic range. Thus phenytoin toxicity may be observed at blood levels between 15 and 20 μg/mL in patients also receiving valproic acid, which displaces phenytoin from protein-binding sites [3]. The occurrence of side effects at total blood levels within the therapeutic range may also be due to a high concentration of a metabolite of the drug. This may occur particularly with carbamazepine, which is metabolized to carbamazepine 10, 11-epoxide, a major metabolite that can cause side effects [4].

C. Tolerance

Tolerance is the reduction in the pharmacologic effect of a drug following repeated administration. Tolerance may develop either to the desired activity or to the adverse effects of a drug. Tolerance to the neurologic side effects of many antiepileptic drugs tends to occur over days or weeks in most individuals. Thus the neurologic side effects of many antiepileptic drugs, particularly the benzodiazepines, phenobarbital, and carbamazepine, can be minimized by starting with a low dose of the drug and increasing the dose gradually every 5 to 7 days.

D. Drug Interactions

The complexity of the metabolic and binding interactions between many of the antiepileptic drugs is one of the major reasons for using monotherapy. Phenobarbital, phenytoin, and carbamazepine induce the hepatic microsomal metabolism of many other drugs, resulting in lower blood levels and decreased efficacy of these drugs [5] (Table 2). In contrast, valproic acid inhibits the metabolism of

Table 2 Nonepileptic Drugs That May Have Reduced Efficacy When Used in Combination with Phenobarbital, Primidone, Phenytoin, or Carbamazepine

Corticosteroids
Oral contraceptives
Cyclosporine
Theophylline
Chloramphenicol
Coumadin
Vitamin K
Digoxin
Quinidine
Haloperidol

phenobarbital, resulting in higher phenobarbital levels. Interactions may also influence protein-binding or specific metabolic pathways, and these may result in toxicity at blood levels within the therapeutic range (see above). Important interactions may also occur with nonprescription medications. Thus acetylsalicylic acid has a complex effect on the protein binding and β-oxidation of valproic acid [6] and may result in valproate toxicity [7].

E. Detection of Adverse Drug Effects

The majority of side effects are recognized by the patient or can be detected on clinical examination. Education of the patient and/or parents is essential. They should be made aware of all serious or life-threatening side effects and of the common side effects of a drug. Provision of a drug information sheet can be particularly helpful. Such a sheet should list the early clinical signs of serious toxicity, the more common side effects, and any important drug interactions.

The value of performing laboratory tests in the hope of early detection of a serious side effect is very doubtful. Whereas severe reactions to antiepileptic drugs occur in approximately 1 in 20,000 to 1 in 50,000 newly treated patients [8], the incidence of clinically insignificant abnormal laboratory tests is relatively high. Elevated serum, glutamic-oxaloacetic transaminase activity was observed in approximately 14% of children on monotherapy in one study, occurring in children on phenobarbital (15%), phenytoin (9%), carbamazepine (9%), and valproic acid (15%) [8]. Although SGOT activities of more than two times the upper end of the normal range were observed in one-third of the patients with elevated enzymes, all repeat measurements were closer to normal and the medication was not required to be discontinued on the basis of abnormal SGOT activity. Similarly, transient leukopenia occurs in approximately 10% of patients receiving carbamazepine [4]. The recognition of these clinically insignificant laboratory abnormalities may also be associated with certain drawbacks. Abnormal laboratory tests are often repeated, rarely alter management,and result in unnecessary anxiety for the parent and child [8]. In addition, the annual cost for measuring a complete blood count, SGOT, and platelet count three times each year in every person with epilepsy in North America has been estimated to be approximately $400,000,000 [8]. A greater awareness on the part of the patient, parents, and physician of the early clinical signs of potentially serious side effects is much more important. The parent and child should be instructed to contact a physician immediately if any of these signs appear [9]. Laboratory monitoring should be performed prior to starting the drug and thereafter if there are clinical concerns. A closer surveillance should be considered for those at high risk, such as children less than 3 years of age who are receiving valproate polytherapy.

III. INDIVIDUAL DRUGS

A. Phenobarbital

1. Serious Side Effects

Erythema multiforme, the Stevens–Johnson syndrome, and toxic epidermal necrolysis are rare but serious complications of phenobarbital therapy, which require that the medication be discontinued [10]. Scarlatiniform or maculopapular rashes occur in 1 to 3% of patients receiving phenobarbital [11] and can be difficult to distinguish from viral exanthemata. The presence of lymphadenopathy, hepatomegaly, eosinophilia, elevated liver enzymes, or an abnormal urinalysis would suggest a hypersensitivity reaction. In contrast, it may be appropriate to observe the patient with only a mild erythema without altering the medication. In one study, the rash that developed during phenobarbital therapy was transient and did not require a change in treatment in 5 of the 13 patients [19].

A hypersensitivity reaction characterized by eosinophilic or granulomatous infiltration of the liver, and presenting with rash, conjunctivitis, lympadenopathy, eosinophilia, and fever is a rare but life-threatening complication of phenobarbital therapy and precludes further use of that drug. In contrast, increased liver enzyme activity occurs in 15% of children receiving phenobarbital [8]. The hepatic histology in such children demonstrates no evidence of specific liver disease [12]. Consequently, the presence of raised liver enzymes in the absence of other evidence of a hypersensitivity reaction should not be considered an indication for withdrawal of phenobarbital.

The teratogenicity associated with phenobarbital appears to be less than that associated with other antiepileptic drugs [10]. A severe coagulation defect has been observed in neonates born to mothers receiving antiepileptic drugs, particularly phenobarbital [13]. This abnormality in coagulation can be prevented by administering vitamin K to the mother prior to delivery [10]

2. Other Side Effects

Adverse effects on behavior, affect, and cognition are common in children receiving phenobarbital, even at serum levels less than 15 μg/mL [14]. Hyperactivity, sleep disturbance, and aggressive behavior are the most common side effects in children. Altered mood and depression may also occur. Tolerance to these side effects may develop in some patients after several weeks. Dysarthria, ataxia, and nystagmus are usually observed at higher serum concentrations. Dyskinesias and Tourette-like symptoms appear to be more common in the neurologically impaired child [15].

Phenobarbital may have subtle effects on memory and cognition and it is important to play close attention to the school performance of any child receiving this drug. The educational difficulties encountered by these children are often greater than would be expected on the basis of standardized psychologic tests [16]. This may represent a lack of sensitivity of such tests to the impairment caused by the phenobarbital. Phenobarbital appears to be associated with more cognitive and behavioral disturbances than does valproic acid [17]. Furthermore, it has been suggested that the effect of phenobarbital on cognitive performance may outlast use of the drug by several months [18].

Phenobarbital has relatively few systemic side effects. Mild leukopenia may occur but is rarely of clinical significance [19]. Gastrointestinal side effects occur less frequently than in patients receiving other antiepileptic drugs [10]. Low serum folate levels have been observed in some patients receiving phenobarbital, but the significance of this abnormality is uncertain and megaloblastic anemia is rare [10]. Patients receiving phenobarbital over a prolonged period, particularly those on polytherapy, may develop mild vitamin D deficiency [20].

3. Interactions

Phenobarbital induces the hepatic mixed-function oxidase system and increases the clearance of many drugs (Table 2). The serum concentrations of phenytoin, valproic acid, carbamazepine, and clonazepam are generally lower in patients receiving phenobarbital comedication. Similarly, the increased clearances of oral contraceptives, warfarin, prednisone, and dexamethasone in patients receiving phenobarbital may be clinically significant and necessitate adjustment of the dosages of these drugs [21]. Valproic acid, acetazolamide, and very occasionally, phenytoin may inhibit phenobarbital metabolism and result in increased phenobarbital blood levels [22].

B. Phenytoin

1. Serious Side Effects

Phenytoin hypersensitivity occurs usually within 2 months of starting treatment [23]. Rash, fever, generalized lymphadenopathy, and hepatitis are the major manifestations of phenytoin hypersensitivity. A morbilliform rash, erythema multiforme, and Stevens–Johnson syndrome are the most common dermatologic manifestation of phenytoin hypersensitivity. The latter two conditions are absolute indications to discontinue phenytoin therapy. The incidence of skin rash appears to be higher in patients receiving an initial high dose of phenytoin, and the rash may resolve if the dose is reduced [24]. However, the risk of developing a more serious drug reaction makes withdrawal of the drug advisable in most patients.

Fatal hepatic involvement is a rare manifestation of phenytoin hypersensitivity. Because raised liver enzyme activity has been described in 9% of children receiving phenytoin, routine measurement of liver enzyme activity is not an effective method of predicting serious hepatotoxicity [8]. The possibilty of a serious hepatitis should be considered if fever, a rash, lymphoid hyperplasia, or clinical signs of liver dysfunction are present.

Pure red cell aplasia, agranulocytosis, and thrombocytopenia are extrememly rare side effects of phenytoin, but mild leukopenia may be observed, particularly in the early months of treatment [25]. Routine laboratory monitoring for these abnormalities has not been demonstrated to be of value.

Children born to mothers receiving phenytoin during pregnancy have an increased incidence of congenital abnormalities. A higher incidence of congenital abnormalities has been observed in mothers who have received phenytoin at higher dosages or in combination with other drugs [26]. A severe coagulation defect, similar to that described with vitamin K deficiency, has been reported in neonates born to mothers receiving phenytoin during the pregnancy [13]. This coagulation abnormality can be prevented by administering vitamin K to the mother prior to delivery [10].

2. Other Side Effects

Blurred vision, nystagmus, ataxia, and sedation are concentration-dependent side effects of phenytoin. One or more of these signs may be absent, particularly in the handicapped child, in whom neurotoxicity may be easily overlooked [27]. The persistence of ataxia after withdrawal of phenytoin has been described in several patients who had experienced prolonged acute toxicity [28]. For this reason, early diagnosis of phenytoin neurotoxicity is important. Phenytoin-related dyskinesias occur more often in children with neurologic handicap and have been described at levels within the therapeutic range [25]. A few reports have described and exacerbation of seizures at phenytoin levels above the therapeutic range [25]. Peripheral polyneuropathy has been reported in patients receiving phenytoin, particularly in patients on polytherapy [25].

Phenytoin may impair concentration, memory, cognitive function, and motor speed. These effects appear to be dose-related and may be difficult to diagnose. Thus careful attention must be made to the developmental and educational performance of children receiving phenytoin. A progressive pseudodementia may also occur in the neurologically impaired child and may be the only manifestation of phenytoin toxicity [29].

Hyperplasia of the gums is observed frequently in children receiving phenytoin. Regular brushing may help to minimize this effect. Hirsutism, acne, pigmentation of the skin, enlargement of the subcutaneous tissues leading to coarsening of the facial features, and radiologic evidence of calvarial thickening are other side effects observed with prolonged phenytoin therapy. These effects can have a marked impact on the self image of patients, particularly girls.

Phenytoin treatment may result in folate deficiency in some patients, possibly by affecting folate absorption or by induction of the enzymes involved in folate metabolism [25]. The incidence of folate deficiency appears to be lower in patients on monotherapy. The significance of folate deficiency in children receiving phenytoin is uncertain, but folate deficiency has been implicated in the neurotoxicity associated with phenytoin [30]. Megaloblastic anemia is uncommon in patients receiving phenytoin. Folic acid supplementation is of uncertain value in the asymptomatic patient, but a daily dose of 1 to 3 mg has been recommended during pregnancy [31]. Metabolic bone disease manifesting as rickets or fractures has been described in patients phenytoin treatment but is rare in patients on monotherapy [25].

3. Interactions

The metabolism of phenytoin is unusual in that at higher concentrations a small dosage increase may result in a disproportionately large rise in the blood level. Thus dosage increases should not exceed 25 mg when the blood level is in the therapeutic range. Phenobarbital and carbamazepine may increase or decrease the phenytoin level. Consequently, blood levels should be monitored in patients on polytherapy if there is a change in the dosage of any of the drugs. Phenytoin enhances the metabolism of certain drugs and may cause a fall in the blood levels of the drugs listed in Table 2. Phenytoin is normally a highly protein-bound drug, but it is displaced from its protein-binding sites by valproic acid. Thus the total phenytoin concentration may not reflect accurately the free phenytoin level. Consequently, patients receiving both drugs may exhibit phenytoin toxicity at phenytoin concentrations between 14 and 20 μg/mL.

C. Ethosuximide

1. Serious Side Effects

Serious adverse effects are rare in patients receiving ethosuximide. The medication should be discontinued in patients who develop a skin rash. Steroid therapy may be required in patients with Stevens–Johnson syndrome or erythema multiforme. A lupus syndrome has been described in children receiving ethosuximide and usually responds to withdrawal of the drug [32]. Asymptomatic children with antinuclear antibodies do not usually develop lupus, but these children should be followed more closely [32].

Agranulocytosis and pancytopenia have been reported in children receiving ethosuximide and monitoring of blood counts at monthly intervals has been recommended [32]. On the other hand, the effectiveness of this approach in preventing serious blood disorders has not been demonstrated, and routine laboratory monitoring appears to be of doubtful value [9]. There is limited information on the teratogenic effect of ethosuximide but experimental studies suggest that this drug is substantially less toxic than the other major antiepileptic drugs [33].

2. Other Side Effects

Nausea and drowsiness are the side effects observed most often in patients receiving ethosuximide [34]. Anorexia, vomiting, epigastric discomfort, and diarrhea may also occur, particularly in the first few weeks of of treatment. These symptoms may diminish if the drug is administered with meals or if smaller doses are used at more frequent intervals.

Drowsiness and cognitive dysfunction appear to be related to serum levels of ethosuximide. Although educational acheivement improves in many children as the absence seizures are controlled, the cognitive side effects of ethosuximide may result in a deterioration in school performance [35]. Adolescents and adults receiving ethosuximide have a high incidence of more serious behavioral and psychiatric effects [36]. The development of psychiatric disturbance following control of absence seizures occurs more frequently in patients receiving ethosuximide than in those on volproate [36]. Those with previous history of emotional or mental illness are more likely to develop this complication. The manifestations include aggresiveness, depression, sleep disturbance, anxiety, and psychosis [36].

When headaches complicate ethosuximide therapy, they tend not to respond to a simple reduction in the dosage and often require that the medication be withdrawn [32]. Acute dyskinesias, similar to those observed in patients receiving phenothiazines, have been described occasionally following treatment with ethosuximide [37].

3. Interactions

Comedication with valproic acid may result in elevated ethosuximide levels, possibly by inhibition of ethosuximide metabolism [38,39]. Carbamazepine induces the metabolism of ethosuximide and results in lower serum ethosuximide levels [40]. Other enzyme-inducing drugs may have a similar effect.

D. Carbamazepine

1. Serious Side Effects

Skin rashes have been described in 2 to 17% of patients receiving carbamazepine and are mild and transient in the majority of patients, even when treatment in continued [41]. On the other hand, exfoliative dermatitis, Stevens–Johnson syndrome, and Lyell syndrome are life-threatening, and carbamazepine should be discontinued immediately if there are features of these disorders. A more generalized hypersensitivity reaction involving fever, skin rash, generalized lymphadenopathy, hepatosplenomegaly, pulmonary symptoms, renal involvement, and myocarditis has been reported in patients receiving carbamazepine. These abnormalities resolve in most patients if the carbamazepine is discontinued, but treatment with corticosteriods may be helpful in patients with more severe involvement [42].

Aplastic anemia, agranulocytosis, and thrombocytopenia are life threatening but rare complications of carbamazepine therapy. Aplastic anemia complicates carbamazepine therapy in approximately 1 in 200,000 patients, agranulocytosis in approximately 1 in 700,000 patients, and death due to either of the above occurs in approximately 1 in 450,000 patients [43]. By contrast, clinically insignificant leukopenia occurs in approximately 10% of children and adults [44] and is transient in the majority [43]. For these reasons, routine monitoring of the white blood count, although advocated frequently, is unlikely to be effective in detecting the rare patient with life-threatening toxicity. Furthermore, abnormalities in the white count are more likely to lead to unnecessary changes in treatment or to further laboratory investigations in the 10% of patients with transient leukopenia. It is the author's practice to advise the patient and parents of the remote possibility of a serious side effect and to educate them about the early clinical features. In addition, a complete blood count is measured prior to starting therapy and thereafter whenever there is clinical concern. A white blood count of less than $2500/mm^{-3}$ or a neutrophil count of less than $1000/mm^{-3}$ should lead to careful clinical assessment, but discontinuation of the medication is rarely necessary. Thus the abnormal white count will be transient and relate to an intercurrent viral infection in most such children.

Serious hepatotoxicity occurs rarely in patients receiving carbamazepine, but the drug should be discontinued in any patient who develops jaundice or other signs of a generalized hypersensitivity. On the other hand, there is no indication to alter the medication in those 5 to 10% of patients receiving carbamazepine who develop elevated serum liver enzymes without clinical signs [8,43].

2. *Other Side Effects*

The majority of the side effects associated with carbamazepine are related to the drug level and can be eliminated by reducing the dose. The serum concentration of carbamazepine may fluctuate markedly during the day. Thus it is important to measure the blood level at the time of day when the patient complains of symptoms. Carbamazepine-10,11-epoxide, a major metabolite of carbamazepine, is not measured by most clinical laboratories but may be responsible for some of the toxicity associated with carbamazepine therapy. Patients on carbamazepine polytherapy appear to have a higher ratio of the 10,11-epoxide to the parent drug. For this reason, adverse effects may occur at blood levels within the therapeutic range, particularly in patients receiving polytherapy.

Drowsiness is one of the most frequently reported side effects of carbamazepine therapy and may be particularly prominent at the start of treatment [44]. The incidence and severity of drowsiness at the start of treatment may be lessened by the use of a low initial dose and small dosage increments at 5- to 7-day intervals. Periods of drowsiness occurring around the same time of day are strongly suggestive of carbamazepine toxicity. This side effect may be eliminated by reducing the daily dose or by administering the drug at more frequent intervals. Although drowsiness may be a problem at the start of treatment in some patients, the cognitive side effects associated with carbamazepine appear to be less than those associated with other antiepileptic drugs, particularly phenytoin and phenobarbital [45].

Nausea, vomiting, diplopia, nystagmus, ataxia, and slurred speech are among the most common manifestations of acute carbamazepine toxicity and respond to total daily dose reduction or to giving smaller doses more frequently. Movement disorders, including tics, chorea, dystonia, and myoclonus, appear to occur more frequently in neurologically impaired individuals and may respond to a reduction in the carbamazepine dose [41].

Carbamazepine may exacerbate seizures in some patients, particularly those with nonconvulsive seizures and those with generalized slow spike and wave on the EEG [46]. The seizures that arise are usually myoclonic, atonic, or absence seizures. Carbamazepine prolongs atrioventricular conduction time in animals, and conduction abnormalities have been described in association with carbamazepine therapy in a few patients [47]. This effect may be dose related, and care should be taken in children with abnormalities of cardiac conduction.

3. Interactions

The metabolism of carbamazepine may be inhibited or induced by other drugs. A marked increase in serum carbamazepine levels sufficient to cause coma has been described in patients receiving erythromycin or propoxyphene, both of which inhibit the metabolism of carbamazepine significantly [48]. Comedication with acetazolamide, isoniazide, cimetidine, imipramine, diltiazem, and denzimol may also increase serum carbamazepine levels [48].

Decreased serum carbamazepine levels may occur following comedication with phenytoin, phenobarbital, primidone, or valproic acid, which induce hepatic microsomal metabolism. However, induction of carbamazepine metabolism may also be associated with increased blood levels of carbamazepine 10,11-epoxide (CBZ epoxide), a major metabolite of carbamazepine [49]. In addition, valproic acid inhibits the further metabolism of the CBZ epoxide and results in an increase in serum CBZ-epoxide levels [49]. Although CBZ epoxide may cause side effects, this metabolite is not measured by the enzyme immunoassay methods used in most medical laboratories. Thus patients receiving carbamazepine in combination with valproic acid and phenobarbital or phenytoin may develop high CBZ-epoxide levels and exhibit toxicity at carbamazepine levels within the therapeutic range.

Carbamazepine induces the hepatic microsomal system, and this may lead to a decrease in the blood levels of a variety of drugs, including phentoin, valproic acid, phenobarbital, coumadin, and doxycycline [48] [Table 2].

E. Valproic Acid

1. Idiosyncratic Effects

a. Severe Hepatotoxicity. Severe hepatotoxicity, occurs most often in the very young child and in those receiving other drugs. The incidence of fatal hepatotoxicity in children under 3 years of age who are taking valproic acid as polytherapy is between 1 in 500 and 1 in 800 [50,51]. By contrast, the incidence of hepatic fatality in patients between 3 and 20 years of age is 1 in 20,000 to 1 in 50,000 in those on monotherapy, and 1 in 8000 to 1 in 17,000 in those on polytherapy [50,51]. The increased incidence of VPA hepatotoxicity in infancy may be related, in part, to the exacerbation of inborn errors of metabolism. Thus fatal hepatic failure has been described in several sets of siblings in whom only one of the siblings has received valproic acid [51–53).

Plasma carnitine levels below the normal range have been described in children receiving valproic acid [54]. The decrease in plasma carnitine levels may relate to the involvement of carnitine in the elimination of valproic acid by the formation of a valproylcarnitine conjugate [55]. The possibility that hypocarnitinemia may play a role in valproic acid–induced hepatotoxicity [56,57] has led to the suggestion that plasma carnitine levels should be measured in patients receiving valproic acid who develop unexplained weakness, lethargy, or hypotonia, and in those with evidence of hepatic dysfunction [58]. Oral carnitine supplementation at a dose of 100 mg/kg per day has been suggested for symptomatic children receiving valproate in whom hypocarnitinemia is demonstrated [58]. Although the evidence that hypocarnitinemia is causatively implicated in valproate hepatotoxicity is circumstantial, the adverse effects associated with carnitine therapy are relatively minor and occur infrequently [54].

Fatal valproic acid hepatotoxicity occurs most often in the first 6 months of therapy, and patients with mental retardation are at highest risk. The prodromal symptoms include lethargy, edema, jaundice, anorexia, nausea and vomiting, and loss of seizure control. The value of routine monitoring of liver enzymes in the early prediction or diagnosis of severe valproic acid hepatotoxicity has not been established. Abnormal liver enzyme activity has been described in up to 44% of patients receiving valproic acid [56]. Thus routine monitoring is likely to be associated with a lot of unnecessary repeat testing and increased anxiety and discomfort for the child and parents. A more important approach is the education of the patient and parents in the early clinical features of valproic acid hepatotoxicity and the advice to contact a physician immediately if any of these occur. On the other hand, it may be prudent to monitor liver enzymes in those at particular risk of developing valproate hepatotoxicity, especially the very young child on polytherapy [59].

b. Pancreatitis. Valproic acid–induced pancreatitis is a rare complication that does not appear to be dose dependent. The pancreatitis develops within the first 6 months of treatment in most patients, although is has occurred as late as 4 years after starting the drug [60,61]. Exploratory laparotomy has been associated with a higher morbidity and mortality, and surgery should be avoided [61]. Pancreatitis has recurred in most patients who have been rechallenged with the drug. Pancreatitis should be suspected in any patient receiving valproic acid who develops abdominal pain and vomiting. The drug should be stopped immediately and serum amylase measured. However, routine monitoring of serum amylase is not necessary in asymptomatic patients [61].

c. Teratogenicity. An increased incidence of congenital abnormalities has been described in children born to mothers receiving valproic acid during pregnancy. Neural tube defects (spina bifida and anencephaly) occur in 1 to 2% of exposed fetuses, and valproic acid monotherapy may be associated with a higher risk than polytherapy [62]. In addition, infants born to mothers receiving valproic acid appear to have a higher incidence of other major malformations and of minor craniofacial and digital anomalies than do those born to mothers receiving other antiepileptic drugs [63]. Finally, developmental delay and behavior disturbance have been reported in infants born to mothers receiving valproic acid [64,65].

In is important to inform adolescent females and those of child-bearing age of the teratogenic risks associated with this drug. The incidence of both major and minor anomalies may be dose dependent [66] and the lowest possible dose should be used during pregnancy. Amniocentesis and ultrasound may permit the intrauterine diagnosis of a neural tube defect.

2. Other Side Effects

The correlation between the serum concentration and pharmacologic effect of valproic acid is not as strong as with certain other antiepileptic drugs. Many of the less serious side effects may be observed at concentrations in the middle of the therapeutic range. However, these side effects usually resolve if the dose is reduced.

Nausea and epigastric discomfort are among the more common side effects associated with valproic acid and relate partly to the formulation used. Some retarded children receiving valproic acid syrup appear to be particularly bothered by these symptoms. A much lower incidence of gastrointestinal side effects has been observed in those receiving the enteric-coated valproic acid formulations.

Excessive weight gain is a well-described side effect that appears to be the result of a central effect on the satiety mechanism [67]. Weight gain occurs in between 20 and 44% of children receiving valproic acid [68,69] and may be a particular problem in young women. This side effect is best dealt with by dosage reduction or by a dietary approach.

Drowsiness is a relatively uncommon side effect of valproic acid monotherapy [70]. The higher incidence of drowsiness in patients receiving valproic acid polytherapy may relate partly to the effect of valproic acid on other drug levels. For example, valproic acid may increase both serum phenobarbital and serum ethosuximide concentrations by impairing the clearance of these drugs; valproic acid increases the levels of carbamazepine 10,11-epoxide, an active metabolite that may cause toxicity, and valproic acid decreases the protein binding of phenytoin, with the result that phenytoin toxicity is common at serum phenytoin concentrations above 15 μg/mL.

Stupor and coma have been described in patients receiving valproic acid at blood levels within the therapeutic range [71]. Hyperammonemia may be the cause of altered consciousness in some patients receiving valproic acid and should be excluded. However, hyperammonemia has not been observed in most affected children [67]. Stupor has also been described in patients receiving valproic acid in combination with acetylsalycilic acid [7]. Acetylsalycilic acid alters the protein binding and inhibits the β-oxidation of valproic acid [6] and should be avoided in patients receiving valproic acid.

Action tremor resembling benign essential tremor has been described in 2% of patients receiving valproic acid [70]. Reduction of the dose of valproic acid is usually sufficient to lessen this side effect. If it is essential to maintain the valproic acid dose, treatment with propanolol may be effective [72]. Intermediary metabolism is affected by valproic acid, and mild hyperglycinemia and hyperammonemia are common. These are not usually associated with clinical symptoms, and routine monitoring of blood ammonia and amino acids is not appropriate. On the other hand, valproic acid may exacerbate certain rare inborn errors of metabolism. Consequently, valproic acid should be used with caution in children in whom such a disorder is suspected and in children with a family history of a metabolic disorder or of unexplained death in childhood [52,53].

Various hematologic abnormalities have been described in patients receiving valproic acid [70]. Thrombocytopenia, abnormalities of platelet aggregation, and hypofibrinogenemia are the abnormalities that have been reported most often. The majority of patients with these changes have been asymptomatic and the hematologic effects of valproic acid have been considered to be of little clinical significance except in patients undergoing surgery [73]. Neutropenia and bone-marrow suppression have also been described but are rare and usually clinically insignificant [74].

F. Benzodiazepines

1. Diazepam

Diazepam administered intravenously may cause sedation. hypotonia, respiratory depression, and hypotension. These side effects occur more often in children also receiving phenobarbital [75]. The respiratory depression and hypotension may relate to the propylene glycol solvent used in the preparation of the intravenous solution [76] and rapid administration of the intravenous solution should be avoided. Clinically significant respiratory depression is extremely uncommon in children receiving diazepam rectally [77]. Children who are markedly underweight, retarded, or are receiving phenobarbital may be at greater risk [78]. Consequently, it may be wise to give a test dose in a hospital or office setting if rectal diazepam is prescribed for the acute treatment of convulsions at home in such children.

2. Lorazepam

Although considered initially to have less toxicity than diazepam, intravenous lorazepam administered with phenytoin has been associated with a similar incidence of cardiorespiratory depression as intravenous diazepam and phenytoin [79]. In addition, the absorption of lorazepam administered rectally is slow and erratic [80]. This limits the usefulness of rectal lorazepam in the acute treatment of status epilepticus [80]. Both lorazepam and diazepam may exacerbate tonic seizures in children with secondary generalized epilepsy, and tonic status epilepticus may be precipitated in some children [81,82].

3. Clonazepam

The neurotoxicity associated with clonazepam has limited the usefulness of this drug. Drowsiness, ataxia, and behavioral changes are the most frequently reported side effects. Patients may develop tolerance to these side effects, Consequently, treatment with clonazepam should be started at a low initial dose and the dose increased by small amounts every 5 to 7 days. Comedication with phenobarbital appears to exacerbate the drowsiness [83] and this drug combination should be avoided if possible. Hypotonia, increased salivation, and bronchial hypersecretion may also occur and increase the risk of respiratory complications, particularly in the immobile handicapped child. Increased appetite and marked weight gain occurred in 9 of 81 children treated with clonazepam [84]. Withdrawal seizures may occur when clonazepam is discontinued rapidly, and a dosage reduction of 0.25 mg/week has been recommended [85].

REFERENCES

1. Shear NH, Spielberg SP. Anticonvulsant hypersensitivity syndrome. J Clin Invest 1988; 82:1826–32.
2. Spielberg SP, Gordon GB, Blake DA, Goldstein DA, Herlong HF. Predisposition to phenytoin hepatotoxicity assessed in vitro. N Engl J Med 1981; 305:722–27.
3. Mattson RH, Cramer JA. Valproate: interactions with other drugs. In: Levy R, Mattson R, Meldrum B, Penry JK, Dreifuss FE, eds. Antiepileptic drugs. New York: Raven Press, 1989:621–32.
4. Gram L, Jensen PK. Carbamazepine: toxicity. In: Levy R, Mattson R, Meldrum B, Penry JK, Dreifuss FE, eds. Antiepileptic drugs. New York: Raven Press, 1989:555–65.
5. Perucca, E. Clinical implications of hepatic microsomal enzyme induction by antiepileptic drugs. Pharmacol Ther 1987; 33:139–44.
6. Abbott FS, Kassam J, Orr JM, Farrell K. The effect of aspirin on valproic acid metabolism. Clin Pharmacol Ther 1986; 40:94–100.
7. Goulden KJ, Dooley JM, Camfield PR, Fraser AD. Clinical valproate toxicity induced by acetylsalicylic acid. Neurology 1987; 37:1393–94.
8. Camfield C, Camfield P, Smith E. Tibbles JAR. Asymptomatic children with epilepsy: little benefit from screening for anticonvulsant induced liver, blood, or renal damage. Neurology 1986; 36:838–41.
9. Camfield P, Camfield C, Dooley J, Farrell K, Humphries P, Langevin P. Routine screening of blood and urine for severe reactions to anticonvulsant drugs in asymptomatic patients is of doubtful value. Can Med Assoc 1989; 140:1303–5.
10. Mattson RH, Cramer JA. Phenobarbital: toxicity. In: Levy Rh, Dreifuss FE, Mattson RH, Meldrum BS, Penry JK, eds. Antiepileptic drugs. New York: Raven Press, 1989:341–55.
11. Schmidt RP, Wilder BJ. Epilepsy. Philadelphia: FA Davis Company, 1968.
12. Aiges HW, Daum F, Olson M, Kahn E, Teichberg S. The effects of phenobarbital and diphenylhydantoin on liver function and morphology. Pediatr 1980; 97:22–26.
13. Mountain KR, Hirsh J, Gallus AS. Neonatal coagulation defect due to anticonvulsant drug treatment in pregnancy. Lancet 1970; i:265–68.
14. Wolf SM, Forsythe AB. Behaviour disturbance, phenobarbital and febrile seizures. Paediatrics 1978; 61:728–31.
15. Sandyk R. Phenobarbital-induced Tourette-like symptoms. Pediatr Neurol 1986; 2:54–55.
16. Stores G. Behavioural effects of antiepileptic drugs. Dev Med Child Neurol 1975; 17:647–58.
17. Vining EPG, Mellits Ed, Dorsen MM, Cataldo MF, Quaskey SA, Spielberg SP, Freeman JM. Psychologic and behavioural effects of antiepileptic drugs in children: A double-blind comparison between phenobarbital and valproic acid. Pediatrics 1987; 80:165–73.
18. Farwell JR, Lee YJ, Hirtz DG, Sulzbacher SI, Ellenberg JH, Nelson KB. Phenobarbital for febrile seizures: effects on intelligence and on seizure recurrence. N Engl J Med 1990; 322:364–69.

19. Matson RH, Cramer JA, Collins JF, Smith DB, Delgado-Escueta AV, Browne TR, Williamson PD, Treiman DM, McNamara JO, McCutchen CB, Homan RW, Crill WE, Lubozynski MF, Rosenthal NP, Mayersdorf A. Comparison of carbamazepine, phenobarbital, phenytoin and primidone in partial and secondarily generalized tonic–clonic seizures. N Eng J Med 1985; 313:145–51.
20. Offermann G. Chronic antiepileptic drug treatment and disorders of mineral metabolism. In: Oxley J, Janz D, Meinardi H, eds. Chronic Toxicity of Antiepileptic Drugs. New York: Raven Press, 1983:175–84.
21. Loiseau P, Duche B. Phenobarbital. In: Dam M, Gram L, eds. Comprehensive Epileptology. New York: Raven Press, 1990:579–91
22. Kutt H, Phenobarbital: interactions with other drugs. In: Levy RH, Dreifuss FE, Mattson RH, Meldrum BS, Penry JK, eds. Antiepileptic Drugs. New York: Raven Press, 1989:313–27.
23. Haruda F, Phenytoin Hypersensitivity: 38 cases. Neurology 1979;29:1480–85.
24. Schmidt D, Adverse effects of antiepileptic drugs. New York: Raven Press, 1982:25–33
25. Reynolds EH, Phenytoin: Toxicity. In: Levy RH, Dreifuss FE, Mattson RH, Meldrum BS, Penry JK, eds. Antiepileptic Drugs. New York, Raven Press, 1989:241–55.
26. Eadie MJ. Anticonvulsant drugs. An update. Drugs 1984; 27:328–63.
27. Trimble MR, Reynolds EH. Anticonvulsant drugs and mental symptoms. Psychol Med 1976; 6:169–78.
28. Reynolds EH. Chronic antiepileptic toxicity: A review. Epilepsia 1975; 16:319–52.
29. Logan WJ, Freeman JM. Pseudo-degenerative disease due to diphenylhydantoin intoxication. Arch Neurol 1969; 21:631–37.
30. Trimble MR, Corbett J, Donaldson D. Folic acid and mental symptoms in children with epilepsy. J Neurol Neurosurg Psychiatry 1980: 43:1030–34.
31. Kutt H. Hydantoins. In: Dam M, Gram L, eds. Comprehensive Epileptology. New York: Raven press, 1990:563–77.
32. Dreifuss FE. Ethosuximide: Toxicity. In: Levy RH, Dreifuss FE, Mattson RH, Meldrum BS, Penry JK, eds. Antiepileptic Drugs. New York, Raven Press, 1989:699–705.
33. Sullivan FM, McElhatton PR. A comparison of the teratogenic activity of the antiepileptic drugs carbamazepine, clonazepam, ethosuximide, phenobarbital, phenytoin and primidone in mice. Toxicol Appl Pharmacol 1977; 40:365–78.
34. Browne TR, Dreifuss FE, Dyken PR, Goode DJ, Penry JK, Porter RJ, White BG, White PT. Ethosuxmide in the treatment of absence (petit mal) seizures. Neurology 1975; 25:515–24.
35. Roger J, Grangeon H, Guey J, Lob H. Incidences psychiatrique et psychologique du traitement par l'ethosuximide chez les épileptiques. Encephale 1968; 57:407–38.
36. Wolf P, Inoue Y, Rodder-Wanner U, Tsai J. Psychiatric complications of absence therapy and their relation to alteration of sleep. Epilepsia 1984; 25(Suppl 1): S56–59.
37. Ehyai A, Kilroy AW, Fenichel GM. Dyskinesia and akathisia induced by ethosuximide. Am J Dis Child 1978; 132:527–28.

38. Mattson RH, Cramer JA. Valproic acid and ethosuximide interaction. Ann Neurol 1980; 7:583–84.
39. Pisani F, Narbone MC, Trunfio C, Fazio A, La Rosa G, Oteri G, Di Perri R. Valproic acid–ethosuximide interaction: Apharmacokinetic study. Epilepsia 1984; 25:229–33.
40. Warren JW, Benmaman JC, Braxton B, Wannamaker BB, Levy RH. Kinetics of a carbamazepine–ethosuximide interaction. Clin Pharmacol Ther 1980; 28:646–51.
41. Gram L, Jensen PK. Carbamazepine: Toxicity In: Levy RH, Dreifuss FE, Mattson RH, Meldrum BS, Penry JK, eds. Antiepileptic Drugs. New York; Raven Press, 1989:555–65.
42. Lewis IJ, Rosenbloom L. Glandular fever-like syndrome, pulmonary eosinophilia and asthma associated with carbamazepine. Postgrad Med J 1982; 58:100–101.
43. Pellock JM. Carbamazepine side-effects in children and adults. Epilepsia 1987; 28(Suppl 3):S64–70.
44. Hart RG, Easton JD. Carbamazepine and hematological monitoring. Ann Neurol 1982; 11:309–12.
45. Trimble MR. Anticonvulsant drugs and cognitive function: A review of the literature. Epilepsia 1987; 28(Suppl 3):S37–45.
46. Snead CO, Hosey LC. Exacerbation of seizures in children by carbamazepine. N Engl J Med 1985; 15:916–21.
47. Durrelli L, Mutani R, Sechi GP, Monaco F, Glorioso N, Gusmaroli G. Cardiac side effects of phenytoin and carbamazepine. A dose-related phenomenon? Arch Neurol 1985; 42;1067–68.
48. Leppick IE. Carbamazepine. In: Dam M, Gram L, eds. Comprehensive epileptology. New York; Raven Press, 1990.
49. Kerr BM, Levy RH. Carbamazepine: carbamazepine epoxide. In: Levy RH, Dreifuss FE, Mattson RH, Meldrum BS, Penry JK, eds. New York: Raven Press, 1989:505–20.
50. Dreifuss FE, Santilli N, Langer DH, Sweeney KP, Moline KA, Menander KB. Valproic acid hepatic fatalities: a retrospective review. Neurology 1987; 37:379–85.
51. Dreifuss FE, Langer DH, Moline KA, Maxwell JE. Valproic acid hepatic fatalities. II. US experience since 1984. Neurology 1989; 39:201–7.
52. Appleton RE, Farrell K, Zaide J, Rogers PC. The high incidence of valproate hepatotoxicity in infants may relate to familial matabolic defects. Can J Neurol Sci 1990; 17:145–48.
53. Lenn NJ, Ellis WG, Washburn ER, Ruebner B. Fatal hepatocerebral syndrome in siblings discordant for exposure to valproate. Epilepsia 1990; 31(5):578–83.
54. Winter SC, Szabo-Aczel S, Curry CJR, Hutchinson HT, Hogue R, Shug A. Plasma carnitine deficiency: clinical observations in 51 pediatric patients. Am J Dis Child 1987; 141:660–665.
55. Millington DS, Bohan TP, Roe CR, Yergey AL, Liberto DJ. Valproylcarnitine: a noval drug metabolite identified by fast atom bombardment and thermospray liquid chromatography–mass spectrometry. Clin Chim Acta 1985; 145:69–76.
56. Coulter DL. Carnitine deficiency: a possible mechanism for valproate hepatotoxicity. Lancet 1984; i:689.

57. Beghi E, Bizzi A, Codegoni AM, Trevisan D, Torri W. Valproate, carnitine metabolism and biochemical indicators of liver function. Epilepsia 1990; 31:346–52.
58. Coulter DL. Carnitine, valproate and toxicity. J Child Neurol 1991; 6:7–14.
59. Haslam RHA, Koren G. Screening of the epileptic patient: Is it worthwhile? Can J Neurol Sci 1989; 16:363–64.
60. Williams LHP, Reynolds RP, Emery JL. Pancreatitis during sodium valproate treatment. Arch Dis Child 1983; 58:543–44.
61. Wyllie E, Wyllie R, Cruse RP, Erenberg G, Rothner AD. Pancreatitis associated with valproic acid therapy. Am J Dis Child 1984; 138:912–14.
62. Lindhout D, Schmidt D. In-utero exposure to valproate and neural tube defects. Lancet 1986; i:1392–93.
63. Jager-Roman E, Deichl A, Jakob S, Hartmann AM, Koch S, Rating D, Steldinger R, Nau H, Helge H. Fetal growth, major malformations and minor anomalies in infants born to women receiving valproic acid. J Pediatr 1986; 108:997–1004.
64. DiLiberti JH, Farndon PA, Dennis NR, Curry CJR. The fetal valproate syndrome. Am J Med Genet 1984; 19:473–81.
65. Massa G, Lecoutere D, Casaer P. Prognosis in fetal valproate syndrome. J Pediatr 1987; 111:308–9.
66. Nau H, Hendrickx AG. Valproic acid teratogenesis. ISI atlas sci pharmacol 1987:52–56.
67. Dreifuss F. Valproate: toxicity. In: Levy RH, Dreifuss FE, Mattson RH, Meldrum BS, Penry JK, eds. Antiepileptic drugs. New York: Raven Press, 1989:643–51.
68. Clark JE, Covanis A, Gupta AK, Jeavons PM. Unwanted effects of sodium valproate in children and adolescents. In: Parsonage MJ, and Caldwell ADS eds. The place of sodium valproate in the treatment of epilepsy. London: Royal Society of Medicine, 1980:223–33.
69. Egger J, Brett EM. Effects of sodium valproate in 100 children with special reference to weight. Br Med J 19 ; 283:577–81.
70. Schmidt D. Adverse effects of valproate. Epilepsia 1984; 25(Suppl 1):S44–49.
71. Sackallares JC, Lee SI, Dreifuss FE. 1979; Stupor following administration of valproic acid to patients receiving other antiepileptic drugs. Epilepsia 1979; 20:697–703.
72. Karas BJ, Wilder BJ, Hammond EJ, Bauman AW. Treatment of valproate tremors. Neurology 1983; 33:1380–82.
73. Loiseau P. Sodium valproate platelet dysfunction and bleeding. Epilepsia 1981; 22:141–46.
74. Jaeken J, van Goethem C, Casaer P, Carchon H, Eggermont E, Eeckels R. Neutropenia during sodium valproate treatment. Arch Dis Child 1979; 54:985–86.
75. Prensky AL, Raff MC, Moore MJ, Schwab RS. Intravenous diazepam in the treatment of prolonged seizure activity. *N Engl J Med* 1967; 276:779–84.
76. Sharer L, Kutt H. Intravenous administration of diazepam. *Arch Neurol.* 1971; 24:169.
77. Knudsen FU. Rectal administration of diazepam in solution in the acute treatment of convulsions in infants and children. Arch Dis Child 1979; 54:855–57.
78. Farrell K. Benzodiazepines in the treatment of children with epilepsy. Epilepsia 1986; 27(Suppl 2):45–52.

79. Leppik IE, Derivan AT, Homan RW, Walker J, Ramsey RE, Patrick B. Double-blind study of lorazepam and diazepam in status epilepticus. JAMA 1983; 249:1452–54.
80. Graves NM, Kriel RL, Jones-Saete C. Bioavailability of rectally administered lorazepam. Clin Neuropharmacol 1987; 10:555–59.
81. Homan RW, Walker JE. Clinical studies of lorazepam in status epilepticus. In: Delgado-Escueta AV, Wasterlain CG, Treiman DM, Porter RJ, eds. Advances in neurology. Vol. 34. Status epilepticus: mechanisms of brain damage. New York: Raven Press, 1983.
82. Tassinari CA, Daniele O, Michelucci R, Bureau M, Dravet C, Roger J. Benzodiazepines: efficacy in status epilepticus. In: Delgado-Escueta AV, Wasterlain CG, Treiman DM, Porter RJ, eds. Advances in neurology, Vol 34. Status epilepticus: mechanisms of brain damage and treatment. New York: Raven Press, 1983:465–75.
83. Browne TR. Clonazepam: a review of a new anticonvulsant drug. Arch Neurol 1976; 33:326–32.
84. Hansen RA, Menkes JH. A new anticonvulsant in the management of minor motor seizures. Dev Med Child Neurol 1972; 14:3–14.
85. Schmidt D. How to use benzodiazepines. In: Morselli PL, Pippenger CE, Penry JK, eds. Antiepileptic drug therapy in paediatrics. New York: Raven Press, 1983:271–78.

12

Genetic Considerations in Convulsive Disorders in Children

W. ALLEN HAUSER
College of Physicians and Surgeons
Columbia University
New York, New York

V. ELVING ANDERSON
University of Minnesota
Minneapolis, Minnesota

I. GENERAL CONSIDERATIONS

The tendency for epilepsy to aggregate in families has long been recognized. This tendency has been described from the earliest Hippocratic writings. While restrictions on marriage and the codification of sterilization practices have been repealed for at least 15 years in the United States, there are still many misconceptions regarding the role of genetics in the expression of epilepsy. There is a general tendency to overestimate the risk for epilepsy in other family members of persons with epilepsy. It is also frequently forgotten that familial aggregation does not necessarily imply a genetic mechanism. Members of a family unit share a number of common environmental exposures which must also be explored as potential mechanisms.

II. THE NEED FOR APPROPRIATE COMPARISONS

The clinical literature continues to provide information on the ''proportion of cases'' with a family history of seizures (epilepsy). This type of information generally does not specify the relationship of affected members or the number of people at risk. In addition, there is seldom a clear indication of what is included as ''seizures'' or as ''epilepsy.'' This type of information is useless for the evaluation of familial or genetic risks since there is no identifiable comparison group.

When information is restricted to first-degree relatives (parents, siblings, offspring) with recurrent unprovoked seizures (epilepsy), 1 in 10 adults will have a "family history" by chance alone. If the definition of affected first-degree relative is expanded to "seizures," almost 1 in 3 adults will have a family history.

Some investigators have defined the relationship of relatives to the proband (e.g., siblings), have provided denominator figures to allow the actual proportion of individuals affected to be determined, and have then used population prevalence to estimate an expected frequency. Prevalence is not an appropriate comparison, however, since it excludes those people with epilepsy who have died or who are in remission. This comparison will underestimate the expected number of cases and thus overestimate the relative risk within families of probands by a factor of 2 to 4.

For a condition such as epilepsy, the *cumulative incidence* is an estimate of the proportion of the population who have ever been affected by a specific age. Since there is little increase in mortality for most cases of epilepsy, the cumulative incidence to a given age will be a close approximation to the prevalence of a *history of epilepsy* whether current or not.

The cumulative incidence of epilepsy (recurrent unprovoked seizures) to age 20 is about 1% and about 1.8% by age 40 [1]. By age 80, about 4% of the population can be expected to have had epilepsy. If the comparison is seizures rather than epilepsy, a bit more than 4% of the population will have been affected by age 20 and over 10% by age 80. It is the expected number of cases based on this age-specific cumulative incidence that should be used in the estimation of the expected number of affected individuals within a family.

III. MODES IN INHERITANCE

A. Mendelian Patterns of Inheritance

There are over 150 disorders that are inherited as a Mendelian single gene disorder and for which seizures or epilepsy are part of the symptomatology [2]. For most of these, epilepsy is not the primary symptom nor are most of these disorders specific for the development of epilepsy. When seizures are present, the clinical characteristics of the seizures (phenotypic expression) tend to be similar, although this is not invariably the case. In some situations, this heterogeneity of symptomatology can cause difficulty in evaluation of the mode of inheritance. For some of these Mendelian disorders a chromosomal locus has been identified through linkage and mapping studies. Again, there is evidence for heterogeneity. Two loci have been identified for tuberous sclerosis [3] and two for neurofibromatosis [4].

B. Linkage Studies and Gene Mapping in Epilepsy Syndromes

There are three epilepsy syndromes for which a single gene locus has been suggested or identified. *Benign familial neonatal convulsions* (BFNG) is a dominantly inherited epilepsy syndrome in which convulsions occur early in life (often on the third or fourth postnatal day) in otherwise normal children [5,6]. For many affected individuals seizures persist beyond the neonatal period, although only about 15% will have epilepsy at an older age. In Caucasian families, the gene for BFNC has been mapped to the long arm of chromosome 20 [7]. This localization have not been confirmed in a Hispanic family [8].

Starting with probands with *juvenile myoclonic epilepsy* (JME) and including affected individuals with epilepsy (not necessarily JME) or abnormal EEG patterns (not necessarily *generalized spike and wave* GSW), linkage to the BF and HLA loci on chromosome 6 has been established [9]. This localization is not specific JME; rather it represents a localization for juvenile onset idiopathic epilepsies [10]. Complex segregation analysis has as yet failed to demonstrate a clear mode of inheritance in these families.

Progressive myoclonus epilepsy of the Baltic type is a recessively inherited epilepsy syndrome [11–13]. Most affected individuals develop symptoms of stimulus-sensitive myoclonus and generalized tonic–clonic seizures between the ages of 8 and 13 years. Based on studies of 12 Finnish families, including 26 affected persons, the gene locus for this syndrome has been localized to the long arm of chromosome 21 [14].

When multiple family members are affected with seizures or with epilepsy in the absence of a clearly identified syndrome, it is important to evaluate mode of inheritance through carefully determined pedigrees. Only a few families will demonstrate clear Mendelian patterns of inheritance. For these unique families, biochemical or other specialized studies are warranted to identify the underlying mechanisms by which seizures occur. Such studies may ultimately lead to clues about underlying mechanisms for all persons with epilepsy. Linkage studies and gene mapping are appropriate to determine the location of the abnormal gene.

C. Chromosomal Abnormalities

Abnormalities of the central nervous system occur in most of the syndromes associated with chromosomal abnormalities, and in this situation epilepsy is frequently included in the constellation of symptoms. Epilepsy may not be manifested at an early age. While the risk for seizures or epilepsy is substantial in individuals with Down syndrome [15], seizures start in adulthood for most, presumably in association with the development of the pathologic changes characteristic of Alzheimer disease.

Chromosomal evaluation in children with a constellation of dysmorphic features and neurologic abnormalities may provide additional clues to potential sites of genes important to the development of epilepsy. In patients with seizures, an inverted duplicated segment of chromosome 15, dysmorphic features are not part of the clinical picture [16,17]. In other situations, such as Angelman syndrome, the parent contributing the abnormal gene may affect the phenotypic expression, a phenomenon known as genome imprinting [18].

D. Mitochondrial Inheritance

Mitochondrial genes are unique in that all are maternally inherited [19]. These genes, which control subunits of oxidative enzymes, have been implicated in the development of some forms of epilepsy, such as Myoclonic Epilepsy with ragged red fibers (MERRF), and have been implicated in other neurologic syndromes in which seizures or myoclonus occur [20]. While a classical maternal pattern is usual in disorders of mitochondrial DNA, some mitochondrial enzymes are under nuclear genetic control, so that Mendelian inheritance may also play a role in these conditions.

E. Polygenic and Multifactorial Inheritance

The chromosomal, mitochondrial, and single-gene disorders are associated with a high risk for seizures in siblings or offspring of affected individuals, but these risks are quite predictable when the mode of inheritance is understood. Unfortunately these diseases and syndromes account for only a small proportion of all epilepsy. For the majority of situations in which multiple members of a family have seizures, the clinical manifestations are heterogeneous, and the patterns of affected individuals within the family structure does not immediately suggest Mendelian inheritance. In this situation, inheritance is either associated with a *polygenic* (multiple genes) and/or *multifactorial* (an interaction between genetic and environmental factors) mechanism. The risk for recurrence of symptoms in family members is modest and factors affecting this risk become important for genetic counseling.

IV. CLINICAL STUDIES OF FAMILIAL AGGREGATION

A. The Electroencephalogram

Electroencephalographic abnormalities are the hallmark of many types of epilepsy and it is clear that genetic factors are important in the determination of general features of the electroencephalogram. In studies of monozygotic (MZ) and dizygotic (GE) twins, EEG characteristics such as frequency spectrum and spatial wave form distribution suggest a substantial proportion of interindividual variation to be genetically determined [21,22]. Variation in EEG recordings in MZ pairs is no greater than that of sequential recordings in the same person. Type of pattern, rate of maturation of the EEG, and age-specific manifestations of specific patterns are similar in MZ pairs, as is the power spectrum on quantitative EEG analysis [23]. This is true even if the MZ siblings are reared apart [24]. In older MZ pairs, there is concordance in degree of slowing of dominant rhythms and increase of temporal theta [11]. In MZ pairs, sleep patterns [25] and responses to activation procedures and to alcohol [26] are also similar.

Nonepileptiform patterns such as alpha variants and some beta patterns may also be under genetic control. When present, low-voltage fast EEG patterns tend to show a bimodal distribution within families, and segregation analysis suggests a single major locus with dominant mode of inheritance [10]. Although rare on a population basis, *slow alpha variant* patterns have shown concordance in MZ twins both for occurrence and for persistence and have also been observed in siblings. The pattern of inheritance of the slow alpha variant (if any) remains elusive [27]. Some beta patterns also may be genetically determined [28].

B. Epileptiform Electroencephalographic Patterns

1. The Generalized Spike-and-Wave Pattern

Based on family and twin studies, Lennox suggested that the risk of manifesting a generalized spike-and-wave EEG pattern (GSW) is in part genetic [29). He reported an 84% concordance for GSW in MZ pairs and no concordance in DZ pairs. The tendency for these patterns to aggregate in families was further elaborated by the Metrakoses [30,31]. In studies of EEG patterns in relatives of probands with "centrencephalic epilepsy" and a 3 per second generalized spike-and-wave EEG pattern, almost 50% of siblings also manifested GSW (although not necessarily 3 per second). They concluded that the centrencephalic EEG pattern (not the epilepsy) was the expression of an autosomal dominant gene with low penetrance at birth, nearly complete penetrance in childhood and disappearance by age 40. Only waking records were obtained, and no distinction was made between the GSW pattern and the photoparoxysmal response (PPR).

a. Population frequency. It is possible that there are major population differences in the frequency of the GSW pattern. In European children with no history of neurologic difficulties, waking records (with hyperventilation activation where possible) demonstrated GSW in from 0.3 to 1.8% of children [32,33]. The frequency of abnormalities in the waking state may be much higher in nonepileptic French Canadian populations (10%), although GSW and PPR were not separately categorized [30]. The age at the time of recording must be taken into consideration, since the manifestation of GSW seems to be age-dependent. In normal German children the waking and hyperventilation-activated records demonstrated a peak prevalence of GSW (2.8%) in 7 to 8-year-olds.

In studies of normal children which included sleep [33,34], 7.9% of normal Swedish children and 16.3% of Japanese children demonstrated GSW. These proportions in fact may not be different since the recordings in Japanese children were obtained only at age 3, whereas the Swedish study included children from ages 1 to 15. In Sweden, 15% of 3 and 4-year-old children demonstrated GSW during sleep.

b. Rates of GSW in Siblings and in Offspring of Patients with GSW and Generalized Epilepsy. For the most part, studies of the familial occurrence of GSW (and other EEG patterns felt to be genetically determined) have been performed in relatives of probands who also have epilepsy. There may therefore be a confounding effect between epilepsy in general and, more important, the proband's specific type of epilepsy on the tendency of relatives to manifest GSW. In a study of siblings of children with all types of epilepsy who demonstrated GSW, 7% of siblings also demonstrated GSW [32], while a study of siblings of probands with generalized minor seizures reported a frequency of 17% [35].

In studies of Doose and associates which limited analysis to waking and hyperventilation-activated recordings, the highest prevalence of GSW in siblings of probands with GSW and with epilepsy occurred in recordings done between ages 3 and 6. In this age group, 13% of siblings of all epilepsy probands also demonstrated GSW. In siblings of probands with generalized minor motor epilepsy, 34% demonstrated GSW at ages 2 to 3, with rates decreasing after that age. In studies of offspring of probands with primary generalized epilepsy and GSW, 24% demonstrated GSW, a rate more than double that in offspring of probands with partial epilepsy [36].

Gender seems important in the manifestation of GSW in family members. In most studies, the frequency of GSW is slightly higher in female siblings or female offspring of GSW probands. The frequency is also higher for siblings of female probands than for siblings of male probands.

All investigators agree that genetic mechanisms are important in the manifestation of GSW, although the actual mode of inheritance remains in question. Metrakos and associates have concluded that the pattern is inherited as a dominant trait [31], while Doose and associates have concluded that the mechanisms are polygenic or possibly recessive. There seem to be no reports which have utilized complex segregation analysis to evaluate the most likely model of inheritance. If epilepsy rather than EEG pattern is used as an outcome, complex segregation analysis suggests that the familial aggregation is most consistent with a dominant trait [37].

c. Other EEG Patterns in Siblings of Probands with GSW. While the frequency of GSW is increased in siblings of epilepsy probands with GSW alone, the frequency of photoparoxysmal patterns (PPR) is not increased. PPR occurred in 7% of siblings of probands with GSW and epilepsy, similar to the 8%

found in siblings of probands with epilepsy and no GSW [38]. It seems from this and other data that GSW and PPR are genetically independent phenomena.

2. Photoparoxysmal Responses

Between 8 and 9% of children with no history of brain disease will demonstrate a photoparoxysmal response (PPR) [33.39]. The prevalence of PPR is significantly higher in females in the early teenage years, when the EEG will manifest PPR in about 20% of normal females and 10% of normal males. The prevalence of PPR may be considerably lower in older teenagers [40], although this has not been a consistent finding [46].

a. Rates of PPR in Relatives of PPR Probands. In a study of siblings of probands with PPR (most probands also had epilepsy), Doose found that 23% of siblings also had PPR [38]. Age-specific trends in the distribution of PPR in siblings of PPR probands were similar to those observed in normal children, although the prevalence in siblings was greater in each age group. The prevalence of PPR in siblings was very low before the fifth birthday and tended to increase with age reaching a maximum in those siblings age 15 and 16, when over 40% demonstrated PPR. The prevalence of PPR was higher in female than in male siblings and was also higher in the siblings of female than in male probands (27% vs. 19.5%) It was assumed that the patterns within families were those of a multifactorial and polygenic trait.

b. Other EEG Patterns in Relatives of Probands with PPR. There is little information on the population frequency of PHOTOMYOCLONIC RESPONSE (PMR). In a study of relatives of probands with epilepsy and a PPR, 11.5% demonstrated PMR. [41,42]. This compared with 2.6% of relatives of probands with generalized-onset epilepsy but without PPR. PMR was noted in the older age groups, and as with PPR, was more frequent in female than in male relatives. The proportion of relatives with PPR or PMR was 20% and was similar within each age stratum. PPR predominated in the younger age groups and the prevalence fell with advancing age. In contrast, PMR prevalence was lowest in the younger and increased in the older age groups. This led to the suggestion that PPR is replaced by PMR in older age groups.

In studies of probands with epilepsy, PPR and GSW occur with a frequency greater than that expected based on general population frequencies. In siblings of PPR probands with epilepsy, GSW may occur at rates higher than those in the general population, although this increased rate would seem attributable to the presence of GSW in some of the probands. As mentioned earlier, PPR and GSW appear to occur independently within families. In siblings of probands with GSW, the proportion with PPR is independent of GSW and determined only by the presence (or absence) of PPR. PPR was demonstrated in 16.6% of siblings of probands with both GSW and PPR, but PPR was noted in only 7.3% of siblings of epilepsy probands with GSW alone. The proportion with PPR among siblings of GSW/PPR probands is similar to that for siblings of any PPR proband, while the rate in siblings of probands with GSW alone is similar to the frequency of PPR in neurologically normal populations. The coexistence of other patterns, such as focal spikes or rhythmic theta, has no influence on the occurrence of PPR in relatives. The presence of an occipital delta pattern (felt by Doose to occur in families) does have an apparent influence on the manifestation of PPR in other family members. When present in probands, only 8.6% of siblings show PPR compared with 31.8% when this pattern is absent in probands.

The mode of inheritance of PPR remains in question. While dominant inheritance has been suggested in some Japanese populations [43], other patterns of inheritance have been suggested by some investigators. If epilepsy is considered as an outcome in probands with epilepsy and PPR, the familial patterns are most consistent with a single major locus [32].

3. *Focal Spikes*

Between 1 and 2% of normal children will demonstrate focal spikes in the waking electroencephalogram [44,16]. This proportion increases to 2.7% when sleeping recordings are also obtained [26]. There seems to be no specific age of selective predisposition for focal spikes. Almost 70% involved the central or temporal areas. Studies of the waking records of siblings of probands with focal spikes revealed a prevalence of 2.9%, a frequency similar to that of the general population.

Benign epilepsy of childhood with centrotemporal EEG foci accounts for up to 20% of childhood-onset epilepsy in the European studies [45]. Localization of spikes to the temporal areas in normal populations may be meaningful in view of the reports of familial aggregation of seizures and of centrotemporal EEG epileptiform abnormalities [46,47]. In a Swedish cohort, rolandic discharges were identified in 34% of siblings and seizures occurred in 15%, all generalized. Seizures had also occurred in childhood in 11% of parents, although only one parent demonstrated an epileptiform abnormality (this was in the centrotemporal area). In an American study, 36% of children or siblings of epilepsy probands with rolandic discharges also demonstrated Rolandic discharges, as did 19% of parents. In this study, over 50% of family members tested between the ages of 6 and 10 demonstrated this pattern. It was concluded that the EEG pattern represented a dominant trait. Only 12% of individuals with the EEG abnormality had a history of seizures.

4. *Other EEG Patterns in Probands with Rolandic Discharges*

About 50% of children with Rolandic epilepsy also demonstrated GSW in deeper stages of sleep [48], and presumed GSW was noted in 13% of siblings and 16% of parents of probands with epilepsy and centrotemporal sharp waves, with even higher percentages in siblings during sleep [49,50]. The relationship between Rolandic discharges and GSW warrants further investigation but suggests that this pattern and the associated epilepsy may represent a transition between the localization-related and the generalized-onset epilepsies.

5. Other Patterns That Aggregate in Families

a. Parietal Theta Rhythms of Doose. A rhythmic 4 to 5-Hz pattern occurring in the parietal region in children has been described by Doose [51,52]. The pattern remains somewhat controversial since it closely resembles hypersynchronous hypnogogic patterns. This pattern occurs in 5.6% of neurologically normal children. Unlike most patterns occurring in families, the Theta pattern is much more prevalent in males than in females. The prevalence is highest at age 3 (10%) and decreases with advancing age. The pattern is of particular interest because of a particularly high prevalence in children with febrile convulsions and with generalized-onset epilepsies.

In epilepsy probands with Theta, 13% of siblings also demonstrated this pattern. The trend in age-specific prevalence is similar to that in the normal population but with a higher prevalence, with a maximum of about 30% in the 3- and 4-year age groups and falling after that age. The frequency of this pattern in siblings of probands with epilepsy but without Theta was similar to that seen in normal populations. [53]

The Theta pattern is of particular interest because of a high frequency of GSW at later ages—upward of 60%—identified in longitudinal studies of children with this pattern. There also may be a high frequency of PPR in these children. There is no increase in the frequency of GSW, PPR, or other patterns in siblings of Theta probands.

b. Posterior Delta Rhythms. Rhythmic occipital delta rhythms, either accentuated with eye closure or continuous, have been described in about 5% of neurologically normal children, with a peak prevalence of about 22.5% in children between the ages 3 and 4 [54]. They are found with maxima at somewhat later ages in epileptic probands. These patterns occur in about 10% of siblings of probands with epilepsy who also demonstrate delta, and in only 3% of siblings of epilepsy probands without delta. This pattern is reported to occur with increased frequency in children with absence seizures.

c. Interaction with Other Patterns. The posterior delta rhythm pattern is of interest in that its coexistence in probands with GSW or with PPR reduced the frequency with which GSW or PPR was identified in siblings. The pattern was interpreted as a reflection of a genetically inherited inhibitory phenomenon.

d. Multiple Independent Spike Foci Pattern (MISF) This pattern must be quite rare and possibly nonexistent in the neurologically normal population. In clinical series, epilepsy occurs in from 84 to 94% of children with this pattern [55,56] and only 30% are without history of neurologic insult. This pattern may also be genetically determined. In studies in Minneapolis, 15% of siblings of epilepsy probands with MISF also had epilepsy, a risk higher than that associated with any other patterns singly or combined.

V. CLINICAL STUDIES OF FAMILIAL AGGREGATION OF CONVULSIVE DISORDERS

A. Epilepsy

In the absence of an identifiable single gene, chromosomal, or mitochondrial disorder, there is an increased risk for first-degree relatives also to have epilepsy. This increase in risk is modest—on the order of two- to threefold over that expected in the general population [57].

Factors associated with differential risk for onset of epilepsy include seizure type or epilepsy syndrome, etiology of seizures, age at onset of epilepsy and gender of the proband, specific relationship of the relative of interest to the affected proband, and whether additional members of the family are also affected. Variables such as EEG may also be important. Unfortunately, many of these factors are hopelessly confounded, so that risk is best assessed using multivariable techniques, an approach seldom used in clinical studies.

1. Seizure Type

There is a general perception that generalized epilepsies are more likely to be genetically determined than are partial epilepsies. There are several reasons for this assumption. Many studies of familial aggregation have identified individuals with a specific seizure type and have determined the proportion of affected relatives. These studies have tended to concentrate on childhood-onset generalized epilepsies which have interictal generalized spike-and-wave patterns (GSW) and which may in some situations be inherited as a Mendelian trait. Such has been the approach of Janz and colleagues [58,59] and of Tsuboi and Christian [60] for impulsive petit mal, of the Metrakoses [30], Matthes [61], and Doose and colleagues [62] for absence seizures, and of Doose and Baier [63] for myoclonic–astatic epilepsy. These authors have selectively studied childhood-onset generalized epilepsies with spike-and-wave patterns, and in many situations the studies may have been initiated because of familial aggregation in index families. Despite this, the proportion of relatives affected was low and similar to the proportion of affected relatives of probands with partial seizures. Further, seizure types in affected relatives are heterogeneous.

When compared with relatives of unaffected controls, a higher proportion of relatives of probands with partial epilepsy also have epilepsy, suggesting some level of familial (genetic) risk [64,65]. Only a few studies have independently reported the proportion of affected relatives of generalized versus partial epilepsy [66,67]. These studies report a slightly higher proportion of relatives of probands with generalized-onset seizures to be affected.

Using epidemiologic analytic methods, a study of epilepsy in offspring of parents with epilepsy failed to demonstrate a difference in risk to offspring of probands with partial seizures compared with generalized-onset seizures. [68]. Among offspring of probands with absence, there is a substantially higher risk than for offspring of the group with partial seizures or with all other generalized-onset seizures.

As is the case with absence seizures in the generalized seizure epilepsy cases, it seems that the risk for epilepsy to relatives with partial seizures who fulfill criteria for benign rolandic epilepsy of Childhood may be substantially higher than for other forms of epilepsy [42,43]. As mentioned in the discussion of EEG phenomena, this idiopathic localization-related epilepsy syndrome may represent a transition between the partial epilepsies and the generalized epilepsies.

2. *Etiology*

There are many antecedent factors that predispose to epilepsy [69]. Two questions may be asked in relationship to etiology. First, it is clear that not all individuals who suffer brain injury in association with events such as trauma develop epilepsy. Does a family history of epilepsy increase the likelihood of epilepsy following major brain insults such as those related to cerebral infarction or central nervous system infection? There are few good studies of this question, and none in children, but there is as yet no clear evidence that family history of epilepsy is associated with an increase in risk for seizures or epilepsy in association with or following specific brain insults. Only the follow-up of the Viet Nam Head injury cohort has systematically studied this question, and no association between the risk for epilepsy in the patients and a family history of epilepsy was found [70]. This cohort, consisting of individuals with penetrating head injuries, clearly represents a group with exceedingly severe injury. It is possible that in persons with less severe injury, genetics may play a role.

A second question is whether a family history of epilepsy associated with brain insults is associated with an increased risk of epilepsy in other relatives. Our studies in Minneapolis have shown a risk for epilepsy to siblings of patients with remote symptomatic epilepsy intermediate to that seen in the general population and that in relatives of patients with idiopathic epilepsy. Using epidemiologic methods, the risk to offspring of patients with epilepsy has been shown to be similar for probands with idiopathic epilepsy compared to those with symptomatic epilepsy [71].

3. *Age at Onset*

In general, relatives of probands with onset of epilepsy in childhood (other than the first year of life) have a higher risk for epilepsy than do relatives of probands with adult onset of epilepsy [63,66,71]. Although there are few studies in which multivariable analysis has been undertaken, this seems true even after taking into account potential confounding factors such as the proband's etiology (idiopathic or cryptogenic vs. symptomatic), epilepsy syndrome, or seizure type (generalized vs. partial). There also is a tendency for concordance of age of onset, with epilepsy starting at an early age in relatives of probands with onset of epilepsy at an early age.

B. Acute Symptomatic Seizures

A distinction must be made between seizures occurring at the time of a systemic metabolic derangement or as the immediate consequences of brain insult such as brain injury or stroke (Acute symptomatic seizures) and Unprovoked seizures which may develop months or years following a brain insult such as infection of the central nervous system or severe head (brain) injury (Remote symptomatic seizures or epilepsy). The former are related to the acute disruption of homeostatic mechanisms, which is presumably reversible; the latter occur in association with the potentially epileptogenic state associated with the static encephalopathy that may follow a severe brain insult. In general, the relationship between family history of seizures or epilepsy and risk for seizures in the context of an acute insult is poorly established. The one exception is in the unique situation of febrile seizures.

C. Febrile Seizures

Febrile seizures clearly aggregate in families, although the mode of inheritance remains in question. While dominant, recessive, and purely environmental factors have been suggested as underlying mechanisms for the occurrence of febrile seizures, it appears that there is again genetic heterogeneity in this situation. In studies from Rochester, Minnesota, the majority of cases are clearly polygenic. Nonetheless, a subgroup characterized by the occurrence of multiple febrile seizures (three or more) in the proband appears to be associated with a dominant mode of inheritance [72]. In some situations, such as with febrile illness, a family history of epilepsy or of febrile seizures may increase the likelihood of a seizure occurrence [63,73] as well as recurrence once a febrile seizure has occurred [74]. The very high frequency of GSW in children with febrile convulsions suggests an interaction with other childhood epilepsies [36,75].

VI. RELATED TOPICS

A. Teratogenesis/Congenital Abnormalities

Clefting disorders are among the most frequent major malformations identified in offspring of probands with epilepsy. It has been suggested that epilepsy and clefting may in some way be linked genetically, but epidemiologic studies of siblings of probands with epilepsy demonstrated no increase in the frequency of clefting over that expected [76,77] and epilepsy occurred no more frequently than expected among descendants of nonepileptic parents of probands with clefting [78].

B. Family History and Prognosis

A family history may be important as a predictor of prognosis, although findings have not been consistent. Among 149 patients with a first unprovoked idiopathic seizure, a history of epilepsy in a sibling was associated with a two fold-increase in the risk for seizure recurrence [79]. In a similar study of seizure recurrence after a first seizure in children, family history was an important predictor only in those with an abnormal EEG. [80,81]. Other studies of first seizures have not found family history important, but have not limited analysis to first-degree relatives or to epilepsy [82]. Family history could not be shown to be a predictor of remission in the general patient with epilepsy [83], and conversely, offspring of individuals with a protracted course of epilepsy do not have a higher risk of developing epilepsy than that of those who go into remission.

VII. STRATEGIES FOR GENETIC COUNSELING

The optimal evaluation of a familial aggregation of seizures or epilepsy requires information about seizures in the proband, including characteristics of the ictus, age of onset, and any relevant clinical or laboratory data that may be necessary to allow appropriate categorization of the case. Similar information regarding seizure manifestation and relevant clinical findings is necessary to allow appropriate classification of cases in relatives. The relationship of the proband to the relative, and the age (or age at death), sex, and relationship of all relatives presumed to be unaffected must also be determined. This will allow the calculation of an age (and sex)-adjusted risk for seizures or epilepsy in relatives for all classes of seizures or epilepsy and for specific seizure types. These rates in relatives can then be compared with the population rate to allow determination of changes in risk within the families of interest.

Risk estimates for epilepsy in relatives (e.g., siblings or offspring) of a patient with epilepsy (proband) should be based on clinical features of the proband's seizure disorder and augmented by knowledge of interictal EEG patterns in both the proband and the relative of interest.

A. Sibling Risk (Figure 1)

If a proband is known to have epilepsy but there is no other available information about clinical features of the proband's convulsive disorder, the risk for epilepsy in siblings of probands is about 5%. Siblings of probands with febrile convulsions have a similar risk for epilepsy. The risk in siblings is lower if the proband has a clearly defined cause for the epilepsy (such as stroke or head trauma) or if

LLYFRGELL U.C.N.W. LIB

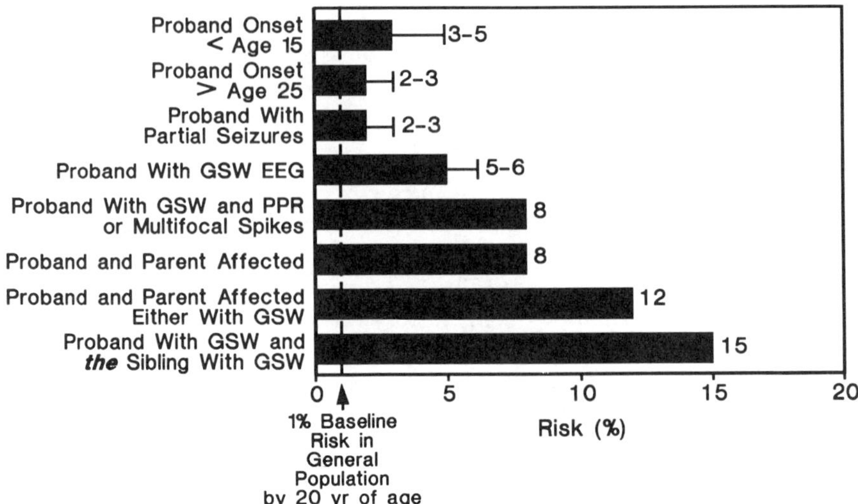

Figure 1 Sibling risk for epilepsy. EEG electroencephalogram; GSW, generalized spike–wave; PPR, photoparoxysmal response. (Modified from Ref. 84.)

the proband is over age 20 at the time of onset of epilepsy. Risk increases to 8% if a parent also has a history of epilepsy. Sibling risk for epilepsy is about 10% if the proband with epilepsy also has had febrile seizures.

There is some information regarding the presence of genetically determined EEG patterns and the sibling risk for epilepsy. Epilepsy will occur in 4%, and seizures in 10 to 12% of siblings of probands with epilepsy and GSW. This risk is higher in siblings of female probands. These proportions seem similar to the general risks for siblings of probands with childhood onset of epilepsy irrespective of the presence of GSW. Epilepsy will occur in 2.8% of siblings of probands with both PPR and epilepsy. This is again a risk similar to that for siblings of probands with epilepsy but with no evidence of a genetically determined EEG pattern, suggesting that the presence of PPR alone does not alter sibling risk for epilepsy. If the proband with epilepsy has both GSW and PPR, the risk for epilepsy in siblings is 10%.

Risk estimates for seizures or epilepsy in siblings may be modified by knowledge of the sibling's EEG. If a proband has benign rolandic epilepsy and both proband and sibling have Rolandic spikes, the sibling risk for seizures (not epilepsy) is 10%. The risk for seizures or epilepsy is probably at population rates if there are no epileptiform abnormalities in the sibling. If the proband has GSW and epilepsy and the sibling also has GSW, that sibling's risk is about 12% for epilepsy and about 33% for seizures of any type.

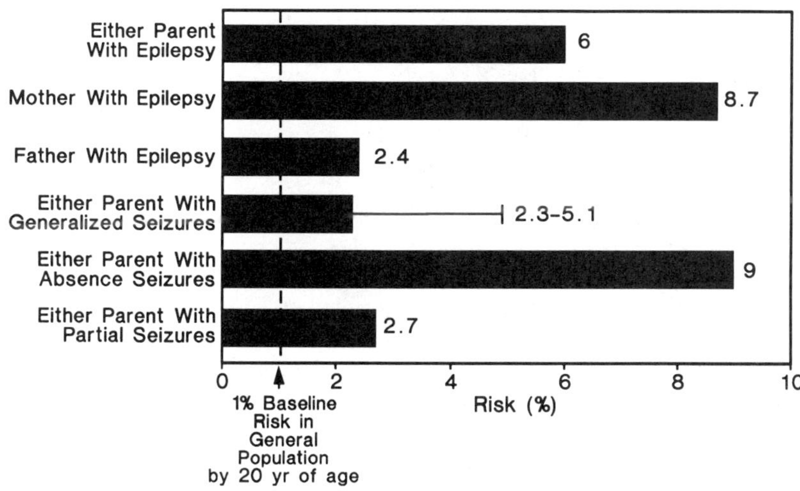

Figure 2 Offspring risk for epilepsy. (Modified from Ref. 84.)

Offspring Risk (Figure 2)

Most studies of the familial aggregation of epilepsy deal with siblings. From a genetic standpoint, offspring are not the same as siblings, although sibling data are frequently used to estimate offspring risks. From the few studies of epilepsy in offspring of parents with epilepsy, risks are similar to those reported for siblings. In offspring, risk for epilepsy is also about 5%. This risk is higher (6% vs. 3%) if the affected parent is female or if there is no known etiology for the partner's epilepsy (5% vs. 2%). If the parent has generalized epilepsy rather than partial epilepsy, the risk in offspring is slightly higher (5% vs. 4%). This difference is accounted for primarily by an offspring risk of 7% if the parent has absence seizures and 15% if the parent has myoclonic seizures. If both the parent and the grandparent have generalized-onset epilepsy, the risk may be 20%. There is little information on how risk in offspring will be modified by EEG patterns in either parent or the offspring.

REFERENCES

1. Hauser WA, Annegers JF. Epidemiologic measures for genetic studies. In: Beck-Mannagetta G, Anderson VE, Doose H, Janz D, eds. Genetics of the epilepsies. Berlin: Springer-Verlag, 1989: 7–12.
2. Anderson VE, Rich SS, Hauser WA, Wilcox KJ. Family studies of epilepsy. In: Anderson VE, Hauser WA, Leppik IE, Noebels JL, Rich SS, eds. Genetic strategies in epilepsy research. Amsterdam: Elsevier, 1991:89–103.

3. Sandkuyl LA, Janssen LAJ, Lindhout D, Merkens EC, Fleury P, Sunde L, Zaremba J, Halley DJJ. Linkage studies in tuberous sclerosis: evidence for genetic heterogeneity. Epilepsia 1990; 31:818.
4. McKusick VA. Mendelian inheritance in man, (9th ed.) The Johns Hopkins University Press, Baltimore, 1990.
5. Bjerre I, Corelius E. Benign familial neonatal convulsions. Acta Paediatr Scand 1968; 57:557–61.
6. Quattlebaum TG. Benign familial convulsions in the neonatal period and early infancy. J Pediatr 1979; 95:257–59.
7. Leppert M, Anderson VE, Quattlebaum T, Stauffer D, O'Connell P, Nakamura Y, Lalouel J-M, White R. Benign familial neonatal convulsions linked to genetic markers on chromosome 20. Nature 1989; 237:647–48.
8. Ryan SG, Wiznitzer M, Hollman C, Torres MC, Szekeresova M, Schneider S. Benign familial neonatal convulsions: evidence for clinical and genetic heterogeneity. Ann Neurol 1991; 29:469–73.
9. Greenberg, DA, Delgato-Escueta AV, Widelitz H, Sparkes RS, Treiman L, Maldonado HM, Terasaki PI, Park MS. A locus involved in the expression of juvenile myoclonic epilepsy (JME) and of an associated EEG trait may be linked to HLA and BF on chromosome 6. Cytogenet Cell Genet 1987; 46:623.
10. Durner M, Sander T, Greenberg DA, Johnson K, Janz D. Localization of idiopathic generalized epilepsy on chromosome 6p in families ascertained through juvenile myoclonic epilepsy patients. Neurology 41:1651–1655.
11. Unverricht H. Die Myoclonie. Leipzig: Franz Deuticke, 1891: 1–128.
12. Lundborg H. Die progressive Myoklonus-Epilepsie (Unverricht's Myoklonie). Uppsala: Almqvist & Wiksell, 1903: 1–207.
13. Norio R., Koskiniemi M. Progressive myoclonus epilepsy: genetic and nosological aspects with special reference to 107 Finnish patients. Clin Genet 1979; 15:382–98.
14. Lehesjoki A, Koskiniemi M, Sistonen P, Miao J, Hastbacka J, Norio R, de la Chapella A. Localization of a gene for progressive myoclonus epilepsy to chromosome 21q22. Proc Natl Acad Sci USA 1991; 88:3696–99.
15. Tangye SR. The EEG and incidence of epilepsy in Down's syndrome. J. Ment Defic Res 1979; 23:17–24.
16. Maraschio P, Zuffardi O, Bernardi F, Bozzola M, De Paoli C, Fonatsch C, Flatz SD, Ghersini L, Gimelli G, Loi M, Lorini R, Peretti D, Poloni L, Tonetti D, Vanni R, Zamboni G. Preferential maternal derivation in inv dup (15). Analysis of 8 new cases. Hum Genet 1981; 57:345–50.
17. Wisniewski H, Hassold T, Heffelfinger J, Higgins JV. Cytogenetic and clinical studies in five cases of inv dup (15). Hum Genet 1979; 50:259–70.
18. Knoll JH, Nicholls RD, Magenis RE, Graham JM Jr, Lalande M, Latt SA. Angelman and Prader–Willi syndromes share a common chromosome 15 deletion but differ in parental origin of the deletion. Am J Med Genet 1989; 32:285–90.
19. Lombes A, Bonilla E, Dimauro S. Mitochondrial encephalomyopathies. Rev Neurol (Paris) 1989; 145:671–89.
20. Berkovic SF, Carpenter S, Evans A, Karpati G, Shoubridge EA, Andermann F, Meyer E, Tyler JL, Diksic M, Arnold D, Wolfe LS, Andermann E, Hakim AM. Myoclonus epilepsy and ragged-red fibres (MERRF). 1. A clinical, pathological,

biochemical, magnetic resonance spectrographic and positron emission tomographic study. Brain 1989; 112:1231–60.

21. Vogel F. The genetic basis of the normal human electroencephalogram. Humangenetik 1970; 10:91–114.
22. Vogel F. Gründlagen und Bedeutung genetisch bedingter Variabilität des normalen menschlichen EEG. Z EEG-EMG 1986; 17:173–88.
23. Stassen HH, Lykken DT, Propping P, Bomben G. Genetic determination of the human EEG. Survey of recent results on twins reared together and apart. Hum Genet 1986; 80:165–76.
24. Juel-Nielson N, Harvald B. The electroencephalogram in monovular twins brought up apart. Acta Genet 1958; 9:57–64.
25. Zung W, Wilson WP. Sleep and dream patterns in twins: Markow analysis of a genetic trait. Recent Adv Biol Psychiatry 1967; 9:119–30.
26. Propping P. Genetic control of ethanol action on the central nervous system. Hum Genet 1977; 33:309–34.
27. Heintel H, Schalt E, Vogel F. The 4–5c/s rhythm: changes in time. Eur Arch Psychiatry Neurol Sci 1986; 235:199–300.
28. Vogel F. Genetic variation of the normal human EEG. In: Beck-Mannagetta G, Anderson VE, Doose H, Janz D. Genetics of the epilepsies. Berlin: Springer-Verlag, 1989: 84–94.
29. Lennox WG. The heredity of epilepsy as told by relatives and twins. JAMA 1951; 146:536–39.
30. Metrolos K, Metrakos JD. Genetics of convulsive disorders. II. Genetic and electroencephalographic studies in centrencephalic epilepsy. Neurology 1961; 11:473–83.
31. Metrakos JD, Metrakos K. Genetic factors in epilepsy. Mod Prob Pharmacopsychiatry 1970; 4:71–86.
32. Gerken H, Doose H. On the genetics of EEG abnormalities. III. Spikes and waves in the resting record and/or during hyperventilation. Neuropaediatrie 1973; 4:88–97.
33. Eeg-Olofsson O, Peterson I, Sellden U. The development of the electroencephalogram in normal children from age of 1 through 15 years. Paroxysmal activity. Neuropaediatrie 1971; 2:375–404.
34. Tsuboi T. Seizures in childhood. A population based and clinic based study. Acta Neurol Scand 1986; 74 Suppl:110.
35. Doose H, Baier WK. Genetic factors in epilepsies with primary generalized minor seizures. Neuropediatrics (1987); 18 (suppl 1): 1–64.
36. Benninger CK, Matthis P, Scheffner D. EEG findings in children of epileptic parents. In: Anderson VE, Hauser WA, Penry JK, Sing CF, eds. Genetic basis of the epilepsies. New York: Raven Press, 1982: 95–99.
37. Hauser WA, Anderson VE, Rich SS. Effect of photoconvulsive response (PCR) on the occurrence of seizures and of generalized EEG patterns in siblings of generalized spike and wave (GSW) probands. Electroencephalogr Clin Neurophysiol 1983; 56:27P.
38. Doose H, Gerken H. On the genetics of EEG abnormalities. IV. Photoconvulsive reaction. Neuropaediatrie 1973; 4:162–71.

39. Doose H, Gerken H. On the genetics of EEG-anomalies in childhood. IV. Photoconvulsive reaction. Neuropaediatrie 1972; 4:162–68.
40. Eeg-Olofsson O, Peterson I, Sellden U. The development of the electroencephalogram in normal adolescents from the age of 16 through 21 years. Neuropaediatrie 1971; 3:11–45.
41. Klepel H, Rabending G. Photosensitivity. In: Beck-Mannagetta G, Anderson VE, Doose H, Janz D, eds. Genetics of the epilepsies. Springer-Verlag, Berlin, 1989: 104–7.
42. Rabending G, Klepel H. Fotokonvulsivreaktion und Fotomyoklonus: Altersabhangige genetisch determinierte Varianten der gesteigerten Fotosensibilität. Neuropaediatrie 1970; 2: 164–72.
43. Takayaski T, Tsukahara Y. Influence of color on the photoconvulsive response. Electroencephalogr Clin Neurophysiol 1976; 41:113–24.
44. Doose H, Gerken H, Kiefer R, Volzke E. Genetic factors in childhood epilepsy with focal sharp waves. Neuropaediatrie 1977; 8:10–20.
45. Blom S, Heijbel J, Bergfors PG. Benign epilepsy of childhood with centrotemporal EEG foci. Prevalence and follow-up study of 40 patients. Epilepsia 1972; 13:609–19.
46. Heijbel J, Blom S, Rasmuson M. Benign epilepsy of childhood with centrotemporal EEG foci. A genetic study. Epilepsia 1975; 16:285–93.
47. Bray PF, Wiser WC. Hereditary characteristics of familial temporal-central focal epilepsy. Pediatrics 1965; 36:207–11.
48. Blom S, Heijbel J. Benign epilepsy of childhood with centrotemporal EEG foci. Discharge rate during sleep. Epilepsia 1975; 16;133–40.
49. Degan R, Degan H-E. Some genetic aspects of Rolandic epilepsy: Waking and sleep EEGs in siblings. Epilepsia 1990; 31:795–801.
50. Bray PF, Wiser WC. The relationship of focal to diffuse epileptiform EEG discharges in genetic epilepsy. Arch Neurol 1965; 13:223–37.
51. Doose H, Gerken H, Volzke E. On the genetics of EEG-abnormalities in childhood. I. Abnormal theta rhythms. Neuropaediatrie 1972; 3:386–401.
52. Doose H, Baier WK. Theta rhythms in the EEG; genetic trait in childhood epilepsy. Brain Dev 1988; 10:347–54.
53. Doose H, Ritter K, Volzke E. EEG longitudinal studies in febrile convulsions. Genetic aspects. Neuropediatrics 1983; 14:81–87.
54. Gerken H, Doose H. On the genetics of EEG-abnormalities in childhood II. Occipital 2–4/s rhythms. Neuropaediatrie 1972; 3:437–54.
55. Blume WT. Clinical and electroencephalographic correlates of the multiple independent spike foci pattern in children. Ann Neurol 1978; 4:541–47.
56. Noriega-Sanchez A, Markand ON. Clinical and electroencephalographic correlation of independent multifocal spike discharges. Neurology 1976; 26:667–72.
57. Annegers JF, Hauser WA, Anderson VE, Kurland LT. The risks of seizure disorders among relatives of patients with childhood onset epilepsy. Neurology 1982; 32:174–79.
58. Janz D, Christian W. Impulsiv-petit mal. Dtsch Z Nervenheilk 1957; 19:155–82.
59. Janz D, Durner M, Beck-Mannagetta G, Pantazis G. Family studies on the genetics of juvenile myoclonic epilepsy (epilepsy with impulsive petit mal). In: Beck-

Mannagetta G, Anderson VE, Doose H, Janz D, eds. Genetics of the epilepsies. Berlin: Springer-Verlag, 1989: 44.
60. Tsuboi T, Christian W. On the genetics of the primary generalized epilepsy with sporadic myoclonias of impulsive petit mal type. Humangenetik 1977; 19:155–82.
61. Matthes A. Genetic studies in epilepsy. In: Gastaut H, Jasper H, Bancaud J, Waltregny A, eds. The physiopathogenesis of the epilepsies. Springfield IL: Charles C Thomas, 1969: 26–35.
62. Doose H, Gerken H, Horstmann T, Volzke E. Genetic factors in spike-wave absences. Epilepsia 1973; 14:57–75.
63. Doose H, Baier WK. Epilepsy with primarily generalized myoclonic-astatic seizures: a genetically determined disease. Eur J Neurol 1987; 146:550–54.
64. Andermann E, Metrakos JD. A multifactorial analysis of focal and generalized cortico-reticular (centrencephalic) epilepsy. Epilepsia 1972; 13:348–49.
65. Lennox WG, Lennox M. Epilepsy and related disorders. Boston: Little Brown and Company, 1960: Vol. 1.
66. Eisner V, Pauli LL, Livingston S. Hereditary aspects of epilepsy. Bull Johns Hopkins Hosp 1959; 105:245–71.
67. Tsuboi T, Endo S. Incidence of seizures and EEG abnormalities among offspring of epileptic patients. Hum Genet 1977; 36:173–89.
68. Ottman R, Annegers JF, Hauser WA, Kurland LT. Seizure risk in offspring of parents with generalized versus partial epilepsy. Epilepsia 1989; 30:157–61.
69. Hauser WA, Annegers JF. Risk factors for Epilepsy. In: Anderson VE, Rich RR, Hauser WA, Leppik IE, Noebels JL, Rich SS, eds. Genetic strategies in epilepsy research. Amsterdam: Elsevier 1991:45–52
70. Salazar AM, Jabbari B, Vance SC, Grafman J, Amin D, Dillon JD. Epilepsy after penetrating head injury. I. Clinical correlates: a report of the Vietnam head injury study. Neurology 1985; 35:1406–14.
71. Ottman R, Annegers JF, Hauser WA, Kurland LT. Higher risk of seizures in offspring of mothers than of fathers with epilepsy. Am J Hum Genet 1988; 43:257–64.
72. Rich SS, Annegers JF, Hauser WA, Anderson VE. Complex segregation analysis of febrile convulsions. Am J Hum Genet 1987; 412:249–57.
73. Hauser WA, Annegers JF, Hauser A, Anderson VE, Kurland LT. The risk of seizure disorders among relatives of patients with febrile convulsions. Neurology 1985; 35:1268–73.
74. Annegers JF, Blakley SA, Hauser WA, Kurland LT. Recurrence of febrile convulsions in a population-based cohort. Epilepsy 1990; 5:209–16.
75. Frantzen E, Lennox-Buchthal M, Nygaard A. Longitudinal EEG and clinical study of children with febrile convulsions. Electroencephalogr Clin Neurophysiol 1968; 24:197–212.
76. Friis ML, Holm NV, Sindrup EH, Fogh-Anderson P. Facial clefts in sibs and children of epileptic patients. Neurology 1986; 36:346–50.
77. Friis ML. Facial clefts and congenital heart defects in children of parents with epilepsy: genetic and environmental etiologic factors. Acta Neurol Scand 1989; 79:433–59.
78. Hecht JT, Annegers JF, Kurland LT. Epilepsy and clefting disorders: lack of evidence of a familial association. Am J Med Genet 1989; 33:244–47.

79. Hauser WA, Rich SS, Annegers JF, Anderson VE. Seizure recurrence after a first unprovoked seizure: an extended follow-up. Neurology 1990; 40:1163–70.
80. Shinnar S, Berg AT, Moshe SL, Petiz M, Maytal J, Kang H, Goldsohn ES, Hauser WA. The risk of seizure recurrence following a first unprovoked seizure in childhood: a prospective study. Pediatrics 1990; 85:1076–85.
81. Hopkins A, Garman A, Clarke C. The first seizure in adult life. Lancet 1988; 1:721–26.
82. Hirtz DB, Ellenburg JH, Nelson KB. The risk of recurrence of nonfebrile seizures in children. Neurology 1984: 34:637–41.
83. Shafer SQ, Hauser WA, Annegers JF, Klass DW. EEG and other early predictors of epilepsy remission: a community study. Epilepsia 1988; 29:590–600.
84. Hauser WA, Hesdorffer DC. Facts about epilepsy. Landover, MD; Epilepsy Foundation of America, 1990.

13

Laboratory Studies in Patients with Epilepsy

FEREYDOUN DEHKHARGHANI
University of Missouri
and Children's Mercy Hospital
Kansas City, Missouri

I. INTRODUCTION

Laboratory studies in the patient with epilepsy are useful in the initial workup, in continued follow-up of the patient, and when antiepileptic drug (AED) withdrawal is being considered. Save for the initial electroencephalogram (EEG), these studies should not be done routinely, but should reflect the questions raised by the specific condition. In the initial workup, these investigations may help to (1) confirm the suspected diagnosis of a seizure disorder, (2) detect a treatable underlying disorder, (3) determine prognosis, (4) classify the type of seizure, and (5) discover precipitation events (e.g., photosensitivity). During the course of the illness such studies may be useful in determining (1) if the therapy is efficacious, (2) side effects of the therapy, and (3) whether or not suspicious events are a sign of a recurrence of seizures.

Finally, some studies (e.g., the EEG) will help to determine the risk of withdrawal of AEDs. As most studies of brain function are expensive, available studies have to be utilized selectively to aid in the diagnosis and treatment. Such studies never replace a precise history and description of the event in question, nor do they substitute for an appropriate physical and neurological examination. The history and clinical examination will help the physician to decide on the extent and type of diagnostic workup to initiate.

It is important to remember the role of the age of the child in laboratory evaluation. A normal 12-year-old with good athletic, academic, and social skills who has generalized tonic clonic seizures (juvenile generalized tonic–clonic epilepsy) needs neither imaging procedures nor metabolic studies in his or her evaluation. These studies have a much higher yield in the infant with frequent generalized seizures. Brain tumors, strokes, and bleeding from a vascular malformation are not uncommon etiologies for seizures in adults, but it is extremely rare that these entities present as seizures in children.

If one sees a child at the time of a first generalized seizure, one needs to consider toxic exposure (e.g., alcohol), hypoglycemia, infection, electrolyte disorders, and so on. The workup is different if the patient is seen for the first evaluation after several seizures have occurred over a period of time.

There are more sophisticated studies for the evaluation of the patient with unusual or refractory seizures. These include telemetry, prolonged video monitoring, intracarotid injection of amobarbital to determine cerebral dominance for language, and positron emission tomography (PET). These studies are generally performed in tertiary care centers and are discussed only briefly in this chapter.

II. ANALYSIS OF BODY FLUIDS

A. Hematological Evaluation and Routine Chemistry

A decision on the type of specific hematological and chemical study is based on suspected underlying cause of seizure, patient's age, associated clinical findings, and general examination. A complete blood count, including differential white cells and platelet count, standard clinical chemistry evaluation, electrolytes, calcium, liver and renal function tests, and routine urinalysis are performed as a baseline for assessing possible side effects of certain antiepileptic drugs. The extent of laboratory workup depends on the history and clinical findings. Electrolyte studies, blood count, and urine tests are not helpful as a routine diagnostic workup. A complete blood count can be performed to check for infection, anemia, and as a baseline laboratory test before antiepileptic drug therapy.

Blood chemistries, such as serum glucose, calcium, magnesium, and electrolytes should be measured in neonates and infants with epilepsy [1]. In older children, certain blood studies are needed when a metabolic etiology of seizure is suspected. Renal function tests are also indicated whenever electrolyte disturbance is assumed to be the cause of seizure.

Acute convulsions can happen due to hypernatremia or hyponatremia. Chromatographic screening of amino acid, organic acids, and blood ammonia is needed when there is clinical evidence of a metabolic disorder in childhood epilepsy, mental retardation, and epileptic patients with progressive central nervous system dysfunction.

Routine chemistry may be of value in patients whose seizures are resistant to antiepileptic drugs. Attention to the patient's fluid balance is important. Calcium and blood urea should be measured before initiation of therapy.

Laboratory investigation may involve serological tests (especially for viral infections), serum protein and amino acid concentration, and chromosome analysis. If intrauterine infection is suspected, appropriate serological tests for common intrauterine encephalopathies are indicated.

Amino acidurias may occasionally be the cause of seizures in young children and newborns. Screening tests and confirmation with chromatography are needed to diagnose amino acid disorders. Appropriate diagnostic workup for organic acidemia, urea cycle dysfunction, and glycogen storage disease is needed when other clinical symptoms suggest metabolic disorders. Blood, urine, liver function tests, and electrolytes, including calcium, glucose, magnesium, and phosphorus, are indicated when toxic encephalopathy is considered as the etiology of the seizure and when the child presents in active seizure.

Blood chemistry, cell count, and AED measurements become more important during pregnancy for early detection of potential side effects of therapy. Investigation for hypoglycemia is indicated if seizures recur after prolonged fasting.

B. Lumbar Puncture

As the cerebrospinal fluid (CSF) is normal in a great majority of patients, there is no need for a routine lumbar puncture in patients with a seizure disorder. However, if there is evidence of central nervous system infection or the underlying cause of epilepsy is known to reflect on the cytochemistry of spinal fluid, a lumbar puncture may prove helpful: examples being degenerative disease, chronic infection, and subarachnoid hemorrhage. A slight rise in protein and pleocytosis is seen following a prolonged seizure when the lumbar puncture is done shortly after convulsion [2].

III. ELECTROPHYSIOLOGICAL TESTING IN THE PATIENT WITH EPILEPSY

A. Electroencephalography

Hans Berger's discovery of the human EEG in 1924 and his later work proved the correctness of Hughlings Jackson's hypothesis that an epileptic seizure is a clinical manifestation of exaggerated discharges of gray matter in an area of the brain related to the clinical symptoms of seizures [3].

Even in the era of sophisticated neuroimaging techniques, EEG remains the only methodology that can physiologically monitor an ongoing cerebral function. The electroencephalogram is noninvasive and can be repeated several times or be recorded continuously and represents the functional state of brain. An abnormal EEG does not make the diagnosis of epilepsy, and a normal EEG does not rule out that diagnosis. The EEG may show paroxysmal nonepileptiform discharges which should be differentiated from true epileptic activities. The EEG can be extremely helpful, but it is not necessarily diagnostic.

The term *epileptiform discharges* has been applied to any paroxysmal discharges containing spikes or sharp waves, either localized or generalized. Spikes are referred to electrical events lasting less than 70 ms that exceed the amplitude of the background rhythms. An epileptiform discharge is not synonymous with an interictal discharge. Epileptiform discharges do occur in persons without seizures. Nonetheless, epileptiform discharges provide important evidence for a diagnosis of epilepsy [4].

The contribution of the EEG in diagnosis, prognosis, and classification of epileptic seizures has been discussed in numerous publications. The EEG is the most informative test for the diagnosis of epilepsy [5–10]. In recent years, the modern technological development has further facilitated investigation of epileptic seizures. The EEG often mirrors the physiological disturbance of an epileptic focus and delineates its location in the brain [11].

Routine electroencephalograms represent a brief slice of time of the life of an epileptic patient. Rarely in a routine study is an epileptic attack captured. The new technique of video-EEG monitoring permits collection of accurate visual data of the patient's "event" and correlation with its simultaneous electroencephalographic changes. Present systems also allow simultaneous collection from multiple channels on different montages and reconstruction of montages for further delineation of an epileptic focus at the onset of a seizure. Studies can be done with cable telemetry or on radio frequency with a time-lapse video-audio system [12]. Prolonged monitoring is essential in the diagnostic workup of patients in whom surgical treatment is being contemplated. The computer prints out information collected and thus facilitates reviewing a large volume of information in a short period of time [13,14].

The clinican should be aware of the limitation of the electroencephalogram, ask specific questions of the electroencephalographer, and provide pertinent clinical and laboratory findings. This information will aid the electroencephalographer to correlate the EEG findings with the patient's clinical condition. Several epileptic syndromes, such as hypsarrhythmia, benign rolandic epilepsy, absence seizures, Lennox–Gastaut syndrome, and SSPE have typical electroencephalographic findings. Their recognition helps to formulate a treatment plan and to project prognosis. The electroencephalogram can give information regarding background activity, presence of an encephalopathic pattern, or presence of focal or diffuse slowing. The background activity of an EEG is normal in benign epilepsies such as febrile convulsions, absence seizure, or benign Rolandic epilepsy.

Precise localization of epileptic discharges on the EEG can help to diagnose the type of epilepsy or epileptic syndrome. The standard placement of electrodes (international 10–20 system) does not adequately cover different cortical segments. When exact localization is *clinically* important, additional electrode placement is needed. For the evaluation of inferior and mesial temporal lobe dysfunction, nasopharyngeal electrodes are inserted through the nose to record from the roof of the nasopharynx. Sphenoidal electrodes are inserted through the skin under the zygomatic arch to record from the region of the foramen ovale representing activities from inferior and mesial aspects of the temporal lobe.

The EEG can demonstrate two main electrophysiological changes in an epileptic focus which can be used for the diagnosis and classification of seizure disorders: (1) interictal changes and (2) ictal changes. Interictal changes are discharges on the EEG without concomitant clinical seizures and can be further divided into nonspecific and specific (clearly, epileptiform) [15]. Of much lesser degree of specificity are slow transients, in the absence of a typical paroxysmal event. Electrographic monitoring of a seizure, preferably combined with synchronized visual and auditory documentation, is the most reliable method to diagnose and classify an epileptic seizure. The history and physical examination is needed to diagnose the epilepsy itself.

B. Correlation of EEG Findings and Type of Seizure

Generalized epileptiform activity is the only EEG abnormality that supports the diagnosis of generalized seizures. There is a correlation between the location of epileptogenic focus and the manifestation of the clinical seizure. For example, Gibbs et al. found that 90% of cases with anterior temporal spikes had complex partial seizures [16]. However, focal spike discharges have a limited value in localizing brain lesions in children [17]. The EEG abnormality is helpful in the selection of appropriate antiepileptic drugs for that type of epilepsy. The response to therapy can be monitored by EEG in absence seizures, as there is good correlation between an EEG finding and a clinical seizure. In general, one would expect that epileptiform activity would be suppressed when the seizure disorder is being treated with an appropriate and effective anticonvulsant. However, this is not always the case. In benign focal epilepsy of childhood an EEG abnormality may continue for several years after seizures are brought under control.

When the clinical diagnosis of epilepsy is made and documentation of the type of seizure is important, the EEG becomes an important method of evaluation. If the first EEG is normal, the recording should be repeated, as it has been shown that serial awake and asleep recordings will increase the likelihood of detecting abnormalities. Approximately 50% of epileptic patients do not demonstrate epileptic abnormalities in their first EEG [18,19]. Ten to 20% remain negative even after serial EEGs [19]. As a result, epilepsy remains a clinical diagnosis: *A normal electroencephalogram does not exclude a diagnosis of epilepsy in the child in whom clinical events appear as epileptic attacks.*

Many epileptologists believe that electroencephalograms have predictive value at the time of withdrawal of AEDs, but a decision to discontinue medication should not be made solely on the EEG findings. Emerson et al.'s study [20] indicated that EEGs are of benefit in predicting which patients can be withdrawn from medication, but according to Thurston et al.'s study [21], the EEG is of no prognostic value. This issue has remained controversial.

Although the role of the EEG concerning discontinuation of antiepileptic therapy in an epileptic patient is controversial, an EEG should be obtained to serve as a baseline for assessing subsequent changes. In a child being treated for epilepsy, there is no justification for routinely repeated EEGs yearly or at any interval. A repeat EEG is indicated if its findings alter management or change the prognosis [22]. A repeat EEG is also indicated in an epileptic child when the clinical picture changes and the cause is not immediately apparent.

The role of the electroencephalogram on initiation of therapy after the first seizure is controversial. In a study of the risk of seizure recurrence following a first unprovoked seizure in childhood, Shinnar et al. [23] found that in children with an idiopathic first seizure, an abnormal EEG was the most important predictor of recurrence of seizures.

The EEG may be useful in the diagnosis of side effects of antiepileptic drugs in looking for background slowing on the recording and drug-induced encephalopathic patterns. The EEG is essential for monitoring the process of therapy during status epilepticus when barbiturate coma, a neuromuscular blocking agent, or a very high dose of multiple AEDs have been used.

The electroencephalogram is helpful in differentiating behavioral changes from an increasing number of seizures, increasing anticonvulsant side effects, or the progression of an underlying encephalopathy. This evaluation is done by looking at the background activity on the EEG in between epileptic discharges, not necessarily on frequency of interictal discharges [24].

There are several neurologic and epileptic syndromes with a chronic progressive course which may present with epileptic seizures or nonspecific clinical findings such as intellectual retardation or developmental slowing. When progressive epilepsy is suspected, serial EEGs may help to document the process of illness. For example, in progressive myoclonic epilepsy and progressive polio dystrophy (Alpers disease), EEGs reflect progression of the disease. The serial EEG in neonatal seizures is important, as a normal interictal EEG is associated with a good prognosis. On the other hand, the persistence of an abnormal EEG correlates strongly with severe cerebral disease.

The EEG is diagnostic only when a characteristic spell is associated with abnormal paroxysmal discharges during the recording. Interictal EEG abnormalities are not diagnostic but may support the clinical diagnosis. In general, 55%

of first EEGs in epileptic children with epilepsy show paroxysmal discharges. These paroxysmal discharges are also seen in 2 to 4% of nonepileptic children; on the other hand, 82% of Trogaborg's 242 children with spike foci had epilepsy [17,25–27].

Interictal abnormalities occur far more commonly than clinical seizures during recording. Interictal discharges should be carefully detected, recognized, localized, and differentiated from artifacts and from nonepileptic discharges [25,28]. Thus there is a good but imperfect correlation between epileptiform activity in resting EEGs and seizure disorders in children [29]. However, a patient could have focal spikes without a seizure disorder, and vice versa. The diagnosis of a seizure disorder does not require the presence of spike discharges on the EEG. Thirty percent of children with partial seizures do not show epileptic discharges on their EEGs [30].

The EEG must be interpreted in conjunction with the patient's history. Abnormalities on the EEG become significant only when they support the clinical impression of epileptic seizures. The persistence of focal spikes for many years after a child has been free of seizures is well known. Thus the EEG plays a complementary role to the clinical impression. When the clinical diagnosis is difficult because of insufficient history or atypical clinical features of the attacks, the EEG may help to further establish a diagnosis [31].

C. Closed Circuit Television/EEG

The simultaneous recording of EEG and clinical event is of particular value in supporting the diagnosis of epilepsy. Sheridan et al. [32] found that the clinical impression was altered in 5 to 17 patients who had one or more seizures reported. Video-EEG monitoring is used when the type of epileptic seizure is unclear or when nonepileptic seizures are suspected but not clear. In nonepileptic events, the electroencephalogram remains normal during attacks. This technique permits identification of nonepileptic disorders and the differentiation of generalized seizures from partial seizures. Video-EEG monitoring provides permanent visual images and simultaneous EEG tracings of patients for future analysis.

By this technique, absence seizures, a form of generalized epilepsy, are easily differentiated from complex partial seizures, which may present with similar symptoms. Ictal and interictal changes on the EEG are helpful to differentiate between petit mal absence and psychomotor attacks with lapse of consciousness. In patients with absence seizures, the background activity on EEG is normal, whereas in psychomotor seizures, this background cortical activity may or may not be normal.

Prolonged monitoring is performed for (1) determining whether a patient has epilepsy, (2) diagnosing the type of seizures, and (3) quantifying and characterizing patterns of seizure activities [33–35]. Combining this technique with radio telemetry gives more freedom for patients to move around, but this technique necessitates the use of multiple cameras. When it is indicated, an EEG recording can be combined with other physiological measurements, such as EKG, respiratory monitoring, and oximetry.

Prolonged electroencephalographic and video monitoring of ictal events is useful in the diagnosis of atypical and complicated seizures. Using this technique, Willmer and Brunet [36], in the study of 48 patients with the preliminary diagnosis of epilepsy, found that the diagnosis changed in 54% of patients, 14% had their diagnosis confirmed, and the remaining patients had inconclusive studies. When psychogenic seizures are suspected, video and EEG recording of a typical episode is frequently necessary to make a definite diagnosis in order to make firm recommendations for discontinuation of antiepileptic medication and initiation of psychiatric treatment [37].

D. Activation Procedures

1. Hyperventilation

Hyperventilation is a specific activation procedure and should be performed during all routine EEG recordings unless medically contraindicated. Hyperventilation is an important activating procedure that should be done whenever absence attack is suspected. Generalized spike–wave discharges by hyperventilation can occur in 50% of patients with absence seizures [29].

2. Sleep

Sleep is another activator, particularly for frontotemporal seizures. When natural sleep cannot be obtained, a hypnotic dose of chloral hydrate (50 mg/kg up to 1 g) is helpful. Deprivation of sleep the night before the EEG also facilitates spontaneous sleep in EEG evaluation, thus activating epileptiform discharges.

A sleep EEG is standard procedure in the investigation of epilepsy, and it should be obtained in all pediatric EEGs. Temporal lobe discharges are specifically sensitive to this stage. As many EEG abnormalities as well as seizures occur when the patient's state of consciousness changes from wakefulness to sleep, it is important to obtain a sleep electroencephalogram with special attention to the state of drowsiness. Sleep has an activating effect in epileptic discharges of some types of epilepsy, such as Lennox–Gastaut syndrome and benign Rolandic epilepsy. A seizure focus may appear only during its transition between waking and sleeping.

3. Pharmacological Activation

In special cases, pharmacological activation can be performed by fractional administration of intravenous barbiturates to cause narcosis and activate interictal spikes by short-acting barbiturates such as methohexital (Brevital). Barbiturate suppression of EEG activities has also been used to determine epileptic location and differentiate secondary generalization from primary generalized epilepsy.

4. Photic Stimulation

Photic stimulation is another important activation procedure. When photoparoxysmal discharges are associated with a seizure, this finding supports the clinical impression of generalized epilepsy. Gastaut et at. [38] found photoparoxysmal response in 40% of patients with absence and in 20% of patients with grand mal epilepsy. Photoparoxysmal discharges may be seen in 10 to 15% of the nonepileptic population.

5. Drug Withdrawal

Withdrawal or reduction of an anticonvulsant is a technique used to increase the chance of recording epileptiform activity, both interictal and ictal. This procedure should be done cautiously under close supervision, as there is risk for status epilepticus.

E. Ambulatory Cassette EEG Recording

In this type of monitoring, the patient wears a cassette-battery-powered EEG recording device. The EEG is recorded during all daily activities of life. This is then transformed into a standard EEG using specialized equipment. Ebersol [39] found that such ambulatory monitoring increases the yield for discovery of epileptiform abnormalities by a factor of 1.5 to 2.5. Major limitations are the limited number of channels, the presence of artifacts, and lack of a clinical picture of the event. Ambulatory cassette recording is also helpful in assessing the effect of therapy. This has been used in patients with absence seizures to quantitate a number of attacks and their response to treatment.

Cassette recording is an effective way to detect epileptiform activities and electrographic changes during the event. The principal value of cassette EEG monitoring is the enhanced opportunity to detect and confirm actual EEG seizure activity during normal activity to support a diagnosis of epilepsy. The sensitivity of this method has been shown by several investigators [39–44]. During recording the EEG signals are amplified and recorded on a small analog magnetic tape recorder carried on the belt or in a pocket. Long-term monitoring provides important information that can lead to a definite diagnosis of epilepsy in specific circumstances, but it is more helpful in determining the number of spells and situations that may provoke them.

F. Magnetoencephalography (MEG)

This technique records the magnetic fields of an epileptic focus. This technique is superior to EEG by demonstrating depth of epileptic focus and the signals are not distorted by the skull. MEG and EEGs are complementary techniques [22]. At the present time, MEG is a research tool. It is anticipated to play a significant role in future for localization of epileptic foci during presurgical evaluation.

G. Quantitative Electroencephalography

Topographic mapping of electroencephalograms in patients with epilepsy defines and localizes electrical abnormalities even when the computerized tomography (CT) scan is normal and conventional EEG shows diffuse discharges or no discharges at all [45]. Brain mapping is not indicated in routine evaluation of epileptic patients.

Application of a routine or special form of EEG recording as mentioned above can be summarized as follows: (1) classification, localization, and distinction of seizure type; (2) classification and diagnosis of epileptic syndrome; (3) presurgical evaluation of epileptic patients; (4) intraoperative monitoring; (5) diagnosis of pseudoseizures; (6) diagnosis of paroxysmal nonepileptic events, (7) evaluation of background rhythm for etiology of epilepsy; (8) quantifying frequency of attacks; (9) monitoring effectiveness of therapy; (10) deciding on discontinuation of therapy and prediction of recurrence; (11) differentiating primary generalized from secondary generalized seizures; (12) differentiating episodic epileptic behavior changes from psychogenic events, (13) separating localization related from generalized epilepsy; and (14) follow-up on patients with suspected progressive encephalopathy.

IV. NEUROIMAGING (ANATOMICAL AND FUNCTIONAL)

In addition to the EEG, a variety of ancillary tests can be useful in pointing to the likely anatomical source of a patient's seizure. This includes a CT scan of the head, magnetic resonance imaging, positron emission tomography (PET), skull x-ray, cerebral angiography, and ultrasonography.

A. Skull X-Ray

Skull x-rays have not shown any real value in evaluation of seizure disorders in infancy and childhood. In one study, skull x-ray abnormality was seen in 6.9% of the cases. Plain skull x-ray is not indicated in patients with chronic epilepsy. Although asymmetry of the skull, increased intracranial pressure, and large cortical calcification can be detected by this test, other neuroimaging techniques are more informative. A few patients with this type of x-ray abnormality benefited from the study [46]. Skull x-ray does not yield useful information in children with febrile seizures, idiopathic, cryptogenic, or primary epilepsy. Of the patients with nonfebrile seizures, the skull x-ray may show a manifestation of microcephaly, cerebral hemiatrophy, and occasionally, an abnormal shape of the calvarium. Intracranial calcifications may be present in some congenital diseases of the brain, such as tuberous sclerosis or intrauterine infections (e.g., toxoplasmosis and cytomegalic inclusion disease). All existing information indicates a low yield of diagnostic information from the skull x-ray in young patients with epilepsy. In most instances, abnormal findings may be anticipated on clinical exams [47].

B. Axial Computed Tomography (CT Scan)

The CT scan is among the most accurate of neurodiagnostic tests for demonstration of anatomical changes. It has very low false negative and false positive rates. A CT scan is an important laboratory test in the evaluation of certain epileptic patients, as one may find a lesion, which may indicate specific therapy and clarify the cause of epilepsy. A high proportion of positive scans is seen when the child's seizures began in neonatal life, when there is an abnormal neurological examination, a focal abnormality in the EEG, and partial epilepsy [48]. A CT-scan abnormality is seen in 5% of epileptic patients with normal neurological and EEG examination. Eight percent of patients with idiopathic grand mal and petit mal seizures have an abnormal CT scan of the head.

Yang et al. [48], in a study of 256 children with seizure disorders, found incidence of abnormal CT scans of the head related closely to the seizure type. Their patients fell into two distinct groups: (1) the low-yield group included children with idiopathic or cryptogenic generalized seizures, normal neurological examination, and electroencephalogram; and (2) the high-yield groups included children with partial seizures and generalized seizures with known etiology and children whose seizures began as neonates. The overall incidence of abnormalities was 33%. An abnormal neurological examination increased the incidence of abnormal CT scans to 64%. Focal abnormality on the EEG also significantly increased the incidence of abnormal CT scan. They found that if the neurological examination and EEG were normal, the yield of abnormal CT scans was only 5%. In primary generalized epilepsies, CT abnormalities are seen in less than 10% of cases [49,50]. In secondary generalized epilepsies, CT abnormalities reach 50% [51], but a higher percent of abnormalities is reported by Lagenstein et al. [52]. Focal hypodensity on the CT scan is reported in patients with partial status epilepticus. This focal abnormality may persist for months [53].

All studies have concluded that in children with focal seizure and focal neurological signs, the scan yield is quite high but the treatment applications are low [54,55]. The greatest incidence of abnormalities is in children with focal motor seizures and in those whose EEG demonstrated focal slowing together with focal spikes [49]. CT scans or other neuroimaging are important diagnostic tools when surgical intervention and removal of epileptic focus are contemplated [52].

In children, the most common abnormality is either focal or generalized atrophy (13%). *Only about 2% of the abnormalities discovered by the CT scan are potentially of therapeutic significance.* The etiology of seizures in children is rarely documented, while the onset of seizures in the adult suggests neoplasia or vascular lesions [49]. Therefore, CT scan of the head is not indicated in children whose history and other examinations indicate a primary epileptic disorder or a nonprogressive lesion [22].

C. Magnetic Resonance Imaging

Magnetic resonance imaging (MRI) is a very useful test for identifying small focal lesions. MRI is more sensitive for regions where bone interference hinders the CT scan. MRI has a greater sensitivity than a CT scan to detect intracranial pathology [56]. MRI has more versatility, as the images can be reconstructed in any plane. This technique allows excellent anatomical evaluation of the brain and produces three-dimensional images with high spatial resolution. T-1 weighted images provide detailed anatomical view, whereas T-2 weighted images represent tissue densities. MRI of the head is better than CT scan for identification of discrete lesions, but areas of calcification are better seen on the CT scan.

An MRI of the head is needed for patients who are candidates for resective surgery. Except for detection of intracerebral calcification, MRI remains the structural test of choice in the evaluation of epileptic patients. A recent report [57] suggests that changes of hippocampal sclerosis can be detected on MRI by the use of correctly oriented slices and appropriate scanning.

D. Ultrasonography

Real-time ultrasonography through the anterior fontanelle is an effective way to evaluate cerebral anatomy in neonates and infants. Its advantage is that it can be brought to the isolette and can be repeated frequently without great cost. Coronal and sagittal planes give visualization of ventricles, parenchyma and vessels. This study is noninvasive, rapid, and there is no risk of harmful radiation. This study is helpful in young infants with partial seizures when anatomical localization is under consideration. Ultrasonography is very helpful in demonstrating hydrocephalus and intraventricular hemorrhage.

E. Positron Emission Tomography

Positron emission tomography (PET) is a noninvasive technique that gives three-dimensional functional images of the brain. Although localized cerebral dysfunction can be evaluated by xenon-133 or single photon emission computed tomography (SPECT), PET provides the highest spatial resolution and anatomical detail, approaching 4 mm resolution [58]. PET scanning visualizes the property of selective short-lived radio isotopes, injected into the patient. Isotope containing tracer will yield a positron ejected from the nuclei when the radio isotope positron encounters an electron. Collision of positrons with electrons from tissue converts both particles to electromagnetic energy of two gamaphotons, the release of which is detected simultaneously by receivers and pinpoints the location of the source from which the image is constructed.

Until recently, functional evaluation of an epileptic focus has been limited to study with electroencephalography, neuropsychological evaluation, and observations of ictal behavior. As PET scan represents metabolic state of the brain, it is sensitive for detection of nonfunctioning regions or areas of the brain with disturbed metabolic state, such as an epileptic zone. PET is a confirmatory test for localization of epileptogenic region [59].

Positron emission tomography (PET) offers another view in the evaluation of epilepsy. During a seizure, PET demonstrates increase in glucose metabolism and blood flow, correlating with the epileptic discharge. In between seizures, the metabolic rate of epileptic focus is decreased below normal levels. This hypometabolism is greatest immediately after a seizure.

During an ictal event, epileptogenic zones change from hypometabolic stage to hypermetabolic zone. In generalized convulsions, and following electroconvulsive shock treatment, diffuse hypermetabolism is seen during the ictal periods and changes to a diffuse hypometabolic region afterward.

False lateralization or localization is much more common with electrophysiological tests than with PET [59]. As the EEG may show widespread electrical activities, the focus in the PET scan represents the area responsible for initiating the episode. The exact localization of an epileptic focus is very important in patients who are undergoing seizure surgery. The site of the hypometabolic zone correlates highly with the epileptogenic region on the EEG. Extratemporal hypometabolic zones are more commonly associated with lesions detected on an MRI or CT scan [60].

Whereas electroencephalography measures the electrical activity of the brain's neurons, PET maps their activity less directly, using radioactive tracers of the brain blood flow and metabolism. By using a specific radioactive tracer that binds to the receptors, it is possible to evaluate the chemical changes during a seizure and to determine whether a drug receptor is increased or decreased in a specific patient.

The cerebral function most commonly studied with PET is glucose metabolism, which is determined by brain uptake and phosphorylation of 18*F*-fluorodeoxyglucose (FDG). This accumulates at active metabolic sites as 18*F*-fluorodeoxyglucose, which is not further metabolized. Other aspects of cerebral function can be measured, depending on the positron-labeled tracer used. Seventy percent of patients with partial epilepsy demonstrate zones of decreased metabolic rate during the interictal state [61].

Although hypometabolic zones refer to abnormal foci, the epileptogenic process has to be documented by an EEG, as any area of damage is hypometabolic but not all areas of damage are epileptogenic. PET scanning has enhanced the accuracy of diagnostic methods and can detect previously unrecognized focal lesions.

PET is currently being utilized in preoperative evaluations of partial epilepsies. Interictal scans may show focal hypometabolism corresponding to EEG findings. Ictal scans, however, may be variable and difficult to interpret. Ictal scans may show a hypermetabolic region produced by propagation of epileptic processes to the neighboring areas. Therefore, the possibility of false localization during ictal scan should be kept in mind [62,63].

PET is helpful in distinguishing secondary partial and generalized seizure disorders from primary seizure disorders. Focal epileptic dysfunction manifests as zones of hypometabolism and decreased blood flow [64,65]. Seventy percent of patients with partial seizures have zones of hypometabolism on their PET scan, while only 20% have lesions identified by MRI [66]. As discussed, the presence of hypometabolic zone on PET scan by itself is not diagnostic for an epileptogenic region. However, if this focus correlates with the ictal EEG or hypermetabolic zone during ictus, it should be pathognomonic for an epileptic focus. Technical difficulty and short half-life of positron-emitting isotopes puts significant limitation on the use of PET scan during seizure.

In a study of five patients with infantile spasms of cryptogenic etiology with a normal CT scan and MRI of the head, Chugani et al. [67] found focal cortical hypometabolism on PET scan. The focal abnormalities corresponded to the location of abnormalities later localized by electrocorticography. Four of these patients underwent surgical removal of the epileptogenic lesion as their seizure had remained refractory to treatment. They remained seizure-free postoperatively.

Depending on the positron-labeled tracer, different functions of the brain can be evaluated. The most commonly used tracers are for measuring glucose metabolism, oxygen metabolism, and blood flow. Various physiological processes, such as tissue blood flow, oxygen consumption, glucose utilization, and protein synthesis may be investigated by this technique.

F. Single Photon Emission Computed Tomography

SPECT utilizes tracers labeled with single-photon-emitting isotopes to produce images of cerebral function [68,69]. In this study, isotopes have relatively long half-lives and does not necessitate an on-site cyclotron. However, this technique has a much lower resolution than that of PET scan. SPECT is used most commonly for the evaluation of cerebral blood flow, and the study has shown an interictal decreased blood flow in partial epilepsy associated with the seizure focus. Ictal SPECT may reveal areas of propagation rather than the primary epileptogenic zone. SPECT does not have the spatial resolution of PET, and the yield of positive studies is relatively low. A recent study has shown that if SPECT is carried out soon after a seizure, it may provide localizing information in a high proportion of patients. This is very cost effective and less invasive than a PET scan [70].

G. Cerebral Angiography and Pneumoencephalography

Cerebral angiography is rarely required in the routine diagnostic workup of children with epilepsy. A new technique, digital subtraction angiography, is safer, faster, and a less invasive technique and can be used instead of cerebral angiography in many cases. Cerebral angiography is generally reserved for preoperative evaluation in selective cases prior to cortical resection in patients whose epilepsy is caused by neoplasm or vascular anomalies (e.g., arteriovenous malformation or aneurysms). Angiography has been supplanted by the CT scan for determination of mass lesions. With the advent of CT scanning and MRI, pneumoencephalography has become obsolete in the diagnostic workup of an epileptic patient.

H. Radionuclide Brain Scans and Flow Studies

The nuclear brain scan has not been very informative in evaluation of a patient with epilepsy [71]. The detection with this test of an abnormality not previously seen on CT scan or MRI of the head is highly unlikely. Radioactive brain scans are now obsolete in the evaluation of patients with recurring seizures.

REFERENCES

1. Freeman JM. Neonatal seizures. In: Dreifuss FE, ed. Pediatric epileptology: classification and management of seizures in the child. Boston; John Wright/PSG, Inc., 1983:159–72.
2. Edwards R, Schmidley JW, and Simon RP. How often does a CSF pleocytosis follow generalized convulsions? Ann Neurol 1983; 13:460.
3. O'Donohoe NV. Epilepsies of childhood. 2d ed. London: Butterworth & Company (Publishers) Ltd., 1985:175–88.
4. Daly DD. Epilepsy and syncope. In: Daly DD, Pedley TA, eds. Current practice of clinical electroencephalography. 2d ed. New York: Raven Press, 1990:269–334.
5. Henry CE, ed. Current clinical neurophysiology: update on EEG and evoked potentials. New York: Elsevier-North Holland, 1980.
6. Kiloh LG, McComas AJ, Osselton JW, Upton ARM. Clinical electroencephalography. 4th ed. London: Butterworth & Company (Publishers) Ltd., 1981.
7. Daly DD, Pedley TA, eds. Current practice of clinical electroencephalography. 2d ed. New York: Raven Press, 1990.
8. Niedermeyer E, Lopes DaSilva F, ed. Electroencephalography: basic principles, clinical applications, and related fields. 2d ed. Baltimore: Urban & Scharzenberg, Inc., 1987.
9. Spehlmann R. EEG primer. Amsterdam: Elsevier/North-Holland, 1981.

10. Tyner FS, Knott JR, Mayer WB Jr. Fundamentals of EEG technology. Vol. 1. New York: Raven Press, 1983.
11. Gloor P. The EEG in seizure disorders. A neurobiological view and some new technological applications. In: Robb P, ed. Epilepsy updated, causes and treatment. Chicago: New York Medical Publishers, 1980:31–50.
12. Ives JR, Gloor P. A long term time-lapse video system to document the patient's spontaneous clinical seizures synchronized with the EEG. Electroencephalogr Clin Neurophysiol 1978;45:412–16.
13. Gotman J, and Gloor P. (1976). Automatic recognition and quantification of interictal epileptic activity in the human scalp EEG. Electroencephalogr Clin Neurophysiol 1976; 41:513–29.
14. Gotman J, Ives JR, Gloor P. Automatic recognition of interictal epileptic activity in prolonged EEG recordings. Electroencephology Clin Neurophysiol 1979; 46:510–20.
15. Ajmone-Marsan C. Electroencephalographic studies in seizure disorders: additional considerations. Clin Neurophysiol 1984; 1(2):143–57.
16. Gibbs EL, Gibbs FA, Fuster B. Psychomotor epilepsy. Arch Neurol Psychiatry 1948; 60:331–39.
17. Trojaborg W. Changes of spike foci in children. In: Kellaway P, Peterson I, eds. Clinical electroencephalography of children. New York: Grune & Stratton, Inc., 1968:213–25.
18. Ajmone-Marsan C, Zivin LS. Factors related to the occurrence of typical paroxysmal abnormalities in the EEG records of epileptic patients. Epilepsia 1970; 11:361–81.
19. Salinsky M, Kanter R, Dasheiff M. Effectiveness of multiple EEG in supporting the diagnosis of epilepsy: an operational curve. Epilepsia 1987; 28:331–34.
20. Emerson R, D'Souza BJ, Vinning EP, Holden RR, Mellits ED, Freeman JM. Stopping medication in children with epilepsy. N Engl J Med 1981; 304:1125–29.
21. Thurston JH, Thurston DL, Hixom RB, Keller AJ. Prognosis in childhood epilepsy. N Engl J Med 1982; 306:831–36.
22. Engel J Jr. Diagnostic evaluation. In: Engel J Jr, ed. Seizures and epilepsy. Philadelphia: F A Davis Company, 1989:303–39.
23. Shinnar S, Berg AT, Moshé SL, et al. Risk of seizure recurrence following a first unprovoked seizure in childhood: a prospective study. Pediatrics 1990; 85:1076–85.
24. Kellaway P, Slatzberg R, Frost JD Jr, Crawley JW. (1979). Relationship between clinical state, ictal and interictal EEG discharges, and serum drug levels: generalized epilepsy/ethosuximide (abstr). Neurology 1979; 29:559.
25. Cavazzuti GB, Capella L, Nalin A. Longitudinal study of epileptiform EEG patterns in normal children. Epilepsia 1980; 21:43–55.
26. Zivin L, Ajmone-Marsan C. Incidence and prognostic significance of epileptiform activity in the EEG of non-epileptic subjects. Brain 1968; 91:751–77.
27. Ajmon-Marsan C, Zivin LS. Factors related to the occurrence of typical paroxysmal abnormalities in the EEG records of epileptic patients. Epilepsia 1970; 11:361–81.
28. Eeg-Olofsson O, Petersen I, Sellden U. The development of the electroencephalogram in normal children from the age of 1 through 15 years. Paroxysmal activity. Neuropediatrie 1971; 2:375–404.

29. Blume WT, Moshé SL, Tharp BR. Electroencephalography and pediatric epilepsy. Cleve Clin J Med 1989; 56(Suppl) Part I:226–33.
30. Deonna T, Ziegler AL, Despland PA, Van Melle G. Partial epilepsy in neurologically normal children: clinical syndromes and prognosis. Epilepsia 1986; 2:241–47.
31. Aicardi J. Diagnosis and differential diagnosis. In: Aicardi J, ed. Epilepsy in children. New York: Raven Press, 1986:287–308.
32. Sheridan PH, Sato S, and Porter RJ. Video monitoring during a single, outpatient, routine EEG recording (abstr). Epilepsia 1984; 25:653.
33. Engel J Jr, Ebersole JS, Burchfiel JL, Gates JR, Gotman J, Homan RW, Ives JR, King DW, Sato S, Wilkus RJ. American Electroencephalographic Society guideline for long-term neuro-diagnostic monitoring in epilepsy. J Clin Neuro Physiol. 1985; 2:419–52
34. Gotman J, Ives JR, Gloor P, eds. Long-term monitoring in epilepsy. Electroencephalogr Clin Neurophysiol 1985; Suppl 37.
35. Gumint RJ, ed. Advances in neurology. Vol. 46. Intensive neurodiagnostic monitoring. New York: Raven Press, 1987.
36. Wilmer JP, Brunet DG. The value of prolonged electroencephalographic and video monitoring in diagnosis of seizure disorders. Can J Neurol Sci 1986; 13:327–30.
37. Wyllie E, Friedman D, Rothner AD, Luders H, Dinner D, Morris H, Cruse R, Erenberg G, Kotagal P. Psychogenic seizures in children and adolescents: outcome after diagnosis by ictal video and electroencephalographic recording. Pediatrics 1990; 85:480–84.
38. Gastaut H, Trevisan C, Naquet R. Diagnostic value of electroencephalographic abnormalities provoked by intermittent photic stimulation. Electroencephalogr Clin Neurophysiol 1958; 10:194–95.
39. Ebersole JS. Ambulatory cassette EEG. J Clin Neurophysiol 1985; 2(4):397–418.
40. Ebersole JS, Leroy RF. An evaluation of ambulatory cassette EEG monitoring. II. Detection of interictal abnormalities. Neurology 1983; 33:8–18.
41. Ebersole JS. (1987). Ambulatory EEG: telemetered and cassette recorded. In: Gumnit RJ, ed. Advances in neurology. Vol. 46. Intensive neurodiagnostic monitoring. New York: Raven Press, 1987:139–55.
42. Ebersole JS, Leroy RF. An evaluation of ambulatory cassette EEG monitoring. III. Diagnostic accuracy compared to intensive inpatient EEG monitoring. Neurology 1983; 33:853–60.
43. Ebersole JS, Bridgers SL. Direct comparison of 3- and 8-channel ambulatory cassette EEG with intensive inpatient monitoring. Neurology 1985; 35:846–54.
44. Bridgers SL, Wade PB, Ebersole JS. Estimating the importance of epileptiform abnormalities discovered on cassette electroencephalographic monitoring. Arch Neurol 1989; 40:1077–79.
45. Gaches J, Gueguen B. EEG mapping in epilepsy. In: Maurer K, ed. Topographic brain mapping of EEG and evoked potentials. Berlin: Springer-Verlag, 1989.
46. Berman W, Johnson BA. The (?) value of routine skull radiography in clinical evaluation of children with recurrent convulsions. J Pediatr 1977; 90:598.
47. Committee of Radiology. Skull roentgenography of infants and children with convulsive disorders. Pediatrics 1978; 62(5):835–37.

48. Yang PJ, Burger PE, Cohen ME, Duffner PK. Computed tomography and childhood seizure disorders. Neurology 1979; 29:1084–88.
49. Bachman DS, Hodges FJ, III, Freeman JM. Computerized axial tomography in chronic seizure disorders of childhood. Pediatrics 1976; 58:828–32.
50. Gastaut H, Gastaut JL. Computerized transverse axial tomography in epilepsy. Epilepsia 1976; 17:325–36.
51. Zimmerman AW, Niedermeyer E, Hodges FJ. Lennox–Gastaut syndrome and computerized axial tomography findings. Epilepsia 1977; 18:463–64.
52. Lagenstein I, Sternowsky HJ, Rothe M, Bentele KH, Kuhne G. CCT in different epilepsies with grand mal and focal seizures. In 309 children. Relation to clinical and electroencephalographic data. Neuropediatrics 1980; 11:323–38.
53. Sammaritano M, Andermann F, Melanson D, Papptus HM, Camfield P, Aicardi J, Sherwin A. Prolonged focal cerebral edema associated with partial status epilepticus. Epilepsia 1985; 26:334–39.
54. Sofijanov NG. Clinical evaluation and prognosis of childhood epilepsies. Epilepsia 1982; 23:61–69.
55. McKinlay I. Hospital investigation of child with epilepsy. In: Ross E, Reynolds E, eds. Paediatric perspectives on epilepsy. Chichester, West Sussen, England: John Wiley & Sons Ltd., 1985.
56. Riela AR, Penry JK, Laster DW, Schartze GM. Magnetic resonance imaging and complex partial seizures. Electroencephalography & clinical neurophysiology supplement. 39:161–73, 1987.
57. Jackson GD, Berkovic SF, Tress BM, Kalnins RM, Falinyi G, Bladin PF. Hippocampal sclerosis can be reliably detected by MRI (abstr). 2d International Cleveland Clinic epilepsy symposium. Epilepsy surgery. Cleveland, Ohio. 1990:63.
58. Phelps ME, Mazziotta JC, Schelbert HR, ed. Positron emission tomography and autoradiography: principles and applications for the brain and heart. New York: Raven Press, 1986.
59. Engel J Jr. The use of positron emission tomographic scanning in epilepsy. Ann Neurol 1984; 15(Suppl 1):S180–91.
60. Engel J Jr, Kuhl DE, Phelps ME, Mazziotta JC. Interictal cerebral glucose metabolism in partial epilepsy and its relation to EEG changes. Ann Neurol 1982; 12:510–17.
61. Engel J Jr, Brown WJ, Kuhl DE, Phelps ME, Mazziotta JC, Crandall PH. Pathological findings underlying focal temporal lobe hypometabolism in partial epilepsy by PCT and EEG. Ann Neurol 1982; 12:529–37.
62. Engel J Jr, Kuhl DE, Phelps ME, Rausch R, Nuwer M. Local cerebral metabolism during partial seizures. Neurology 1983; 33:400–13.
63. Engel J Jr, Kuhl DE, Phelps ME. Patterns of human local cerebral glucose metabolism during epileptic seizures. Science 1982; 218:64–66.
64. Bernardi S, Trimble MR, Frackowiak RSJ, Wise RJS, Jones T. (1983). An interictal study of partial epilepsy using position emission tomography and the oxygen-15 inhalation technique. J Neurol Neurosurg Psychiatry 1983; 46:473–77.
65. Theodore WH, Newmark ME, Sato S, DeLapaz R, DiChiro G, Brooks R, Patronas N, Kessler RM, Munning R, Margolin R, Chaunning M, Porter RJ. 18 F-fluorodeoxyglucose positron emission tomography in refractor complex partial seizures. Ann Neurol 1984; 14:429–37.

66. Sperling MR, Wilson G, Engel J Jr, Babb TL, Phelps ME, Bradley W. Resonance imaging in intractable partial epilepsies. Correlative studies. Ann Neurol 1986; 20:57–62.
67. Chugani HT, Shields WD, Shewmon DA, Olson DM, Phelps ME, Peacock WJ. Infantile spasm. 1. PET identifies focaL cortical dysgenesis in cryptogenic cases for surgical treatment. Ann Neurol 1990; 27:406–13.
68. Bonte FJ, Stokely EM, Devous MD Sr, Homan RW. Single-photon tomographic study of regional cerebral blood flow in epilepsy: a preliminary report. Arch Neurol 1983; 40:267–70.
69. Lee BI, Markand ON, Wellman HN, Siddiqui AR, Park HM, Mock B, Worth RM, Edwards MK, Krepshaw J. IIIPDM-SPECT in patients with medically intractable complex partial seizures. Arch Neurol 1988; 45:397–402.
70. Duncan R, Roberts R, Patterson J, Hadley DM, Bone I, Lindsay K. Postictal/interictal SPECT as a lateralizing and localizing investigation in complex partial epilepsy. 2d International Cleveland Clinic epilepsy symposium. Epilepsy surgery. Cleveland, Ohio 1990:63.
71. Yalaz K, Treves S. Brain scanning and cerebral radioisotope angiography in children. Pediatrics 1974; 54:696.

14

Surgical Treatment of Partial Seizures: Cortical Resection

FEREYDOUN DEHKHARGHANI
University of Missouri
and Children's Mercy Hospital
Kansas City Missouri

I. INTRODUCTION AND OVERVIEW ON EPILEPSY SURGERY

The history of the surgical treatment of epilepsy began with the pioneering work of Victor Horsley in 1886 when he relieved the focal motor seizures of a young Scotsman by resection of a cortical scar [1]. In 1930, Foerster and Penfield's work on posttraumatic epilepsy and their surgical report on temporal lobectomy widened the scope of epilepsy surgery [2]. By 1947, the EEG was widely used in clinical evaluation of epileptic patients. At this time Bailey and Gibbs introduced intraoperative EEG monitoring [3]. Penfield and Flanigan made important contributions to the surgical management of epilepsy [4]. Falconer [5,6] was among the first to recommend early surgical intervention in patients with intractable epilepsy. In 1954, Penfield and Jasper from the Montreal Neurological Institute reported their experiences in epilepsy and the functional anatomy of the human brain [7]. Interest in surgical treatment of epilepsy has increased recently with the availability of more precise electrodiagnostic localization and neuroimaging procedures.

Despite the advancements in medical therapy for epilepsy, there are still a substantial number of patients whose seizures are unresponsive to the present anticonvulsant drugs. Accumulated information over the last two decades indicates that carefully selected children with intractable seizures have benefited from surgical intervention.

The prevalence of patients with severe epilepsy who could be considered for surgery is about 80 to 90 per 100,000 patients with epilepsy. Recent data also suggests that patients who are likely to develop severe epilepsy may be identified earlier than was thought initially [8].

The value of surgery for intractable epilepsy in children is stressed in several recent publications [9–13]. In Lindsay et al.'s [13] reports of 100 children with temporal lobe epilepsy, 32 went into spontaneous remission, 13 underwent temporal lobectomy, 11 of these 13 patients became seizure-free. Of the remaining 55 patients, one-half remained with frequent seizures and showed deterioration. Surgery is therefore a logical option for the patient with intractable epilepsy.

Henriksen [9] reports on 38 children who underwent epilepsy surgery; 17 became seizure-free and 9 of them showed markedly reduced seizure frequency. Several investigators have shown that to prevent sequelae of long-standing seizure disorder and adverse effects of chronic medications, surgery should be done as early as possible [9].

Problems of chronic intractable epilepsies are manyfold. Side effects of drug therapy in this group of children are a major concern. There is risk of kidney, liver or other organ dysfunction, overdosage, encephalopathy, irritability, hyperactivity, and potential teratogenicity during childbearing, to mention a few. Among other problems with long-standing epilepsy, low self-esteem, depression, and psychiatric disorders are more common in children with epilepsy than in other chronic diseases [14,15]. It has been shown that parents' emotional reaction to the children's failures at school or among peer groups is picked up by children and incorporated into their preexisting battered self-images [16].

Presently, surgical treatment is used for only a small minority of children. Epilepsy surgery below the age of 6 is generally limited to those with discrete structural abnormalities, such as arteriovenous malformations, tumors, and children with hemiparesis [9]. Some epileptologists believe that in view of poor responses to drug therapy in many patients, surgical treatment of the epilepsies of childhood deserves more widespread use [17]. In recent years, emergence of interest in the surgical approach for intractable epilepsy in childhood represents acceptance of this view. Duchowny et al. [18] reported five infants under 1 year of age with frequent partial seizures, unresponsive to antiepileptic drugs (AEDs), who underwent resective surgery and have experienced a significant reduction in seizure frequency. The remission in three of five infants parallels the success rate for older subjects undergoing excisional surgery [19,20]. Their results support the view that even in young children, surgery plays an important, although somewhat limited role in the management of epilepsy. The patient considered for resection surgery should have a clearly definable epileptic focus in order to benefit from appropriate surgery.

As the key to successful surgery is patient selection, referral to an epilepsy center is necessary to investigate the type of patient seizure and to determine that the patient's epilepsy is intractable to medical therapy. Then the decision as to whether or not the child could possibly benefit from surgery is made by a team of neurologists, electroencephalographers, and neurosurgeons.

The purpose of seizure surgery is twofold: (1) to eliminate the origin of the seizures, and (2) to improve the patient's well-being [21]. If elimination of epileptic focus is not possible due to location of the focus or multiplicity of foci, the patient may benefit from other surgical intervention. Subpial transection (discussed later) and surgical division of corpus callosum have been used successfully in these cases. Corpus callosotomy is performed in children with bihemispheric seizures and drop attacks or when no single focus can be identified (see Chapter 15). Before attempting surgery, it should have been documented that medical therapy in maximum dosage has failed and that the attacks interfere with the patient's normal living. Other factors, such as the patient's age, the type of epilepsy, and the localization of the epileptogenic zone should also be taken in consideration [17]. Opinions differ as to what represents an adequate trial of antiepileptic drugs and what represents the optimum age for surgery. In recent years, the interval between onset of seizures and operation has been reduced [13,22]. Surgery for epilepsy has now become an option that should be considered in patients who are not completely free of seizures or who do not tolerate the AEDs necessary for control of their seizures.

The duration of observation for reaching a conclusion that the seizures are intractable and will not stop spontaneously or become clinically tolerable is not established. This has to depend on the frequency and severity of the seizures. When a habitual seizure pattern shows no sign of improvement over the years, it suggests that the likelihood of lasting remission is very small. When neuroimaging studies demonstrate a lesion that corresponds to the site of the epileptogenic focus, the possibility of spontaneous remission is less likely [23–25]. Andermann [26] believes that progressive deterioration of behavior and cognitive function, when documented to be secondary to intractable seizures, is an indication for surgical intervention. In this case there is no reason to insist on numbers of years of observation before surgical intervention. Some authorities consider a minimum of 4 years of observation before considering a surgical approach [26]. Others recommended at least a 2-year treatment with the latest standards of treatment before considering medical intractability [27,28]. *Therefore, the character of the patient's lifestyle and interaction of the seizure with the patient's daily activities are more important than the patient's type, timing, and the number of seizures per week or per month* [29,30]. What constitutes a disabling seizure frequency is dependent on the patient's current social, educational, or professional circumstances.

Many authorities believe that if epileptic seizures cannot be controlled by 2 years with adequate, appropriate, first-line antiepileptic drugs, the likelihood of eventual seizure control with other medications or combinations of medications is extremely small [27,28,31]. Complete control of seizures by surgery is more likely if the epileptogenic focus has not been very chronic. Therefore, surgical treatment should be offered before irreversible behavioral disturbances and cognitive deficits are established as a result of many years of treatment of intractable seizures [32–35]. The best outcome is seen in adolescence or young adults with short duration of illness [31].

As surgical resection is an irreversible approach and because of the natural tendency for some seizures to improve with age, strict criteria should be used for the selection of surgical cases [29]. Surgery should be performed when the following criteria are documented:

1. There is sufficient evidence of a localized lesion in an area whose resection would not produce significant neurological deficits in terms of speech, memory, and movement following cortical resection.
2. The family understands the purpose of surgical treatment, extent of presurgical evaluation, and their potential side effects.
3. A precise clinical history with documentation of frequency of seizures and lack of response to adequate therapy is recorded.
4. There is evidence that the intractable epilepsy interferes with the patient's social, physical, or psychointellectual life.
5. The patient does not have a progressive central nervous system disorder.
6. No significant medical or psychiatric disease exists.
7. The patient and family should be willing to accept surgical intervention, recognizing the risks and lack of guarantee [11,36].

Many investigators have shown that lower intellectual scores have been associated with poor seizure control following surgery [37]. This has been explained on the possibility of diffuse and bilateral cerebral damage and multifocal seizures. An IQ of less than 70 is considered a contraindication for surgical treatment in some centers. The validity of such a restriction is questionable, as it has been shown that retarded children also show improvement in their daily activity after corpus callosotomy. Psychosis is another contraindication for surgical treatment of seizures because surgery does not improve the psychosis and the patient does not have adequate motivation and insight [38]. These criteria may be waived depending on the potential beneficial effect of surgery on the patient's well-being.

The presence of bilateral epileptic discharges is not a contraindication for focal cortical resections if it is documented that one hemisphere is active and the bilateral discharges are secondary phenomena [29]. If a noninvasive approach fails to clearly document an epileptic focus, an invasive recording may be necessary. Many authorities require that evidence of localized epileptic focus on the EEG coincide with other evidence for *focal*, *functional*, or *structural* abnormality of cortical region. The CT scan and MRI are excellent tests for this purpose, but focal pathology is seen in only a small percent of epileptic patients [39,40]. Other diagnostic studies are discussed later.

Although concordance of abnormal tissue and neuroimaging with interictal and ictal seizures would increase the chance of postoperative seizure control, existing neuroimaging does not have the resolution necessary to demonstrate microscopic changes in some epileptic foci [13]. Even postoperatively, only 50% of temporal lobe specimens demonstrate some degree of histopathology; most epileptogenic foci are anatomically and histologically normal [41,42].

As an interictal EEG may be nondiagnostic, documentation of clinical seizures and their site of origin is very important. In this case, video-EEG monitoring is essential for close evaluation of behavior, clinical changes, and their correlation with ictal changes on the EEG. Before surgery, the physician should reach concordance between clinical presentation of seizures, ictal and interictal EEG findings, and other neuroimaging. Ictal manifestations are more reliable than interictal.

II. PREOPERATIVE EVALUATION IN PARTIAL EPILEPSIES

Presurgical diagnostic evaluation has three goals: (1) determining the type of seizure, (2) determining the origin of seizures, and (3) evaluating the risk/benefit ratio of possible surgical intervention. Decisions for the use of more invasive studies, such as extensive surface electrode placement, intraoperative electrocorticography, depth electrode placement, subdural grids or strips, and epidural pegs, depend on the accuracy of localization by other procedures and the availability of the individual's experience in utilization of such procedures and orientation of the epilepsy center. Special studies may be necessary to determine the lateralization of language, memory, and delineation of sensory motor cortex to avoid injury to these regions [20,43–45].

The most reliable information for classification of patient's seizure type arrives from a description of the patient's habitual seizure by a reliable observer or on video monitoring. It should also be kept in mind that an epileptic focus may spread to a neighboring region; then clinical symptoms become evident, giving false localization. This is known especially for extratemporal seizures invading the temporal lobe, secondarily, and some types of partial seizures in which the initial presentation may go undetected until manifested as a secondary generalization.

The preoperative evaluation consists of extensive electrophysiology studies, anatomical neuroimaging, functional neuroimaging, neurophysiology testing, and other diagnostic modalities. When these studies are inconclusive, there may be the need for more invasive studies, such as cortical functional mapping localization, intraoperative mapping, speech, and memory cerebral dominance. Neuropsychological information should also be obtained during presurgical evaluation.

Some centers use the categories phase I to phase III to refer to their surgical protocol from the time a potential surgical candidate is identified through the postoperative phase. Phase I is carried out in an attempt to localize the site of onset of the epileptic focus. The potential candidate is admitted to the EEG telemetry unit. One to 2 weeks of recording may be needed to obtain sufficient ictal data [31]. A scalp and sphenoidal EEG with video monitoring, neurophysiological testing, pharmacological activation of seizures, intracarotid sodium amytal testing, and different neuroimaging testing, including a PET scan, is performed.

Phase II consists of intracranial recording. The patient enters phase II when phase I tests are nondiagnostic or conflicting. Subdural electrode placement, depth electrode recording, and other invasive investigation is carried out during this phase. Phase III consists of surgical resection and intraoperative studies. Then the patient will enter the postoperative and follow-up period. Although all patients need phase I of extracranial study, only some patients need phase II.

The first step in presurgical evaluation is electrophysiological identification of the site of the epileptic focus, including appropriate activation procedures such as hyperventilation, photic stimulation, and pharmacological activation. Every attempt should be made to classify the patient's epilepsy, since primary epilepsy is not considered an indication for focal surgical resection. This may necessitate direct recording of epileptic discharges from cortex by surface or depth electrodes. If epidural or subdural grids are used, craniotomy is necessary [46,47]. Location of the epileptogenic tissue should also be confirmed by identification of focal dysfunction, such as an aura, which is the best indicator of the site of seizure onset in partial seizures, ictal behavior, and structural deficits. Functional mapping by direct brain stimulation will identify and delineate essential primary cortical areas. This procedure can be done intraoperatively under local anesthesia [48] or by using a chronic implanted cortical grid outside the operating room [49,50]. False lateralization can happen both on ictal and interictal recording, which may necessitate the use of confirmatory tests [31].

A. Neuroimaging in the Surgical Treatment of Epilepsy

Neuroimaging with CT scan, MRI, PET, or single photon emission computed tomography (SPECT) increase the confidence of localization and aid in developing appropriate strategy for more invasive study [31]. Although an epileptogenic zone can be localized by extracranial or intracranial recording by ictal or interictal discharges, wide propagation of discharges can give rise to false lateralization and localizing information [51]. When intensive monitoring by the EEG and simultaneous video recording of the seizure do not sufficiently define-the seizure type and its localization, anatomical or physiological neuroimaging, neuropsychological profile, and more invasive techniques are needed for localization of epileptic focus. Magnetic resonance imaging (MRI) gives better qualitative and quantitative information, and 40% of patients with complex partial epilepsy have abnormal MRIs, as opposed to 26% with abnormal CT scans. Unilateral temporal horn dilation suggests atrophy of temporal lobe structures. An MRI is sensitive for detection of mesial temporal sclerosis. When cerebral vascularity or neoplasm is suspected, a gadolinium-enhanced MRI may be even more useful.

Functional brain imaging studies, such as PET scanning and SPECT, may be indicated for documentation of epileptic focus. PET is a versatile technology, but it is expensive and requires ready access to a cyclotron. During PET scan, the injected glucose analog accumulates in areas of high glucose uptake, correlating in turn with the metabolic rate in the brain. During the interictal period, epileptogenic areas are hypometabolic, and during the ictal phase they become hypermetabolic. PET scan shows areas of hypometabolism during interictal stage in up to 70% of patients with complex partial seizures [52]. PET scan is helpful in the identification of extratemporal epileptogenic zones [53], but it can give a falsely localizing impression, demonstrating hypometabolism in injured, nonepileptogenic areas (see Chapter 13).

Single photon emission computerized tomography (SPECT) allows the measurement of regional cerebral blood flow. Regional hypoperfusion has been demonstrated in 47% of the patients during the interictal state of complex partial seizures. In 73% of patients, this hypoperfusion region changes to hyperperfusion during the ictal state [54]. The exact clinical utility of SPECT in epilepsy has not yet been defined, but it seems promising in partial epilepsies by measuring regional cerebral blood flow [55].

In a study that compared an EEG, MRI, and SPECT in patients with temporal lobe epilepsy, in 18 patients with refractory complex partial seizures of temporal lobe origin, it was found that perfect agreement between EEG, MRI, and SPECT was obtained in only 5 patients. The MRI correlated better than interictal SPECT with an EEG focus. SPECT provides complementary data but is less distinct than MRI [56]. Whatever the mode of investigation, there should be convergence of evidence of localization and lateralization of epileptic focus by different modalities before surgical intervention is attempted. When there are conflicting lines of evidence for confident localization, a more invasive recording by depth electrode or grid placement is necessary.

B. Electrophysiology Recording

The EEG remains the fundamental technique for localization of the seizure focus. Localization on EEG basis is not completed until several EEGs have been taken, indicating a localized interictal or ictal focus [57]. If the ictal tracing does not give adequate information, surgical resection should be done only if serial interictal EEGs are congruent with neuropsychological, clinical, and radiological findings. Sphenoidal electrodes may be useful. These are inserted by a simple technique and have been shown to be useful in detecting discharges arising from the mesial–basal aspect of the temporal lobe [58,59].

Structural imaging can demonstrate focal lesions, but this does not necessarily mean that this lesion is a source of the epileptogenic process; for example, a patient with focal occipital lesion from an old head trauma may have active complex partial seizure of temporal lobe origin [60,61]. The EEG can show interictal and ictal evidence for epileptiform discharges. Interictal discharges are not always reliable for the purpose of localization [58,60]. For example, bilateral interictal discharges in an EEG of a patient with complex partial seizures rarely indicates bilateral areas of ictal onset [31,62]. Extra-axial recordings of deep hemispheric activity can be done by using grid, strip, or depth electrodes [63].

1. Subdural Grids

Subdural grids consist of sheets of stainless steel or platinum disk electrodes embedded in Silastic. Grids or strips are placed over or under the dural space. This method of recording has improved the localization of neocortical foci. The advantage of grids over depth electrodes is that cerebral tissue is not invaded. Limited sampling is still a problem. Hemorrhagic and infectious complications are reported in about 2% of patients [64,65]. Subdural electrodes can be put over the tentorial edge and under the surface of the medial temporal lobes. Grid electrode placement is used frequently in frontal lobe epilepsy to define posterior extent of frontal neocortical epileptogenic focus and its relationship to primary motor and speech areas. Subdural electrodes are also used for functional mapping of brain by electric stimulation [66]. The disadvantage of the subdural grid is that a craniotomy is required for placement.

2. Depth Electrode Placement

This is the only way to accurately localize the epileptogenic site located in the deep frontal or limbic region. This invasive procedure is performed only if other modes of recordings and investigations have not reasonably localized the site of ictal onset. Depth electrodes are placed stereotactically through a burr hole. Depth electrodes are also used in the evaluation of patients with a generalized or multifocal epileptic discharge where a focal onset is suspected but not confirmed or when the exact site of onset in a specific lobe, such as the temporal area, has to be defined.

A recent study by Walczak et al. [66a] has shown that morbidity associated with depth electrode insertion was higher than morbidity associated with temporal excision itself. Other studies have also shown that depth electrodes often provide crucial information but that they carry a definite risk of neurologic morbidity [67–69].

The most important indication for depth electrode recordings is the presence of bilateral epileptic abnormalities such as bitemporal ictal and interictal discharges, or the discrepancy between the site of clinical presentation and the site of EEG abnormality. Depth electrodes are used in frontal and especially in temporal lobe epilepsy to define laterality and anterior–posterior extent of mesial temporal epileptogenesis. Depth electrode placement is done primarily in adults. Sampling limitation is even more of a problem with depth electrodes than with subdural electrodes. Not all areas can be sampled, and lateral neocortical foci, particularly, are not easily recorded by such a procedure. The risk of major complications include hemorrhage in about 2% by various reports [70,71]. The mortality of depth electrode is less than 1% and serious morbidity occurs in 4%. By comparison, resective surgery by itself is associated with a mortality of less than 0.5% [72,73].

The extent of electrophysiologic and other diagnostic workup depends on the consistency of anatomical location of epileptogenic focus, its clinical symptomatology, and information obtained from routine noninvasive electroencephalography. When no lesion is detected or there is a conflict in routine diagnostic study, a more elaborate workup is needed to obtain convergence between laboratory and clinical findings [74,75]. Despite all these studies, occasionally the interictal abnormalities are on different sides from the ictal EEG findings. If this is the case, surgical resection is done based on ictal findings.

Electrocorticography consists of recording from exposed cortical regions in the operating room during surgery. With this method, information is limited to interictal activities and is confined to the site of surgery. It could be used intraoperatively to establish the site of resection and to decide on the extent to be removed. Electrocorticography is useful to pickup after discharges induced by cortical stimulation, to demonstrate residual activity following resection, and to further delineate the epileptogenic zone. Intraoperative electrocorticography is used for tailoring the resections in the nondominant side and to obtain functional mapping in the dominant side.

C. Neuropsychological Testing

Neuropsychological evaluation plays an important role in the presurgical evaluation of a child who is considered for epilepsy surgery. The patient's intellectual function, memory, emotional stability, behavioral response, and scholastic potential should be established before surgical intervention. Many patients do not need invasive and extensive study if neurophysiological, neuroimaging finding, history, and interictal EEGs are congruent. However, in temporal lobectomy there should be adequate evidence that the temporal lobe contralateral to the resection side can sustain memory.

Reviewing neuropsychological and psychosocial outcome of temporal lobectomy in children suggests that temporal lobectomy is not associated with detrimental effects on cognitive functioning and there is some evidence for improved general intellectual status at follow-up. The postsurgical results also suggest that children operated on under the age of 10 years were less disturbed than children who underwent surgery in early and late adolescent [76]. Similar information is not available on other cortical lobe resections.

D. Functional Localization of Sensory Motor Area

This is an important step in the preoperative evaluation of a child who is going to have surgical resection of epileptic lesion. The goal of the study is to map areas such as motor cortex, language centers, visual, and memory regions. Most of this procedure in adults can be done intraoperatively under local anesthesia. In the pediatric age group, it is difficult to do this test intraoperatively. Recent use of epidural or subdural grid has made it possible to carry out this procedure preoperatively.

The WADA test consists of intracarotid injection of amobarbital and pharmacological inactivation of each hemisphere separately to ascertain that resective surgery will not produce a permanent cognitive or language dysfunction [77–80]. By the injection of sodium amobarbital into the internal carotid artery, that cerebral hemisphere is anesthetized and the patient becomes hemiplegic contralateral to the injection for 5 min. During this time, speech function is examined. If the patient can speak despite the hemiplegia, it is assumed that hemisphere does not play a significant role in speech formation.

III. CORTICAL RESECTION

Localized resection of epileptogenic focus is the most common surgical approach in epileptic patients whose illness has remained refractory to anticonvulsant therapy. Temporal and extratemporal neocortical epileptogenic foci can be removed surgically, but the results of extratemporal resection is less impressive than temporal lobe resection [31,32,81].

A. Temporal Lobectomy

The majority of surgical procedures and experiences in surgical management of epilepsy, in both adults and children, is derived from temporal lobectomy for complex partial seizures. It constitutes 85% of all surgical procedures for epilepsy surgery [19,82].

An epileptic focus may be anywhere in the temporal lobe. The epileptogenic zone is frequently along the length of the hippocampus. A temporal lobectomy can be done on both dominant and nondominant lobes. In the dominant lobe, the speech area should be mapped, and resection of the language areas should be avoided. Dominant or nondominant temporal lobectomy has a high rate of success, ranging from 60 to 95% of complete seizure control [4,20,65,75,83,84].

Complex partial seizures are more common in children than had previously been thought. Among adults with epilepsy, approximately 50% of complex partial seizures are first experienced before the age of 20 and may be refractory before that age. Complex partial seizures occur in 18 to 30% of all children with epilepsy [85]. Typical symptoms of complex partial seizures of temporal lobe origin consists of amygdaloid symptoms, such as fear or an epigastric rising sensation; experimental symptoms, such as a feeling of strangeness or familiarity; complex visual hallucination; and gustatory or olfactory sensations. In one study, the spontaneous remission rate for complex partial seizures was only 17% [86]. These children should be considered for temporal lobe surgery if (1) focal onset of epilepsy is clearly established, (2) intractable handicapping seizures are documented, and (3) location of seizure onset is in a relatively silent area of the brain that could be removed with a low risk of neurological deficit [87].

Temporal resections may be divided into three general categories: (1) en block, (2) selected amygdalohippocampectomy, and (3) temporal lobe resection based on identification of the small area of ictal origin. During an en block resection, the anterior temporal and the medial portion of the temporal lobe, including the amygdala and anterior hippocampus, are removed. The en block resection extends 4 cm posteriorly from the tip of the temporal lobe in the dominant hemisphere and 5 to 6 cm posteriorly in the nondominant hemisphere.

Prior to resection, functional evaluation of the dominant hemisphere is needed. This procedure is done by awakening the patient from deep anesthesia for mapping of the speech and motor areas. Since this procedure is not feasible in young children due to lack of tolerance or cooperation, functional mapping should be done by implanted subdural electrodes. The final stage of localization is by direct electrocorticography in the operating room before excision to confirm the seizure focus [88].

1. Outcome of Temporal Lobectomy

About 50% of patients will have complete control of seizures and 25% will show improvement in their seizures [89,90]. Olivier reports an 80% success rate in patients with temporal lobectomy. However, success was defined as anything from a seizure-free state to a worthwhile improvement. The latter was considered as more than a 50% reduction in their attacks. There are no data to suggest a difference in the incidence of side effects in childhood [91]. Other reports show that at least two-thirds of carefully selected children will benefit from surgery [6,11,92].

In a study of 100 patients (age range from 3 to 51 years) who had undergone an anterior temporal lobectomy for intractable complex partial seizures,

Walczak et al. [66a] found that in the second year after surgery, 63% of the patients were seizure-free, 16% had significant improvement, and 21% were considered not significantly improved. They also found that the surgical result did not change significantly in subsequent postoperative years and that good outcomes tended to persist over the longer time. The average follow-up in this study was 9 years. Some patients are seizure-free for several years and then relapsed. Some patients have seizures postoperatively that eventually will stop [31]. Rasmussen has shown that the results of temporal lobectomy carried out in children are similar to those obtained in adults [12].

2. Postoperative Complications

In a review of complications in a series of 560 consecutive craniotomies for surgery of epilepsy, Olivier found the mortality to be nil and the morbidity to be very low [93]. Multicenter data on mortality of temporal lobectomy has shown mortality of less than 0.5% and morbidity of 3 to 10%. [70,75,94].

Several postoperative neurologic deficits relate to tissue removal. A contralateral superior homonymous quadrantanopsia is secondary to interruption of the fibers of Meyers loop in the resected temporal lobe [95]. This problem usually goes unnoticed by the patient. Minor declines in verbal function may be detected after dominant temporal lobectomy but do not interfere with normal functions of the patient. If preoperative screening of memory function with intracarotid amytal injection has shown bilateral representation of memory on hippocampal region and intactness of contralateral side, the patient will not develop a memory deficit [77]. The patient may experience transient contralateral hemiparesis, dysphasia, anomia, depression, and more rarely, psychosis [96–98]. These symptoms disappear in a few months.

When these results are compared with extratemporal surgery by Goldring, 62% of children have good results. In this study, good results were defined as being seizure-free or enjoying a reduction in seizure frequency. He concludes that the results of surgery need to be related to the pathologic entity causing the seizures. Among his failure cases were children with varying degrees of mental retardation and children with diffuse and focal brain pathology [99].

Reviewing the results of the temporal lobectomy in children and comparison to the predominantly adult series suggests that children are more likely than adults to obtain either complete freedom from seizures or a significant reduction [91]. Several studies suggest that psychosocial adaptation, language, and perceptual skill improvement after successful surgery is age dependent. This observation would encourage corrective surgery as early as possible [37,100,101]. Psychotic behavior is refractory to surgical intervention [38].

B. Frontal Lobe Resection

Extratemporal resection of an epileptic focus is limited to those regions that are functionally silent or foci associated with removable brain tissue abnormality that resulted from trauma, phakoma tumors, or congenital malformations. Frontal lobe epilepsies are responsible for 10 to 30% of complex partial seizures intractable to medical management [101,102]. Large frontal resections can be carried out safely in front of the precentral gyrus [57,103]. In the dominant hemisphere, to prevent speech disturbance, 2 cm of the posterior extent of the third frontal gyrus should be left undisturbed.

The success rate in frontal lobe surgery is much lower than in the temporal lobe, probably due to the difficulty in accurate definition of the focus and difficulty in lateralization of responsible epileptic focus. This is further complicated by limitation of resection, secondary to postoperative language disorder, ocular dysfunction, or muscle weakness. Complications depends on the proximity of the epileptic focus to functional cerebral areas.

Frontal lobe resections for intractable seizures ranks second to temporal lobe resection in large neurosurgical series [102,104]. Depending on the location of the epileptogenic focus, the patient may have predominantly motor, postural, or behavior changes. Frequently, the seizure presents with the association of these symptoms followed by a disturbance of consciousness. Frontal lobe seizures may produce little or no distinctive ictal behavioral manifestation until the seizures spread to the temporal lobe, and then the seizures would manifest themselves with ictal automatic behavior, wrongly suggesting a temporal lobe seizure [104].

Patients with frontal lobe foci need an extensive study for delineation of the epileptic focus. Ictal recording with extracranial electrodes is usually unsatisfactory and does not give reliable localization or lateralization. Bifrontal interictal or ictal epileptic abnormalities are commonly seen in patients with unilateral frontal lobe seizures. Secondary bilateral synchrony may be due to the location of epileptogenic focus in the frontal lobe or extent of epileptogenic brain tissue [104]. In these patients the problem of localization may be solved by a prolonged intracranial recording with depth electrodes, subdural grids, and PET scanning.

The motor area must be identified in frontal resection to avoid inadvertent injury. Especially important is the demonstration of the hand area, as there is no recovery of finger function if cortical injury has happened in this area. The same applies to the cortical representation for toes and ankle movements. Three opercular gyri in the front of the lower end of the precentral gyrus must be preserved [105].

C. Central Resections

Topectomies or focal cortical resections for small localized lesions have been carried out for several decades. Resection of the pre- and postcentral gyri for focal motor-sensory seizure is a challenging task for the surgery of epilepsy [57]. This resection can be done without additional deficit in patients who already have a hemiparesis. Resections of the lower central area of both sensory and motor have been performed in the case of focal motor seizures, even in the dominant hemisphere. This is performed when the seizure involves the face [106].

D. Parietal Resections

On the dominant hemisphere, the resection is limited to the superior parietal lobe. The post-central gyrus should remain intact. This surgical approach should be based on strong congruence of clinical, electrophysiological, and neuroimaging data [106]. Here again, identification of the post-central gyri is essential.

E. Occipital Lobe Resection

Occipital resection can be carried out, provided that all presurgical investigation has given evidence for local onset in the occipital lobe. The patient frequently needs depth electrode evaluation. The side effect of this procedure is hemianopsia. Minimal information is available regarding the long-term effect of surgery in these areas. According to Williamson et al., seizures arising from this area of the brain comprise a small proportion of the patients with uncontrolled focal epilepsy [107].

In the surgery of parieto-occipital lobe, loss of cortical representation of the hand is a serious handicap. In the dominant hemisphere, there is a speech representation about the temporoparieto-occipital junction, including the angular gyrus. This segment occupies a large part of the parietal field. If a visual field defect is to be avoided, parietal resection should remain limited to gray matter, as injury to the white matter at this region causes inferior quadrantanopsia with significant handicapping for the patient [96].

F. Multiple Subpial Cortical Transections

In extratemporal resection, there is controversy as to the extent of the surgical resection [31,108,109]. Some authorities believe that in addition to the site of ictal onset, adjacent tissue in areas of interictal spots should be removed [110,111]. When surgical removal of primary cortex puts a limitation on focal resection, multiple subpial cortical transections are recommended [112].

This procedure is based on the principle that the cortex functions in vertical columns of neurons, and that epileptic impulses spread perpendicularly to these vertical columns or across the surface of the brain. This surgical intervention is aimed at disruption of the surface spread of epileptic impulses by slicing, or transecting, the cortex from bottom to top, thereby preserving the vertical columns of neurons and preserving most of the function of that area of cortex.

The technique is used in medically intractable, localization-related epilepsies and when the epileptic focus is in a vital area of brain (e.g., Wernicke's area of the left temporal lobe). Removal of this cortex could be devastating. Remarkable success has been reported using subpial transections in the Landau–Kleffner syndrome or epileptic aphasia [113].

Were the cortex to be sliced through the pia mater from above, epileptic glial nodules could be introduced into the cortex. Therefore, a small hole is placed in the pia in a sulcus and a small right-angle Morrell knife is introduced. The cortex is then sliced from below to the surface, every 5 mm, until the epileptic focus is no longer evident in surrounding cortical electrodes. At present this technique is in use at a limited number of epilepsy centers.

G. Hemispherectomy

Hemispherectomy involves the removal of most or all of the cortex on one side. Infants and young children with intractable seizures from one hemisphere and contralateral hemiplegia benefit from resection of cortex and subcortical white matter [114–116]. Presurgical evaluation must document that (1) the patient is not a candidate for a more restricted surgery, and (2) the epileptic discharges are limited to one hemisphere with an abnormal contralateral hemisphere. With proper selection, complete relief from surgery is seen in 75% of the patients after a hemispherectomy [31].

This procedure has been reported in acute infantile hemiplegia, Sturge–Weber syndrome, and congenital hemiparesis. Earlier surgery is associated with a greater potential for functional reorganization of the intact hemisphere. Cognitive function is usually preserved or improved. Hemispherectomy has also been performed in patients with frequent focal seizures and epilepsia partialis continua associated with extensive hemispheric damage and hemiparesis.

Hemispherectomy is effective in arresting seizures, but in a high percentage of patients this leads to cerebral hemosiderosis and hydrocephalus [116]. Mental retardation is not a contraindication for this surgical treatment, as care and supervision may be facilitated and the quality of life may be improved when their seizures are controlled [117]. The standard hemispherectomy is now replaced by a functional hemispherectomy that is anatomically incomplete but physiologically complete. By this technique, frontal and occipital lobes are isolated but not removed, resulting in global central disconnection of hemisphere [57,118].

Among the complications of this surgical procedure, bleeding into the operative cavity with later deterioration in the patient's course was reported in 9 of 20 hemispherectomized patients in the Montreal series [119]. Deposition of hemosiderin and intracranial hemorrhage are late sequelae of the hemispherectomy using the standard resection [120,121]. Cerebral hemosiderosis, which may develop 4 to 25 years after the operation, is caused by repeated, small hemorrhages into the hemispherectomy cavity, due to abnormal movement of the unsupported residual brain [122]. Aseptic meningitis is a relatively minor complication and is seen in about 15% of patients following cortical resection [73]. This condition subsides within 2 to 3 weeks.

IV. CONCLUSION

Epilepsy surgery is an alternative treatment if antiepileptic drugs fail. Epilepsy surgery is a costly technology and involves highly specialized personnel. It should be considered only after a thorough investigation is performed. The National Institute of Neurological Disorders and Stroke and the Office of Medical Applications of Research of National Institute of Health convened a consensus development conference on surgery for epilepsy in 1990 and came to useful recommendations before considering a patient for epilepsy surgery: (1) nonepileptic attacks should have been excluded; (2) the epileptic seizure type and syndrome have been clarified; (3) diagnostic tests have been performed to rule out a metabolic or structural cause of the epileptic attacks; (4) the patient has had a reasonable trial of appropriate antiepileptic drugs with adequate monitoring; and (5) the patient and family have received detailed information regarding drug treatment and alternative treatment such as surgery. Although the precise definition of intractable epilepsy is not given, it is specified that in addition to seizure frequency, seizure type, and severity of attacks, the impact on the quality of life should be taken into consideration [123].

REFERENCES

1. Tayler D. (1987). One hundred years of epilepsy surgery: Sir Victor Horsley's contribution. In: Engel J Jr, ed. Surgical treatment of the epilepsies. New York: Raven Press, 1987:7–11.
2. Foerster O, Penfield W. The structural basis of traumatic epilepsy and results of radical operations. Brain 1930; 53:99–119.
3. Bailey P, Gibbs FA. The surgical treatment of psychomotor epilepsy. JAMA 1951; 145:365–70.
4. Penfield W, Flanigan H. Surgical therapy of temporal lobe seizures. Arch Neurol Psychiatry 1950; 64:491–500.
5. Falconer MA. Place of surgery for temporal lobe epilepsy during childhood. Br Med J 1972; 2:631–35.
6. Morrison G. Surgical management of epilepsy in children. Int Pediatr 1988; 3(2):143–47.
7. Penfield WP, Jasper H. Epilepsy and the functional anatomy of the human brain. Boston: Little, Brown and Company, 1954.
8. Kerannen T, Riekkinen P. (1988). Severe epilepsy: diagnosis and epidemiological aspects. In: Surgical treatment of epilepsy. Acta Neurol Scand (Suppl) 1988; 78:7–14.
9. Henriksen O. Clinical aspects in children. In: Surgical Treatment of Epilepsy. Acta Neurol Scand (Suppl) 1988; 78:47–51.

10. O'Donohoe NV. (1985). Epilepsies of childhood. London: Butterworth & Company (Publishers) Ltd., 1985:227–31.
11. Davidson S, Falconer MA. Outcome of surgery in 40 children with temporal lobe epilepsy. Lancet 1975; 1:1260–63.
12. Rasmussen T. Cortical resection in children with focal epilepsy. In: Parsonage M, Grant RHE, Craig AG, Ward AA Jr, eds. Advances in epileptology. 14th Epilepsy international symposium. New York: Raven Press, 1983:249–54.
13. Lindsay J, Ounstead C, Richards P. Long-term outcome in children with temporal lobe seizures. Indication and contraindications for neurosurgery. Dev Med Child Neurol 1984; 26:25–32.
14. Hoare P. Psychiatric disturbances in the families of epileptic children. Dev Med Child Neurol 1984; 26:14–19.
15. Brent DA. Over-representation of epilepsies in a consecutive series of suicide attempters seen at children's hospital 1978–1983. J Am Acad Child Psychiatry 1986; 25(2):242–46.
16. Bjornaes H. Consequences of severe epilepsy: psychosocial aspects. In: Surgical treatment of epilepsy. Acta Neurol Scand (Suppl) 1988; 78:28–31.
17. Aicardi J. General aspects of prognosis. In: Aicardi J, ed. Epilepsy in children. New York: Raven Press, 1986: 309–40.
18. Duchowny MS, Resnick TJ, Alvarez LA, Morrison G. Focal resection for malignant partial seizures in infancy. Neurology 1990; 40:980–84.
19. Jensen F. Temporal lobe surgery around the world: results, complications and mortality. Acta Neurol Scand 1975; 52:354–73.
20. Rasmussen T. Cortical resection in the treatment of focal epilepsy. In: Neurosurgical management of the epilepsies. Advances in neurology. Vol. 8. Purpura DP, Penry JK, Walter RD, eds. New York: Raven Press, 1975: 139–54.
21. Dasheiff R. Epilepsy surgery: is it an effective treatment? Ann Neurol 1989; 25:506–10.
22. Lindsay J, Glaser G, Richards P, Ounstead C. Developmental aspects of focal epilepsies of childhood treated by neurosurgery. Dev Med Child Neurol 1984; 26:574–87.
23. Aicardi J. Epilepsy in brain injured children. Dev Med Child Neurol 1990; 32:191–202.
24. Lindsay J, Ounstead C, Richards P. The long-term outcome in children with temporal lobe seizures. I. Social outcome and childhood factors. Dev Med Child Neurol 1979; 21:285–98.
25. Lindsay J, Ounstead C, Richards P. The long-term outcome in children with temporal lobe seizures. VI. Genetic factors, febrile convulsions and the remission of seizures. Dev Med Child Neurol 1980; 22:429–39.
26. Andermann F. Identification of candidate for surgical treatment of epilepsy. In: Engel J Jr, ed. Surgical treatment of the epilepsies. New York: Raven Press, 1987:51–70.
27. Elwes RD, Johnson AL, Shorvon SD, Reynolds EH. The prognosis for seizure control in newly diagnosed epilepsy. N Engl J Med 1984; 311:944–47.
28. Dreifuss FE. Goals of surgery for epilepsy. In: Engel J Jr, ed. Surgical treatment of the epilepsies. New York: Raven Press, 1987:31–50.

29. Dreifuss FE. Surgical management of epilepsy in childhood. In: Dreifuss FE, ed. Pediatric epileptology. Boston: John Wright/PSG, Inc., 1983:261–64.
30. Aicardi J. Epilepsies with affective-psychic manifestations and complex partial seizures. In: Aicardi J, ed. Epilepsy in children. New York: Raven Press, 1986:140–75.
31. Engel J Jr. Alternative therapy. In: Engel J Jr, ed. Seizures and epilepsy. Philadelphia: FA Davis Company, 1989:443–74.
32. Engel J Jr, Cahan L. Potential relevance of kindling to human partial epilepsy. In: Wada J, ed. Kindling. Vol. 3. New York: Raven Press, 1986:37–51.
33. Crandall PH, Rausch R, Engel J Jr. Preoperative indicators for optimal surgical outcome for temporal lobe epilepsy. In: Weiser HG, Elger CE, eds. Methods of presurgical evaluation of epileptics: basics, techniques, implications. Berlin: Springler-Verlag, 1987:325–34.
34. Meyer FS, Marsch WR, Laws ER, Sharbrough FW. Temporal lobectomy in children with epilepsy. J Neurosurg 1986; 64:371–76.
35. Morrell F. Secondary epileptogenesis in man. Arch Neurol 1985; 42:318–35.
36. Spencer SS. Surgical treatment of epilepsy. Presented in American Academy of Neurology Annual Course 212, 1986:145–57.
37. Rausch R, Crandall PH. Psychological status related to surgical control of temporal lobe seizures. Epilepsia 1987; 23:191–202.
38. Taylor DC. Mental state and temporal lobe epilepsy: a prospective account of 100 patients treated surgically. Epilepsia 1972; 13:727–65.
39. Engel J Jr, Crandall P, Rausch R. The partial epilepsies. In: Rosenberg RN, Grossman RG, Schochet S, Heinz ER, Wilis D, eds. The clinical neurosciences. Vol. 2. London: Churchill Livingstone, 1983:39–80.
40. Engel J Jr., Kuhl DE, Phelps ME. Functional imaging of the epileptic brain with positron emission tomography. In: Rose FC, ed. Research progress in epilepsy. London: Pitman Books Ltd., 1983:301–314.
41. Babb TI, Brown WJ. Pathological findings in epilepsy. In: Engel J Jr, ed. Surgical treatment of the epilepsies. New York: Raven Press, 1987:511–40.
42. Mathieson G. Pathology of temporal lobe foci. In: Penry JK, Daly DD, eds. Advances of Neurology. Vol. II. New York: Raven Press, 1975.
43. Rossi GF. Considerations on the principles of surgical treatment of partial epilepsy. Brain Res 1975; 95:395–402.
44. Jensen I. Temporal lobe epilepsy. On whom to operate and when? In: Penry JK, ed. Epilepsy 8th International symposium. New York: Raven Press, 1977:325–30.
45. Ward AA Jr, Penry JK, Purpura D., eds. Epilepsy. New York: Raven Press, 1983.
46. Engel J Jr, Crandall PH. Falsely localizing ictal onsets with depth EEG telemetry during anticonvulsant withdrawal. Epilepsia 1983; 24:344–55.
47. Ojemann GA, Engel J Jr. Acute and chronic intracranial recording and stimulation. In: Engel J Jr, ed. Surgical treatment of the epilepsies. New York: Raven Press, 1987:263–88.
48. Ojemann GA. Intraoperative functional mapping at the University of Washington, Seattle. In: Engel J Jr, ed. Surgical treatment of the epilepsies. New York: Raven Press, 1987:635–39.

49. Goldring S, Gregorie EM, Picker S. Placement of epidural grid electrodes at Washington University Medical Center, St. Louis. In: Engel J Jr, ed. Surgical treatment of the epilepsies. New York: Raven Press, 1987:629–34.
50. Luders H, Lesser RP, Dinner DS, Morris HH, Hahn JF, Friedman D. Commentary: chronic intracranial recording and stimulation with subdural electrodes. In: Engel J Jr, eds. Surgical treatment of the epilepsies. New York: Raven Press, 1987:297–322.
51. Engel J Jr. The role of neuro-imaging in the surgical treatment of epilepsy. In: Surgical treatment of epilepsy. Acta Neurol Scand. (Suppl) 1988; 78(117):84–89.
52. Engel J Jr, Kuhl DE, Phelps ME, Crandall PH Comparative localization of epileptic foci in partial epilepsy by PCT and EEG. Ann Neurol 1982; 12:529–37.
53. Engel J Jr. Approaches to localization of the epileptogenic lesion. In: Engel J Jr, ed. Surgical treatment of the epilepsies. New York: Raven Press, 1987:75–96.
54. Matsuda K, Yagi K, Mihara T, Tottori T, Watanabe Y, Seino M. Does unilateral temporal hyperperfusion on SPECT indicate epileptic focus localization? International Cleveland Clinic epilepsy symposium. Epilepsy surgery. Cleveland, Ohio, 1990.
55. Andersen AR, Gram L, Kjaer L, Fugisang-Frederiksen A, Herning M, Lassen NA, Dam M. SPECT in partial epilepsy: identifying side of the focus. In: Surgical treatment of epilepsy. Acta Neurol Scand (Suppl) 1988; 78(117) 90–95.
56. Kuzniecky R, Brown J, Dubovsky E, Faught E. Temporal lobe epilepsy: a comparison of EEG, MRI and SPECT (abstr). 2d International Cleveland Clinic epilepsy symposium. Epilepsy surgery. Cleveland, Ohio, 1990.
57. Olivier A. Commentary: cortical resections. In: Engel J Jr, ed. Surgical treatment of the epilepsies. New York: Raven Press, 1987:405–416.
58. Morris HH, Luders H. Electrodes. In: Gotman J, Ives JR, Gloor P. eds. Long-term monitoring in epilepsy. New York: Elsevier Science Publishing Company, Inc., 1985:3–26.
59. Sharbrough F. (1987). Complex partial seizures. In: Luders H, Lesser RP, eds. Epilepsy. Electroclinical syndromes. Berlin: Springer-Verlag, 1987:280–302.
60. Engel J Jr, Rausch R, Lieb JP, Kurl DE, Crandall PH. Correlation of criteria used for localizing epileptic foci in patients considered for surgical therapy of epilepsy. Ann Neurol 1981; 9:215–24.
61. Gloor P. Contribution of electroencephalography and electrocorticography to the neurosurgical treatment of the epilepsies. Adv Neurol 1975; 8:59–105.
62. Engel J Jr, Driver MV, Falconer MA. Electrophysiological correlates of pathology and surgical results in temporal lobe epilepsy. Brain 1975; 98:129–56.
63. Quesney LF. Extracranial EEG evaluation. In: Engel J Jr, ed. Surgical treatment of the epilepsies. New York: Raven Press, 1987:129–66.
64. Goldring S. A method for surgical management of focal epilepsy; especially as it relates to children. J Neurosurg 1978; 49:344–56.
65. Laxer K, Needleman R, Rosenbaum T. Subdural electrodes for seizure focus localization. Epilepsia 1984; 25:651.
66. Luders H, Lesser RP, Dinner DS, Hahn J, Solonga V, Morris HH. The second sensory area in man: Evoked potentials and stimulation studies. Neurology 1983; 33(Suppl 2):185.

66a. Walczak TS, Ratke RA, McNamara JO, Lewis DV, Luther JS, Thompson E, Wilson WP, Friedman AH, Nashold BS. Anterior temporal lobectomy for complex partial seizures: evaluation, results and long-term follow-up in 100 cases. Neurology 1990; 40:413–18.
67. King DW, Flanigan HF, Gallagher BB, et al. Temporal lobectomy for partial complex seizures. Evaluation, results and 1-year follow-up. Neurology 1986; 36:334–39.
68. Cahan L, Sutherling WW, McCullough M, Rausch R, Engel J Jr, Crandall PH. Review of the 20 year UCLA experience with surgery for epilepsy. Cleve Clin Q 1984; 51:313–18.
69. Delgado-Escueta AV, Walsh GO (1983). The selection process for surgery of intractable complex partial seizures: surface EEG and depth electrography. In: Ward AA Jr, Penry JK, Purpura D, eds., Epilepsy. New York: Raven Press, 1983:295–326.
70. Spencer SS. Depth electroencephalography in selection of refractory epilepsy for surgery. Ann Neurol 1981; 9:207–14.
71. Talairach J, Bancaud J. Stereotaxic approach to epilepsy. Prog Neurol Surg 1973; 5:297–354.
72. Jensen I. Temporal lobe epilepsy. Late mortality in patients treated with unilateral temporal lobe resections. Acta Neurol Scand 1975; 52:374–80.
73. Van Buren JM. Complications of surgical procedures in the diagnosis and treatment of epilepsy. In: Engel J Jr, ed. Surgical treatment of epilepsies. New York: Raven Press, 1987:465–76.
74. Wyler AR, Ojemann GA, Lettichi E, Ward AA. Subdural strip electrodes for localizing epileptogenic foci. J Neurosurg 1984; 60:1195–1200.
75. Rasmussen TB. Surgical treatment of complex partial seizures; results, lessons and problems. Epilepsia 1983; 24(Suppl 1):S65–76.
76. Wrennall J. (1990). The neuro-psychological and psychosocial outcome of temporal lobectomy in children (abstr). 2d International Cleveland Clinic epilepsy symposium. Epilepsy surgery. Cleveland, Ohio, 1990.
77. Blume WT, Grabow JD, Darley FL, Aronson AF. Intracarotid amobarbital test of language and memory before temporal lobectomy for seizure control. Neurology 1973; 23:812–19.
78. Lesser RP, Dinner DS, Luders H, Morris HH. Memory for objects presented soon after intracarotid amobarbital sodium injections in patients with medically intractable complex partial seizures. Neurology 1986; 36:895–99.
79. Wada J, Rasmussen T. Intracarotid injection of sodium Amytal for the lateralization of cerebral hemisphere dominance. Experimental and clinical observations. J Neurosurg 1960; 17:266–82.
80. Silfvenius H, Christianson SA, Nilsson LG, Saisa J. Preoperative investigation of cerebral hemisphere speech and memory with the bilateral intracarotid Amytal test. In: Surgical treatment of epilepsy. Acta Neurol Scan (Suppl) 1988; 78(117):79–83.
81. Engel J Jr. Outcome with respect to epileptic seizures. In: Engel J Jr, ed. Surgical treatment of the epilepsies. New York: Raven Press, 1987:553–72.
82. Crandall PH. Recent developments in the diagnosis and therapy of epilepsy: surgery for epilepsy. Ann Intern Med 1982; 97:590–91.

83. Crandall PH. (1975). Developments in direct recordings from epileptogenic regions in the surgical treatment of partial epilepsies. In: Purpura AP, Penry JK, Walter RD, eds. Advances in Neurology. Vol. 8. Neurosurgical management of the epilepsies. New York: Raven Press, 1975: 265–80.
84. Spencer SS, Spencer DD, Williamson PD, Mattson RH. The localizing value of the depth electroencephalography in 32 refractory patients. Ann Neurol 1982; 12:248–53.
85. Wyllie E, Luders H. Complex partial seizures in children. Clinical manifestations and identification of surgical candidates. Cleve Clin J Med 1989; 56(Suppl) Part 1:S43–52.
86. Kotagal P, Rothner AD, Erenberg G, Cruse R, Wyllie E. Complex partial seizures of childhood onset. A five-year follow-up study. Arch Neurol 1987; 44:1177–80.
87. Wyllie E, Rothner AD. Complex partial seizures in children. Merritt-Putnam quarterly. Vol. 4. Morris Plains, NJ: Warner-Lambert Company, 1987:3–13.
88. Ludwig B, Ajmone-Marsan C, Van Buren JM. Depth and direct cortical recording in seizure disorders of extratemporal origin. Neurology 1976; 26:1085–99
89. Uematsu S. (1990). Surgical management of complex partial seizures. JAMA 1990; 264(6):734–37.
90. Taylor DC, Falconer MA. Clinical, socioeconomic and psychological changes after temporal lobectomy for epilepsy. Br J Psychiatry 1968; 114:1247–61.
91. Duchowny M. The role of surgery in childhood epilepsy. Int Pediatr 1987; 2:205–11.
92. Vaernet K. Temporal lobectomy in children and young adults. In: Advances in epileptology. 14th Epilepsy international symposium. New York: Raven Press, 1983:255–61.
93. Olivier A. Risk and benefit in the surgery of epilepsy: complications and positive results on seizures tendency and intellectual function. In: Surgical treatment of epilepsy. Acta Neurol Scand (Suppl) 1988; 78 (117):N114–21.
94. Falconer MA. Reversibility by temporal lobe resection of the behavioral abnormalities of temporal lobe epilepsy. N Engl J Med 1973; 289:451–54.
95. Falconer MA, Wilson JD. Visual field changes following anterior temporal lobectomy: their significance in relation to "Meyer's loop" of the optic radiation. Brain 1958; 81:1–18.
96. Van Buren JM. Complications of surgical procedures in the diagnosis and treatment of epilepsy. In: Engel J Jr, ed. Surgical treatment of the epilepsies. New York: Raven Press, 1987:465–77.
97. Crandall PH. Postoperative management and criteria for evaluation. In: Purpura DP, Penry JK, Walter RD, eds. Advances in neurology. Vol. 8. Neurosurgical management of the epilepsies. New York: Raven Press, 1975:265–79.
98. Horowitz, MJ, Cohen FM. Temporal lobe epilepsy: effect of lobectomy on psychosocial functioning. Epilepsia 1968; 9:23–41.
99. Goldring S. Surgical management of epilepsy in children. In: Engel J Jr, ed. Surgical treatment of the epilepsies. New York: Raven Press, 1987.
100. Lindsay J, Ounstead C, Richards P. Long-term outcome in children with temporal lobe seizure III: psychiatric aspects in children and adult life. Dev Med Child Neurol 1979; 21:630–36.

101. Cavazzuti V, Winston K, Baker R, Welch K. Psychological changes following surgery for tumors in the temporal lobe. J Neurosurg 1980; 53:618–26.
102. Williamson PD, Spencer DD, Spencer SS, Novelly RA, Mattson RH. Complex partial seizures of frontal lobe origin. Ann Neurol 1985; 18:497–504.
103. Rasmussen T. Surgical therapy of frontal lobe epilepsy. Epilepsia 1963; 4:181–98.
104. Quesney LF, Olivier A. (1988). Preoperative EEG evaluation in frontal lobe epilepsy. In: Surgical treatment of epilepsy. Acta Neurol Scand (Suppl) 1988; 78(117):61–72.
105. Rasmussen T. Surgery of frontal lobe epilepsy. In: Purpura DP, Penry JK, Walter RD, eds. Advances in neurology. Vol. 8. Neurosurgical management of the epilepsies. New York: Raven Press, 1975:197–295.
106. Olivier A. Surgery of epilepsy: methods. In: Surgical treatment of epilepsy. Acta Neurol Scand (suppl) 1988; 78(117):103–113.
107. Williamson PD, Spencer SS, Spencer DD, Mattson RH. Complex partial seizures with occipital lobe onset. Epilepsia 1981; 22:247–48.
108. Goldring S, Rich KM, Picker S. Experience with gliomas in patients presenting with a chronic seizure disorder. Clin Neurosurg 1986; 33:15–42.
109. Wyllie E, Luders H, Morris HH III, Lesser RP, Dinner DS, Hahn J, Estes ML, Rothner AD, Erenberg G, Cruse R, Friedman D. Clinical outcome after complete or partial resection for intractable epilepsy. Neurology 1987; 37:1637–41.
110. Munari C, Bancaud J. (1985). The role of stereo-electroencephalography (SEEG) in the evaluation of partial epileptic seizures. In: Porter RJ, Morselli PL, eds. The epilepsies. London: Butterworth & Company (Publishers) Ltd., 1985:267–306.
111. Ojemann GA, Engel J Jr. Acute and chronic intracranial recording and stimulation. In: Engel J Jr, ed. Surgical treatment of the epilepsies. New York: Raven Press, 1987:263–88.
112. Morrell F, Whisler WW, Bleck TP. Multiple subpial transection. A new approach to the surgical treatment of focal epilepsy. J Neurosurg 1989; 70:231–39.
113. Morrell F, Whisler WW, Smith MC, Pierre-Louis SJC, Schmitt J, Brocken C, Ali A, Cooper M, Andrews RV. Landau–Kleffner syndrome: treatment with multiple subpial transection (abstr). Epilepsia 1989; 30:693.
114. Krynauw RA. Infantile hemiplegia treated by removing one cerebral hemisphere. J Neurol Neurosurg Psychiatry 1950; 13:243–67.
115. Till K. Hemispherectomy for infantile hemiplegia. Dev Med Child Neurol 1967; 9:773–74.
116. Rasmussen T. Hemispherectomy for seizures revisited. Can J Neurol Sci 1983; 10:71–78.
117. McNaughton FC, Rasmussen T. Criteria for selection of patients for neurosurgical treatment. In: Purpura DP, Penry JK, Walter RD, eds. Advances in neurology. Vol. 8. Neurosurgical management of the epilepsies. New York: Raven Press, 1975:37–48.
118. Rasmussen T. Commentary. Extratemporal cortical excisions and hemispherectomy. In: Engel J Jr, ed. Surgical treatment of the epilepsies. New York: Raven Press, 1987:417–24.
119. Rasmussen T. Postoperative superficial hemosiderosis of the brain, its diagnosis, treatment and prevention. Trans Am Neurol Assoc 1973; 98:133–37.

120. Brett E. Second thoughts on hemispherectomy in infantile hemiplegia. Dev Med Child Neurol 1969; 11:374–76.
121. Falconer MA, Wilson PJE. Complications related to delayed hemorrhage after hemispherectomy. J Neurosurg 1969; 30:413–26.
122. Adams CBT. Hemispherectomy, a modification. J Neurosurg Psychiatry 1983; 46:617–19.
123. National Institutes of Health Consensus Conference. Surgery for epilepsy. JAMA 1990; 264(6):729–33.

15

Surgical Treatment of Seizures: Corpus Callosotomy

JEROME V. MURPHY
*University of Missouri
and Children's Mercy Hospital
Kansas City, Missouri*

I. BACKGROUND

The performance of corpus callosotomies for the control of intractible seizures developed from two observations: (1) that epileptic discharges spread through the corpus callosum, and (2) that section of the corpus callosum produced no major clinical deficits. Seizures propagate through the brain via known neuronal pathways, and this has been demonstrated by electrical and metabolic studies [1,2]. Spread of a focal epileptic discharge from one cerebral hemisphere to the other occurs through the corpus callosum and the hippocampal commisure to produce generalization and synchronization of the epileptic discharge. Other commisures are also involved, and intractible seizures may use several commisural pathways [3]. In addition, the corpus callosum is essential for the synchrony of bilateral spike and wave discharge in the feline model of penicillin-induced generalized epilepsy. This synchrony persists with isolation of the cortex and corpus callosum and is abolished with section of the corpus callosum [4].

Dandy was the first to report that the corpus callosum could be divided without major neurologic deficits [5]. The first corpus callosotomies for the surgical control of intractible seizures were reported in 1940 [6]. Two of the 10 reported patients were children, 10 and 14 years of age. Both children had generalized convulsions, with loss of consciousness attributed in the 10-year-old to a difficult delivery during which his head was "bashed in" with forceps. The second patient had a left hemiplegia following diphtheritic laryngitis. Both children had excellent seizure control postoperatively, and one child required continued phenobarbital therapy to achieve this control. The parents of the boy with forceps trauma insisted that his mental function had improved concurrent with the surgery.

In this early series, one woman noted postoperatively that there was lack of coordination of motor activity between her two sides. One hand would try to open a door and the other to shut it. The lack of this complication in children is probably explained by the continued reliance in children of ipsilateral pathways until the corpus callosum reaches functional maturity [7].

The first series of pediatric patients whose intractable epilepsy was treated by a corpus callosotomy was reported in 1970 by Luessenhop et al. These patients, ages 4 months to 7 years, had focal cerebral lesions, and therefore had secondarily generalized seizures. Three of the four experienced remarkable improvement in seizure control and function postoperatively. Of the three improved patients, two remained on antiepileptic drugs (AEDs). The 4-month-old child continued to have hourly seizures [8]. A postoperative split-brain syndrome was not described in this pediatric series.

The early commisurotomies were associated with a significant operative morbidity. In the series of eight patients reported by Wilson et al. [9], one died and three experienced aseptic meningitis and hydrocephalus following callosotomy, leaving a 12.5% mortality and a 37.5% morbidity. Two innovations have reduced the morbidity of this procedure: avoidance of penetration of the third ventricle and use of the operative microscope [9,10]. Nevertheless, in one recent series of 18 pediatric patients, 3 suffered aseptic meningitis postoperatively (17% morbidity), and one of these 3 patients required a ventriculoperitonal shunt. In a very recently reported series of 80 patients, there were 2 intraoperative deaths [11]. It is not clear if the deaths occurred in children or adults. Based on these observations there still is a significant morbidity associated with corpus callosotomies.

II. INDICATIONS

A. Partial Seizures

The indications for corpus callosotomy in patients with seizures intractible to medical therapy are unclear. Initially, it was used to seemingly disrupt the generalization of a seizure from one cerebral hemisphere to the other. However, some partial seizures are more severe after corpus callosotomy (see below). In this section the available information on patient benefit will be reviewed briefly. The division into indications for partial seizure disorders and indications for generalized seizure disorders is somewhat arbitrary, as many patients who have been reported had both partial and primary generalized seizures.

In her 1988 review of corpus callosum section for intractible seizures, Spencer accumulated reports on 67 adults and 11 children with partial seizures, both simple and complex, who had undergone partial or complete callosotomy. Sixty percent of the adults had either no change in their seizures or were worse following corpus callosotomy. Of the 11 children collected in this review, 7 had either no change or were worse [3]. Based on this review, corpus callosotomy for intractible partial seizures carries a low benefit/risk ratio. Yet, as described above, the procedure was originally conceived as an intervention to prevent the secondary generalization of partial seizures.

In a later 1988 series of 22 patients undergoing corpus callosotomy for intractible seizures, all patients had partial seizures and 14 of these 22 patients had focal lesions by neuroimaging. Postoperatively, 9 of the 22 patients had either simple partial seizures alone, or no seizures, indicating benefit in partial seizures [12]. In a more recent series, of 18 patients aged 16 years and younger, 12 had partial seizures with or without primary generalized seizures. Only one patient of the 12 did not benefit from the surgery; that one patient died in status epilepticus 3 months after surgery [10]. Similarly, two patients with Sturge–Weber syndrome and intractable secondary generalized seizures improved remarkable after corpus callosotomy [13]. Following surgery both patients exhibited only unilateral seizures, and even these events were very infrequent.

In all these patients the etiology of the epilepsy was variable and the etiology had no relationship to the outcome. It was rare in all the series of children with partial seizures that the seizures resolved or that they could be withdrawn from antiepileptic drugs (AEDs) after corpus callosotomy. The sizable reduction in number of seizures and the prevention of generalization of the partial seizures was most impressive and stands in contrast to Spencer's review, in which a significant number of patients with partial seizures did not improve [3].

Stimulation of the corpus callosum can also inhibit firing of pyramidal cells, indicating that the corpus callosum carried fibers that inhibit neuronal firing [14]. Rovit et al., using rabbits with penicillin-induced epileptic foci, demonstrated that under certain conditions a seizure focus could become more intense when amobarbital was injected into the contralateral internal carotid artery [15]. This amobarbital effect must be mediated by its action on inhibitory neurons in the cerebral hemisphere contralateral to the seizure focus. These neurons project to the opposite hemisphere via a commisural tract, probably the corpus callosum.

More directly, Mutani et al. demonstrated that section of the corpus callosum had no effect on the epileptic activity of a single estrogen-induced epileptic focus. Animals with bilateral and asymmetrical estrogen-induced epileptic foci had increased epileptic activity following resection of the corpus callosum [16]. Thus the corpus callosum must carry fibers that inhibited epileptic discharges.

If this is clinically significant some partial seizures may deteriorate after corpus callosotomy, and such has been reported [18]. Predicting which patients are

Table 1 Effect of Corpus Callosotomy on Generalized Seizures[a]

Seizure	Number of patients	Number remarkably improved (%)
Atonic	14	12 (85)
Tonic-clonic	33	28 (85)
Absence	14	8 (57)
Myoclonic	5	3
Tonic	9	7 (78)

[a]See text for specific references.

at risk for such worsening is difficult. Patients with bilateral asymmetrical seizure foci, and patients with evidence of diffuse brain abnormalities, i.e. severe mental retardation, may carry a higher risk for this deterioration following corpus callosotomy [17]. The EEG recorded during the Wada test may be helpful in predicting which patients are at risk for such worsening. If the seizure focus becomes more active with the contralateral injection of amobarbital, then inhibitory fibres may originate in the contralateral hemisphere [15].

In summary, corpus callosotomy has a role in the treatment of intractible partial seizures if the primary focus cannot be surgically removed. The best candidates for improved control of their partial seizures appear to be patients with secondarily generalized seizures originating from a single epileptic focus. Patients with bilateral, homotopic epileptic foci also appear to benefit from this surgery. Patients with multiple heterotropic foci from which secondary generalization occurs and patients with severe mental retardation may not benefit from corpus callosotomy and may be at higher risk for deterioration of their epilepsy. This rule cannot be applied to all patients with medically intractible partial seizures, as several such patients have benefited from corpus callosotomy [17].

B. Generalized Seizures

Many pediatric patients with medically intractible primarily generalized seizures have improved following corpus callosotomy. The generalized seizures for which corpus callosotomy has been performed are atonic, tonic–clonic, absence, myoclonic, and tonic. (A breakdown in the benefit from corpus callosotomy, according to seizure type, is presented in Table 1.) As most patients considered for corpus callosotomy have multiple seizure types, it is difficult to determine the benefit of the procedure on an isolated and specific seizure type.

The most commonly improved seizure is the *atonic seizure* [10,11,18–20]. The observation that atonic seizures responded favorably to corpus callosotomy was first made by Wilson et al. [18], but the reason why this seizure type responds so favorably is not known. In atonic seizures the child suddenly loses postural tone and, lacking protective reflexes during the seizure, strikes the ground forcefully, frequently leading to cutaneous, boney, brain, or dental damage.

In the series in which ages of patients are included, 14 pediatric patients with atonic seizures are available for evaluation [9,10,18]. Almost all these patients had other seizure types as well, a common observation in patients with atonic seizures. Of these 14 patients, 2 did not have a significant reduction in the number of atonic seizures following corpus callosotomy. The improvement is similar if adult and pediatric patients are combined, and almost all patients operated on as adults had the onset of seizures in childhood. Reduction of AEDs is not always possible following surgery [18]. Therefore, corpus callosotomy seems to be a responsible procedure to perform in children with atonic seizures intractible to available medical therapy.

In three reports a total of 33 patients with intractible *generalized tonic–clonic seizures* underwent corpus callosotomy [10,21,22]. Five (15%) did not improve. (In the second series, by Gates et al. [21], the ages of the patients are not stated. Nevertheless, they are included here.) In this second series all 24 patients with generalized tonic clonic seizures also had partial complex, and generalized atonic and tonic seizures, and all improved following corpus callosotomy. One can conclude that patients with a mixture of seizure disorders, including generalized tonic–clonic seizures, who are refractory to medical therapy, should respond favorably to corpus callosotomy.

Geoffrey included three children with only generalized tonic–clonic seizures in his report on the efficacy of corpus callosotomy [20]. In all three there was a reduction in seizure frequency, and this reduction was 67 to 96%. Our experience with three children who had only generalized tonic–clonic seizures is not as favorable. None responded to a two-thirds corpus callosotomy, and noting no improvement after the initial procedure, completion of the callosotomy was not attempted.

In two reports the effect of this surgery specifically on *absence seizures* is available. In Geoffrey et al.'s article, four patients had absence seizures as part of their medically intractible epilepsy, and none had absence seizures postoperatively [20]. In the series of Nordgren et al., five patients had absence seizures as one of their seizure types [10]. Postoperatively, three experienced a dramatic improvement in the frequency of this seizure, and two had no change. Purves et al. reported five patients with absence as one of their seizure types, one had an excellent response, three had a moderate reduction in absence seizures, and one did not respond favorably to the surgery [23]. (The patients reported by Purves et al. were all more than 16 years old at the time of surgery, but all had the onset of their seizures in early childhood). In summary, of 14 patients with absence seizures, 8 (57%) experienced dramatic improvement postoperatively.

The effect of corpus callosotomy on *myoclonic seizures* is more difficult to determine. Most series do not include this seizure type [11,12,17,18,21,23]. In the two reports in which myoclonic seizures are specified, five patients are reported. In one report all three patients had resolution of their myoclonic seizures, and the two patients in the other report, had persistence of myoclonic seizures [10,20]. Therefore, the evidence for or against the efficacy of corpus callosotomy on the reduction of myoclonic seizures is inadequate.

The effect of corpus callosotomy on nine patients with *tonic seizures* as part of their epilepsy is available in three reports [12,20,23]. Of these nine patients, seven had no further tonic seizures postoperatively, one patient had only focal seizures, and one had no change. Therefore, patients with medically intractible tonic seizures are good candidates for corpus callosotomy.

Based on the summary above, patients with medically intractible mixed and generalized seizure disorders who have predominantly atonic, tonic, or tonic–clonic seizures should respond favorably to corpus callosotomy (see Table 1). If the predominant seizure type that is impairing the patient is absence, the outcome does not appear to be favorable. Insufficient data are available to predict the response of myoclonic seizures to this intervention. A deterioration of seizure frequency after corpus callosotomy, as reported in partial seizures, has not been observed in patients with generalized seizures. In all these reports the number of children with a single type of seizure is insufficient to draw conclusions as to the benefit of corpus callosotomy when only one type of seizure is present and intractible to medical therapy.

III. THE PARTIAL VERSUS COMPLETE CORPUS CALLOSOTOMY

If data were available to indicate which part(s) of the corpus callosum carried fibers permitting either secondary generalization or synchronization of the epileptic discharge, and which carried inhibitory fibers, the resection would be simplified by restricting it to specific fibers. Available laboratory studies do not permit this. Therefore, some reports have advocated complete resection of the corpus callosum, and others that an anterior two-thirds resection would be sufficient to reduce seizure frequency dramatically. In one recent review of this subject, 47% of patients who underwent a partial corpus callosotomy achieved an excellent response, whereas 74% of patients who underwent a complete corpus callosotomy achieved an excellent response [3].

In the report of Purves et al., 24 patients had 40 types of intractible seizures. Following an anterior callosotomy, 37% of the intractible seizures had an excellent response, 45% of the seizures had a moderate or good response, 15% had no change, and aversive seizures worsened in one patient [23]. In another series, including a similar number of patients, 65% of patients experienced no improvement after an anterior callosotomy, and only 23% of patients were left with no improvement after a total section of the corpus callosum [12]. Therefore, if a corpus callosotomy is planned for a patient with intractible seizures, a complete corpus callosotomy should be performed unless satisfactory improvement is observed after dividing only the anterior corpus callosum.

Given that a complete resection of the corpus callosum is optimal for the control of certain intractible seizures, its performance as a one- or two-stage procedure varies from one center to another [11,18,19]. Claims are made that two stages will reduce operative morbidity [19]. Comparisons of operative complications between series where complete corpus callosums are performed in either one or two stages do not support this claim [25].

IV. COMPLICATIONS

Five deaths have been reported in patients during the corpus callosotomy [11,22,24,25]. One was secondary to an air embolism that occurred when the saggital sinus was inadvertently penetrated. Other medical complications are transient or treatable. These included wound infection, subdural or epidural hematomas, aseptic meningitis, shunt-dependent hydrocephalus, hemipareses, and diabetes insipidus [10,11,23]. Worsening of partial seizures has been described in Section II.A and is not considered as a complication of the operative procedure.

If a hemisphere contains an anatomic lesion, a callosotomy may result in lessening of dexterity of the limbs contralateral to the anatomic lesion. Apparently, callosal fibers had compensated for this deficit before their disruption [26].

Functional impairments after corpus callosotomy have involved speech and bimanual dexterity and are reported almost exclusively in adults. Consistent declines in language skills have been observed in patients whose speech-dominant hemisphere is ipsilateral to the dominant limb [24,25]. Stuttering has also been reported as a complication of this procedure [21].

Surprisingly, certain skills improve following corpus callosotomy. Double discrimination tasks (e.g., simultaneously sorting cards for brightness with one hand and for color with the other) are performed relatively more rapidly following commisurotomy than in patients with an intact corpus callosum. This is also true in the split monkey brain [25].

A split-brain syndrome has been described in patients after corpus callosotomy. The nondominant hand has difficulties responding to verbal commands having been disconnected from fibers arising in the dominant hemisphere and crossing to the opposite hemisphere in the corpus callosum. When it has been observed, it is a transient syndrome that rarely persists [3].

It is not clear if these complications occur in children as well as adults, or only in adults, as the age of patients with postoperative impairments is not always reported. In the only large series of pediatric patients who underwent corpus callosum section, the only recognized language complication was a transient mutism, associated with paresis of the nondominant leg [10]. The persistence of a severe language disability has not been reported in children, and this probably relates to bilateral organization of speech and the use of other commisures in the younger brain [7].

Deterioration in behaviors has not been reported in children after callosotomy. Most parents of such patients have noted postoperatively that their children are more attentive and have improved behaviors [10].

Utilizing present operative techniques in appropriately selected patients, major operative complications in children are infrequent. Considering (1) the more frequent presence of language difficulties and split-brain syndromes in adults after undergoing corpus callosotomy, and (2) that many of the seizures for which adults undergo this type of surgery begin, and have been intractible, in childhood, children with intractible seizures need to be considered as candidates for this surgery in order that it can be done at a time of diminished potential for functional morbidity.

V. CRITERIA FOR PATIENT SELECTION

The crucial issue in doing corpus callostomies is the selection of appropriate candidates for this procedure. Once selected, an appropriate candidate needs to be referred to a center with experience in the surgical treatment of epilepsy for a second opinion concerning the potential yield of the procedure and for the actual corpus callosotomy.

The seizures themselves should be sufficiently frequent and severe to impair the child's function. Examples of intractible seizures that may not warrant surgical intervention are (1) those occurring every 6 months and only during sleep, or (2) brief and randomly occurring seizures in a nonambulatory wheelchair-confined child who is at no risk for injury from these seizures.

In addition, there should be evidence that the likelihood of spontaneous remission is small compared to the impairments produced by the persistence of the seizures and their treatment. In one recent report, children without mental retardation and with intractible seizures had a spontaneous remission rate of about 4% annually. This did not occur in children who were mentally retarded [27]. This spontaneous remission rate is slow and the patient could suffer irreversible side effects from the frequent seizures or their therapy.

The seizures have to be medically intractible to available AEDs, or the patient has to be intolerant of any effective AED. This intractibility means that the patient has to have been exposed at least to phenobarbital, carbamazepine, phenytoin, and valproic acid/divalproex sodium with both therapeutic and elevated (as tolerated) serum concentrations of the AED, before being considered refractory to these AEDs. Depending on seizure frequency, this intractibility may take only several months of intensive follow-up to demonstrate.

Other primary AEDs to which the patient should be exposed, depending on seizure type and AED tolerance, include primidone, clonazepam, and ethosuccimide. Secondary AEDs that may be useful additives if partial control is achieved with one of the primary AEDs above include chlorazepate, acetazolamide, nitrazepam, or valium. Recent reports have indicated successful medical control of previously intractable seizures using bromides or methsuximide, and their use will depend on the experience of the treating physician.

In our center all patients considered as candidates for surgical intervention have to have been exposed to at least one research AED. The use of such compounds will depend on the availability of research protocols when the patient is being evaluated. Research AEDs presently undergoing clinical trials in this country include vigabatrin, gabapentin, felbamate, nitrazepam, and progabide.

Nonmedicinal therapies that may be useful are the ketogenic diet and a vagal nerve stimulator. The ketogenic diet has been useful in very young children, requires hospitalization, and should be used only in centers with nutritional expertise [28]. The vagal nerve stimulator is still undergoing clinical trials in adults [29].

If the measures above are not successful in providing adequate control of seizures, and that definition varies with each patient, surgical intervention needs to be considered. If a seizure focus can be demonstrated, and if that area of brain can be resected without significant adversity, a resection of the focus, as opposed to a corpus callosotomy, is the procedure of choice.

In the patient with secondary generalization from a focus in whom the focus cannot be resected, a corpus callosotomy may be a recommended to limit or eliminate the secondary generalization. If the seizures are primarily generalized, the likelihood of satisfactory control will depend on the seizure type(s). All these deliberations must take into account which type of seizure is most disabling to the patient, the expected improvement in seizure control after corpus callosotomy, and the improvement in general patient well-being and function if improved control of seizures is achieved.

It should be obvious to the reader that experience with corpus callostomies in children is still limited by the small numbers thus far reported. In some reports the ages, both of patients under corpus callosotomy and of those suffering complications, are not reported, rendering application of results to pediatric populations difficult. In the reports limited to children [10,20], numerous seizure types are reported and the numbers of patients with one specific epilepsy are small. In the next few years, as more data accumulates, better selection criteria should be available.

REFERENCES

1. Mars NJI, Thompson PM, Wilkns RJ. Spread of epileptic seizure in humans. Epilepsia 1985; 26:85–94.

2. Collins RC. Use or cortical circuits during focal penicillin seizures: an autoradiographic study with [^{14}C]deoxyglucose. Brain Res 1978; 150:487–501.
3. Spencer SS. Corpus callosum resection and other disconnection procedures for medically intractable epilepsy. Epilepsia 1988; 29 (Suppl 2):S89–99.
4. Musgrave J, Gloor P. The role of the corpus callosum in bilaterally interhemispheric synchrony of spike and wave discharge in feline generalized penicillin epilepsy. Epilepsia 1980; 21:369–78.
5. Dandy, WE. Operative experiences in cases of pineal tumors. Arch Surg 1936; 33:19–46.2.
6. Van Wagenen WP, Herren RY. Surgical division of commisural pathways in the corpus callosum: relation to spread of an epileptic attack. Arch Neurol Phychiatry 1940; 44:740–59.
7. Lassonde M, Sauerwein H, Geoffrey G, Decarie M. Effects of early and late transection of the corpus callosum in children. Study of tactile and tactuomotor transfer and integration. Brain 1986; 109:953–67.
8. Luessenhop AJ, dela Cruz TC, Fenichel GM. Surgical disconnection of the cerebral hemispheres for intractible seizures. Results in infancy and childhood. JAMA 1970; 213:1630–36.
9. Wilson DH, Reeves A, Gazzaniga M, Culver C. Cerebral commisurotomy for control of intractible seizures. Neurology 1977; 27:708–15.
10. Nordgren R, Reeves AG, Viguera AC, Roberts DW. Corpus callosotomy for intractible seizures in the pediatric age group. Arch Neurol 1991; 48:364–72.
11. Fuiks KS, Wyler AR, Hermann BP, Somes G. Seizure outcome from anterior and complete corpus callosotomy. J Neurosurg 1991; 74:573–78.
12. Spencer SS, Spencer DD, Williamson PD, Sass K, Novelly RA, Mattson RH. Corpus callosotomy for epilepsy. I. Seizure effects. Neurology 1988; 38:19–24.
13. Rappaport ZH. Corpus callosum in the treatment of intractible seizures in the Sturge–Weber syndrome. Child's Nerv Syst 1988; 4:231.
14. Eidelberg E. Callosal and noncallosal connections between the sensory–motor cortices in cat and monkey. Electroencephalogr Clin Neurophysiol 1969; 26:557–64.
15. Rovit RL, Hardy J, Gloor P. Electroencephalographic effects of intracarotid amobarbital on epileptic activity. An experimental study of rabbits. Arch Neurol 1960; 3:642–55.
16. Mutani R, Bergamini L, Fariello R, Quattrocolo G. An experimental investigation on the mechanisms of interaction of asymmetrical acute epileptic foci. Epilepsia 1972; 13:597–608.
17. Spencer SS, Spencer DD, Glaser GH, Williamson PD, Mattson RH. More intense focal seizure types after callosal section: the role of inhibition. Ann Neurol 1984; 16:686–93.
18. Wilson, DH, Reeves AG, Gazzaniga MS. "Central commisurotomy" for intractible generalized epilepsy: series two. Neurology 1982; 32:687–97.
19. Gates JR, Leppik IE, Gumnit RJ. Corpus callosotomy: clinical and electrographic effects. Epilepsia 1984; 23:308–16.
20. Geoffrey G, Lassonde M, Delisle F, Decarie M. Corpus callosotomy for control of intractible epilepsy in children. Neurology 1983; 33:891–97.

21. Gates JR, Rosenfeld WE, Maxwell RE, Lyons RE. Response of multiple seizure types to corpus callosum section. Epilepsia 1987; 28:28–34.
22. Murro AM, Flanigin HF, Gallagher BB, King DW, Smith JR. Corpus callosotomy for the treatment of intractible epilepsy. Epilepsy Res 1988; 2:44–50.
23. Purves SJ, Wada JA, Woodhurst WB, Moyes PD, Strauss E, Kosaka B, Li D. Result of anterior corpus callosum resection in 24 patients with intractible seizures. Neurology 1988; 38:1194–1201.
24. Murro AM, Flanigan HF, Gallagher BB, King DW, Smith JR. Corpus callosotomy for the treatment of intractible epilepsy. Epilepsy Res 1988; 2:44–50.
25. Gazzanigo MS, Bogen JE, Sperry RW. Dyspraxia following division of the cerebral commisures. Arch Neurol 1967; 16:606–12.
26. Sass KJ, Spencer DD, Spencer SS, Novelly RA, Williamson PD, Mattson RH. Corpus callosotomy for epilepsy. II. Neurologic and neuropsychologic outcome. Neurology 1988; 38:24–28.
27. Huttenlocher PR, Hapke RJ. A follow-up study of intractable seizures in childhood. Ann Neurol 1990; 28:699–705.
28. Schwartz RH, Eaton J, Bower BD, Aynsley-Green A. Ketogenic diets in the treatment of epilepsy: short-term clinical effects. Dev Med Child Neurol 1989; 31:145–51.
29. Uthman BM, Wilder BJ, Hammond EJ, Redi SA. Efficacy and safety of vagus nerve stimulation in patients with complex partial seizures. Epilepsia 1990; 3/ (Suppl 2):S44–50.

16

Epilepsy, the Adolescent Female, and Pregnancy

R. EUGENE RAMSAY
University of Miami School of Medicine
Miami, Florida

VALERIE LYNN CURTIS
University of Texas Health Science Center at Houston
Houston, Texas

INTRODUCTION

Epilepsy is a common neurological disorder with a prevalence of approximately 6 in 1000 [1]. This is the most frequently encountered significant neurological disorder in the fertile and gravid female. There are an estimated 800,000 women with epilepsy of childbearing age in the United States today. They account for 1 of every 200 pregnancies [2]. Over the years, changing social attitudes toward epileptics, improved medical therapy, and other factors have resulted in an increased number of women with epilepsy marrying and having children. These patients present special management problems. The treating physician must understand the influences that pregnancy, seizures, and antiepileptic drugs (AEDs) have on one another. One must be aware of the physiological, psychological, and pharmacokinetic factors that change with pregnancy. In this chapter we focus on the problems of the woman with epilepsy, particularly during pregnancy. The problems of preeclampsia and toxemia are not discussed.

II. MENARCHE AND EPILEPSY

Epilepsy has been anecdotally reported to worsen in many women at the time of menarche. Few investigations to this effect have been conducted. The only systematic study reported failed to demonstrate a provocative effect of menarche on seizures. Partial seizures are equally likely to improve, worsen, or to remain unchanged [3]. Any change evident at menarche is, in part, dependent on the type of epilepsy present. Benign rolandic epilepsy of childhood begins around age 5 and usually remits spontaneously during adolescence. Petit mal epilepsy, which also begins in childhood, continues through menarche and does not remit until the mid to late teens. Benign occipital epilepsy starts in adolescence usually prior to the onset of menses and continues until late teens. Excluding these and other specific seizure syndromes with an age-dependent change in seizures, menarche has no predictable effect on partial or primary generalized seizures.

Catamenial epilepsy, on the other hand, is likely to have its onset at or near menarche [4–6]. In one study, 16 of 25 patients with catamenial epilepsy had onset of their seizures within 3 years of menarche [6]. The electroencephalogram (EEG) of girls has been found to fluctuate in relation to the menstrual cycle and is also attributed to hormonal effects [7]. Generalized spike–wave discharges and photoconvulsive responses are most prevalent between the ages of 5 and 16, declining in occurrence into adulthood [5]. Primary generalized epilepsies are genetically transmitted, with equal distribution of spontaneous spike–wave abnormality between boys and girls. However, the photoconvulsive response is more commonly found in girls, peaking between 14 and 16 years of age. Two factors, genetics modified by the hormone balance, interact to explain the occurrence of the photoconvulsive response. Maturational factors may also be involved, as this is an age-dependent finding [5], declining in incidence as adulthood is reached.

III. CATAMENIAL SEIZURES

Fluctuation in seizures has been suggested to be related to the menstrual cycle [4,5,8,9]. Catamenial epilepsy is the exacerbation or restricted occurrence of seizures during menstruation [4]. A specific relationship does exist in many women, at least during some cycles [5]. The incidence has not been clearly established. Results of studies have varied depending on the relation of seizures and menses used to define a seizure as being catamenial, the type of seizure studied, the length of follow-up, and the care used to select ovulatory cycles [5]. A calendar must be kept documenting seizures over several menstrual cycles in order to establish a pattern. When this is done, a catamenial relationship is substantiated less frequently than reported historically by the patient. Hormone changes differ between ovulatory and nonovulatory cycles; thus a catamenial effect may not be evident with each menses. Premenstrual exacerbation of seizures in ovulatory cycles has been estimated to occur in up to 50 to 80% of women with epilepsy [10,11]. Absence seizures may behave differently. Anecdotally, patients have reported premenstrual increase in absence seizures. In the only well-documented study reported using ambulatory EEG recordings, the number of 3-per-second spike–wave discharges longer than 3 s was greatest during the luteal phase and rapidly decreased after onset of menses. Greatest seizure occurrence did not correlate specifically with the expected time of the estrogen peaks [8]. However, hormone levels have not been measured in patients with absence seizures. Thus the reason for this difference in behavior of partial and absence seizures has not been explained. [4].

There is no evidence to suggest that catamenial changes are more prominent in any specific type of seizure or epilepsy syndrome. Rather, the effect appears to be more dependent on changes within the individual. During the monthly cycle a number of physiological changes occur, including (1) hormone levels (progesterone and estrogen), (2) fluid balance, and (3) hepatic enzyme activity.

Fluid balance, specifically water retention, may affect the seizure frequency. Administration of a fluid load and pitressin was used years ago to precipitate seizures. Many women report swelling of hands and feet as well as premenstrual weight gain. However, total body water does not differ in women with catamenial epilepsy from female epileptics without premenstrual seizure exacerbation [12]. An alteration in the intra- to extracellular water balance could still be the mechanism underlying premenstrual seizure exacerbation, but this has not been definitely established.

Hormones have a prominent effect on seizures. Estradiol has a proconvulsant effect and decreases the electroshock seizure threshold in rats [8]. Application of estrogen directly on the cerebral cortex of an animal [8] produces an active spike focus. In humans, an increase in EEG spike frequency can be seen after an intravenous infusion of estrogen [6]. Conversely, progesterone raises the electroshock seizure threshold in animals and protects mice against pentylenetetrazol-induced seizures [13]. Progesterone also decreased the EEG spikes in cats with a penicillin-induced focus as well as in women with partial epilepsy [8]. In high doses, progesterone may even induce anesthesia in animals and humans [8].

Serum estradiol and progesterone are at their lowest levels at the onset of menses [14]. Estradiol reaches its highest level just prior to the lutinizing hormone (LH) surge at ovulation, which occurs at midcycle. 17-Hydroxyprogesterone, progesterone, and estradiol climb gradually in the serum during the second half, or luteal phase, of the cycle, then drop off precipitously prior to onset of menses. Estradiol's midluteal rise is less than the ovulatory peak. Progesterone, which is secreted by the ovarian corpus luteum, reaches its peak activity midway in the luteal phase (Fig. 1). Backstrom [8,9] studied women with partial epilepsy through six ovulatory cycles and three 1-month nonovulatory cycles. Two periods of increased generalized seizure frequency were noted, the first after the rapid decline of the progesterone level in the early menses and the second during the preovulatory estrogen rise. During the luteal phase with the high progesterone, the number of generalized seizures was very low. The greatest estrogen effect (highest estrogen/progesterone ratio) occurs at the time of the menses (Fig. 1). In nonovulatory cycles, increasing numbers of seizures were noted during

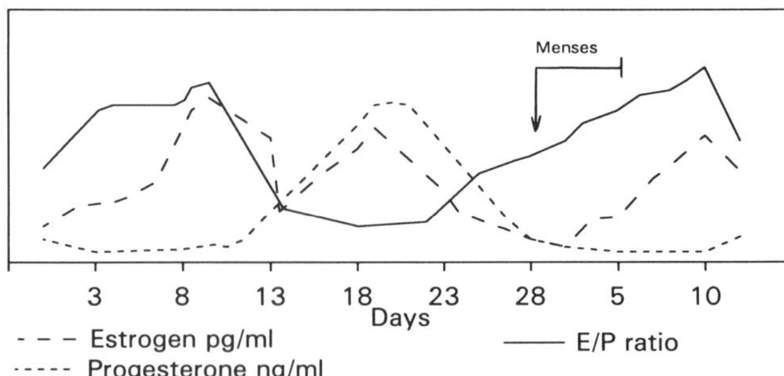

Figure 1 Estrogen and progesterone plasma levels and estrogen/progesterone ratio during a normal menstrual cycle.

estrogen peaks [8,9]. A balance exists between epileptogenic effect of estrogen and protective effect of progesterone. Fluctuation in hormone levels is a major reason that seizure frequency fluctuates over the menstrual cycle [4,8,9,11,15,16]. Seizures increase when the estrogenic effect predominates or when progesterone levels drop rapidly [8,9]. The lowest seizure frequency is evident when the progesterone effect dominates. These facts are important when treating the female with birth control pills (BCPs) or hormone replacement therapy.

A. Treatment of Catamenial Epilepsy

The report by Locock [17] on the effectiveness of bromides in hysteroepilepsy heralded the beginning of the present era of pharmacological treatment of epilepsies. Although bromide therapy has been shown to be helpful in catamenial seizures, this is considered neither a first- nor a second-line drug in this situation [5]. Catamenial seizures can usually be controlled by the proper selection and use of the primary AEDs [carbamazepine (CBZ), phenytoin (PHT), and valproate]. Care must first be taken to document that seizure frequency increases in relation to the menses. If a relationship exists, several treatment options can then be considered.

Antiepileptic drug metabolism changes during the menstrual cycle. Serum phenytoin levels have been shown to be lower in some women at the onset of the menses. Plasma levels have been found to fluctuate less in women with noncatamenial seizures [18]. Protein binding does not change over the menstrual cycle. Thus the difference in blood levels is due to an increase in drug clearance. This effect has only been established for phenytoin. However, the other AEDs that are principally metabolized by the hepatic P450 enzyme system (CBZ, PRM, and PB) should have a similar premenstrual increase in clearance. Although found consistently, the reduction in plasma level is usually small and not clinically significant. Measuring the AED level in midcycle and prior to the menses will establish the degree of change. However, occasionally, a patient will be encountered in which the premenstrual AED level may be reduced by as much as 50% or more. In this instance, increase the dosage of the AED for 7 days beginning 5 days before the start of the menses. Only when the primary anticonvulsants have been optimized and premenstrual exacerbations continue, should other options be considered, such as a second-line AED (e.g., primidone, celontin) or other rational therapies.

Several logical treatment approaches for catamenial seizures have been explored with variable success. Trials with BCPs have yielded considerable interpatient differences in effectiveness. Available BCPs vary in relative proportion and in the total milligrams of hormones contained. Most consist of an estrogen and progesterone combination, but single estrogen or progesterone compounds are available. Exacerbations typically occur during the 7-day period when hormones are stopped [4]. Animal and clinical studies have demonstrated a protective effect of progesterone [8,9,16]. Acutely, the frequency of focal cortical spikes can be reduced with intravenous infusion of progesterone [16]. Chronic high-dose medroxyprogesterone has been used to control seizures. Of the 11 who completed the study successfully, Mattson et al. [19] reported that seven women averaged 50% fewer seizures over baseline. Medroxyprogesterone may be administered orally at a dosage of 10 mg four times daily, or as a depot injection of 120 to 150 mg every 6 to 12 weeks [4]. The dose must be sufficient to eliminate the menses. It is not clear whether the efficacy of medroxyprogesterone is attributable to elimination of menstrual cycle and lower estrogen levels or the presence of relatively constant and high progestin concentrations [20]. This approach may reduce the seizure frequency but is unlikely to result in complete seizure control. Because of the mild subjective report of not feeling right, many women often do not want to continue this route of therapy. Hormonal therapy should be undertaken in conjunction with an obstetrician–gynecologist or endocrinologist. The use of progestin-only BCPs may be efficacious [4], but this has not been studied adequately. BCPs are typically given for 21 days and stopped for 7 days. Seizure increase may still be seen with progesterone-only BCPs during the 7-day withdrawal phase. Hormone supplementation may be considered in medically refractory patients but should be used only as adjunct therapy.

Acetazolamide (Diamox) has been used and seems to be most effective when taken premenstrually. This should be given for 7 days, starting 5 days before the menses. Acetazolamide has a mild diuretic effect for the first few days and thus should be taken in the morning. There is some indication that acetazolamide may have diminishing efficacy over time [4] which is most evident when it is given continuously. Drugs that inhibit carbonic anhydrase activity, such as acetazolamide, have mild anticonvulsant activity. The authors have tried other diuretics premenstrually with limited success. Diamox seems to be more effective and the primary mechanism does not appear to be related to a diuretic effect. Maximum carbonic anhydrase inhibition is usually obtained with doses of 500 mg/day. Higher doses usually do not provide additional anticonvulsant effect, and thus its anticonvulsant effect is probably related to inhibition of carbonic anhydrase activity.

Anecdotally, seizure frequency decreases in some women at menarche. Although estrogens and progesterone affect seizure frequency, loss of these circulating factors at menarche and with oophorectomy does not reliably result in seizure improvement. Most women do not experience improvement, and oophorectomy is therefore not an accepted treatment [5].

Clomiphene is an estrogen analog with both estrogenic and antiestrogenic properties. This was given to 12 women with menstrual and endocrine disorders who also had complex partial seizures [21]. Ten of the women improved, developing normal cycles as well as experiencing an 87% decline in frequency of both complex partial and secondarily generalized seizures. Possible reasons for the observed anticonvulsant effect include (1) drug interaction resulting in increased AED blood level, (2) reduced protein binding of the concurrent AED, (3) normalization of the estradiol and progesterone fluctuations, and (4) direct cerebral anticonvulsant effects. Although this report is suggestive, the results must be interpreted cautiously. The patients were treated openly, involving no control or blinded design. The impressive results with this small group, despite the study limitations, provide encouragement for pursuing a larger investigation with this type of drug and possibly extending it to patients with catamenial epilepsy [21].

IV. EFFECT OF PREGNANCY ON SEIZURES

A significant change in seizure frequency is observed in some women when pregnant. The consensus of most of the literature indicates that an increase in seizures will occur in one-fourth to one-third of women, one-third to one-half have no change, and one-fourth to one-third have fewer seizures [22–29]. Changes in seizure frequency with pregnancy cannot be predicted from the pregestational frequency [23–26,30], sex of the child, or seizure type [23–27]. Change in seizure activity in prior pregnancies is also not predictive of seizure frequency in subsequent pregnancies. In one study of 50 women, those with well-controlled seizures had a better course during their pregnancies, whereas those with frequent pregestational attacks were more likely to have continued or increased seizures during their pregnancy [31]. In another prospective study of 154 pregnancies in 140 epileptic women, Bardy found fewer seizures in women with a shorter duration of their epilepsy [24,25]. This lends support to the intuitive conclusion that good preconception seizure control is important to good seizure control during pregnancy. Analogous to what is observed in catamenial seizures, primary generalized and partial seizures seem to behave differently during pregnancy. Remillard et al., in a prospective study, found that secondarily generalized and partial complex epilepsies are more likely to worsen than primary generalized seizures [28]. This finding suggests that the primary epilepsies respond differently to hormone changes but may also reflect the more benign course often seen with generalized epilepsies as compared to symptomatic or secondary epilepsies. Prior history of catamenial epilepsy is not helpful in predicting the effects of pregnancy [27]. Anecdotally, women have reported the loss of a catamenial occurrence of their seizures after a pregnancy.

In those women with gestational increase in seizures, the tendency to worsen in certain stages of pregnancy has varied in different studies. Canger et al. [26] and Knight and Rhind [27] found that the exacerbation was greatest in the first trimester, whereas Remillard et al. found the third more problematic, with the first trimester ranking second in severity [28]. Similarly, Bardy also found tonic–clonic seizures increased in the second and third trimesters, whereas complex partial seizures worsened in the last trimester and especially the puerperium [25]. In a prospective study of 36 patients and 40 pregnancies, Ramsay found that seizures did not increase in the first 8 weeks of pregnancy [30]. Worsening in seizures was observed most frequently at the end of the first trimester and the beginning of the second trimester (gestational weeks 9 to 16). Through the rest of pregnancy, progressively fewer patients experienced an exacerbation of their seizures.

Factors that may affect seizures during pregnancy include psychological issues and physiological changes. As the fetus grows larger and more active, some women may find it more difficult to sleep well. Sleep deprivation is known to exacerbate seizures and may also play a role during pregnancy [29]. However, sleep deprivation is common in the months after delivery when seizure exacerbation is not usually encountered. Other factors very likely play more important roles during pregnancy.

Out of fear of drug-induced teratogenesis, patients may be noncompliant with their AEDs, resulting in lower blood levels and increase in seizures. Counseling the patient about the relative risks is imperative. Consideration must be given to the fact that having a seizure is not without risk. A brief complex partial seizure while walking down stairs could result in a fall. Low AED levels increase the risk of seizure exacerbation and status. These factors must be balanced against the possible teratogenic effect of the AEDs. The patient must be counseled about all aspects. Any decision to alter a dose or switch AED must be made jointly by the physician and an informed patient. Better compliance and improved seizure control usually results [29].

Plasma progesterone and estrogen, and urinary estradiol, estriol, and estrone all gradually increase during pregnancy, reaching maximum values at parturition

[4]. A dominant estrogenic effect, which lowers seizure threshold, occurs early in pregnancy [30]. The highest estrogen/progesterone ratio is found in weeks 9 to 16, which is the same time that seizures have been reported to exacerbate [26,27,31]. In a prospective study of 30 pregnant epileptic women, significantly higher serum estrogen levels, lower progesterone levels, and lower AED levels were found in patients with increased seizure frequency than in those with no change in seizure frequency [32]. However, other authors have suggested that increased seizure frequency can be attributed only to low AED levels secondary to increased AED metabolism [33].

V. GESTATIONAL EPILEPSY

A small proportion of women have tonic–clonic seizures confined only to the period of their pregnancy, labor, or puerperium. This is called gestational epilepsy, with the seizures usually occurring between the twenty-sixth and thirty-second weeks of pregnancy [27]. In the nonpregnant period, these women remain seizure-free without anticonvulsant treatment. Recurrence in subsequent pregnancies is unpredictable [27]. On the other hand, some women will experience their first seizure during pregnancy and then continue to have more in the nonpregnant state [27]. Women with gestational epilepsy usually have only one or two convulsive seizures. The evaluation of a woman who has her first seizure during pregnancy should be the same as if she were not pregnant. Magnetic resonance imaging (MRI) has been used extensively during pregnancy without apparent risk to the fetus. If the evaluation is negative, careful consideration must be given to whether treatment should be initiated. This must be based on social and medical consideration as well as the patient's willingness to risk having another convulsion. The occurrence of partial seizures, multiple seizures, epileptiform findings on EEG, or significant findings on an MRI increase the chances that the patient has more than gestational epilepsy and thus should be treated.

VI. ANTIEPILEPTIC PHARMACOKINETICS IN PREGNANCY

Plasma levels of all the AEDs gradually decline during pregnancy [34]. Several physiologic changes occur in pregnancy which contribute to alterations in plasma AED levels [35]. These include increases in body weight, body size, intravascular volume, total body water, and a fall in serum albumin, all which result in a larger volume of distribution (V_d). With all other factors remaining constant, an increase in V_d will produce a lower steady-state plasma level and possibly a reduction in seizure control.

As the protein binding decreases, the concentration of unbound or free drug increases. Free drug crosses the blood-brain barrier and determines the concentration that equilibrates at the site of action in the brain. Free drug is also delivered to the liver for metabolism. Clearance of a drug increases as the free level becomes greater. This may ultimately result in lower plasma levels and impaired seizure control. Protein binding of the AEDs is reduced during pregnancy and has been partially attributable to a physiologic gestational hypoalbuminemia. However, the change in binding is often greater than can be explained by low protein and albumin levels. In rats, the decreased binding of salicylic acid, sulfisoxazole, phenytoin, dexamethasone, diazepam, and bilirubin was found to result from an endogenous inhibitor [36]. A similar mechanism is postulated to occur in humans. An intrinsic factor is produced during pregnancy that competes for protein-binding sites, resulting in higher free AED levels. Thus pregnancy is one situation where monitoring of free AED level is clinically indicated, as total plasma level may be misleading.

Drug absorption may be affected by gastrointestinal changes, including delayed gastric emptying and reduced peristaltic activity, resulting in prolonged intestinal transport [14,35,37]. Physiologic increases in gastric pH also occur [14], potentially influencing bioavailability of the AEDs. A case of pronounced phenytoin malabsorption has been described in which over half of the daily dose was recovered unmetabolized in the stool. Plasma phenytoin levels were very low and the patient went into status epilepticus during the second trimester of her pregnancy [38]. Clinically significant malabsorption occurs infrequently during pregnancy, but if encountered, may produce significantly low plasma levels. This is potentially more problematic with the AEDs that are relatively water insoluble or have a high pK_a value (PHT and CBZ). This can be treated by using higher doses given multiple times a day.

As the fetus enlarges, the abdominal contents are displaced. This may distort the anatomy of the gastroesophageal junction and product esophageal reflux. Antacids are frequently prescribed because of heartburn. Simethicone and kaolin have been demonstrated to alter phenytoin absorption significantly [37]. This may be important at labor, when antacids are routinely prescribed [37]. This is also a time when seizure exacerbation is more likely to occur [25,28]. In general, however, absorption changes are not thought to be the most important factors in reducing AED levels during pregnancy, since apart from phenytoin, malabsorption of other AEDs has not been reported. [37].

Gestational enlargement of the liver and an increase in hepatic blood flow occurs. Concurrent with liver enlargement, microsomal enzymes are induced, as evidenced by proliferation of smooth endoplasmic reticulum seen on biopsy specimens [35]. All this results in enhanced drug metabolism but is most significant for AEDs cleared by microsomal enzymes. Despite this increased enzyme activity, liver function measurements usually remain normal in human pregnancies [14].

Increased cardiac output improves renal function by enhancing renal blood flow and glomerular filtration rate. For most AEDs this does not significantly alter metabolism because of the high degree of protein binding: the exception being phenobarbital, primidone, and ethosuximide, which have protein binding of approximately 50%, 50%, and 0%. Increased renal elimination of the unmetabolized form of these drugs may occur in later stages of pregnancy and result in lower plasma levels [35].

All these factors can affect the steady-state plasma level. A gradual increase in effect becomes apparent over the 40 weeks of pregnancy, with maximal impact at time of parturition. The overall outcome of these physiological changes is incorporated in the pharmacokinetic parameter of clearance. This is calculated by dividing the daily dose by the average steady-state plasma level. The intrinsic clearance utilizes free rather than total serum levels with body weight [39] and is a measure of (1) the activity of drug-metabolizing enzyme systems and/or (2) the excretory pathways for unmetabolized drug [36]. Clearances of phenytoin, phenobarbital, carbamazepine, primidone, and valproic acid all increase during pregnancy [35,37,39,40]. These gradually return to the usual nonpregnant value by 8 to 12 weeks postpartum [40]. Plasma levels should be monitored during this postpartum time, particularly if a dosage increase has been made during pregnancy. Reduction in dosage will probably be necessary to prevent clinical toxicity from developing in the second and third postpartum months as the plasma level rises. The change in plasma level is greatest for valproic acid and phenobarbital, intermediate for phenytoin, and least for carbamazepine. However, because multiple factors are operative, the degree of change can vary considerably between individuals.

A. Phenytoin

The most extensively studied of the AEDs, phenytoin is a weak acid, poorly soluble in water, and is not absorbed in the stomach but rather in the small intestine [37]. It is converted to the inactive metabolite *para*-hydroxyphenylphenytoin (p-HPPH) by the hepatic microsomal system, which accounts for most of its elimination [37]. Phenytoin is highly plasma protein bound, making it susceptible to the altered protein binding that occurs in pregnancy. Protein binding may be reduced by 20% and return to normal 2 to 8 weeks postpartum. Monitoring free and total blood levels during pregnancy and the puerperium may be helpful in deciding dosage adjustments [41]. The V_d value increases by approximately 25% during pregnancy, which is much greater than the change in body weight observed [42]. Other studies have found that the half-life of phenytoin is reduced by as much as 50%. From measuring the output of the major metabolite, p-HPPH, enhanced hepatic metabolism by the cytochrome P450 system is a major contributor to the increased clearance observed [37]. Phenytoin levels have been shown to decrease dramatically in some patients, with absorption, metabolism, and binding all playing roles [37]. The drug clearance was shown to increase gradually throughout the first 32 weeks of pregnancy, reaching twice the preconception value during the last 8 weeks. The plasma level returns to normal in the first three postpartum months [38]. Approximately half of the patients will require dosage increases during pregnancy to combat increased seizure frequency [43].

B. Carbamazepine

Carbamazepine is metabolized primarily to its 10,11-epoxide, which is subsequently transformed to a dihydrodiol metabolite by epoxide hydrolase. Increased levels of the epoxide have been documented in pregnancy. This is thought to be due to inhibition of the epoxide hydrolase activity rather than to an increased rate of epoxide formation [44]. This may be important, as epoxide intermediates may play a role in teratogenesis.

Carbamazepine is absorbed slowly, has a wide variability in its bioavailability, and is 75% protein bound [37]. Altered absorption during pregnancy have not been reported [37]. Decline in CBZ plasma concentrations is not as dramatic as with PHT [38], and some patients have minimal or no change [44]. The increased clearance observed has been attributed to accelerated hepatic metabolism [45].

C. Primidone and Phenobarbital

Primidone is metabolized to phenobarbital and phenylethylmalondiamide (PEMA). Primidone levels decline with pregnancy to about the same extent as carbamazepine [38,45]. Accelerated conversion to phenobarbital and PEMA has not been found to be important in the increased clearance observed. Increase in V_d, decreased gastrointestinal (GI) absorption, and an increase in renal clearance are felt to be responsible [45].

Phenobarbital is 45 to 50% protein bound. Of the total daily dose, 20 to 40% is excreted in the urine as unmetabolized drug [37]. The decrease in plasma levels with pregnancy is similar to that seen with primidone. GI absorption does not change with pregnancy. A decrease in protein binding along with an increase in GFR and renal blood flow result in enhanced phenobarbital clearance. Hepatic metabolism may also be increased, but the relative role of these two mechanisms of elimination has not been defined. The overall effect is lower steady-state blood levels as the pregnancy progresses.

D. Valproic Acid

Total serum levels decrease progressively during pregnancy, especially in the third trimester [39]. Valproate has concentration-dependent binding. In low levels, valproate is highly protein bound (95%). The free fraction may be 20% or

Table 1 Ratio of Concentration of the AEDs in Breast Milk Compared to the Total Plasma Level

Anticonvulsant	% Protein binding	Milk/plasma
Valproic acid	95	0.03
Phenytoin	90	0.10
Carbamazepine	75	0.30
Phenobarbital	45	0.40
Primidone	30	0.70
Ethosuximide	05	0.90

more with high plasma levels. Valproate has concentration-dependent binding. With high plasma levels, the protein binding sites become saturated and the free fraction increases. Independent of this concentration-dependent change, the free fraction of valproate increases during pregnancy and is highest at time of delivery. Although total plasma clearance increases, intrinsic clearance remains constant, which suggests that the metabolism of valproate is not altered by pregnancy. The change in total clearance is due to reduction in protein binding and a larger V_d. GI absorption does not seem to be significantly affected by pregnancy [37]. Monitoring of free plasma levels is helpful to avoid seizure exacerbation as well as postpartum toxicity, when binding returns to normal [39].

E. Ethosuximide

Ethosuximide (ESM) is used to treat absence seizures, which occurs predominantly in childhood and adolescence. It is used infrequently in adults. ESM does not bind significantly to serum proteins. Although renal blood flow and glomerular filtration rate increase, no significant alterations in serum levels of ESM have been reported. ESM crosses the blood-brain barrier rapidly and fetal and maternal concentrations are approximately equal [37].

VII. BREAST FEEDING

The concentration of AED in breast milk is directly related to the free plasma concentration. Protein concentration in breast milk is very low. Thus highly bound AEDs are in low concentration in breast milk compared to the plasma (Table 1) [37]. Valproic acid is the most highly protein bound of all the AEDs (95%), and several studies have reported the breast milk concentration to be 2 to 3% of that in the serum [37,46]. Phenytoin is about 90% protein bound and the concentration in breast milk is on the order of 10 to 20% of serum values [37,47]. The protein binding of the other AEDs range from 75 to 0%, resulting in a higher milk/blood ratio [37,47]. Ethosuximide has negligible protein binding and the concentration in milk is about the same as that in the plasma [37,47].

In varying proportions, all antiepileptic drugs appear in breast milk. With the exception of the barbiturates, the AEDs generally do not pose a problem for the nursing infant. Considering the volume of milk ingested, the infant is exposed to only a few milligrams of an AED daily. Breast feeding may usually be undertaken by the epileptic mother without any concerns for adverse effects in the child [48]. Because of the slow metabolism and larger amount to which the infant is exposed, clinically significant phenobarbital levels may develop, resulting in irritability and sedation [49]. The effect is accentuated in infants as the free fraction of phenobarbital may be increased (as high as 90% in some infants) [49]. If the infant demonstrates signs of sedation, plasma level should be obtained. Dosage reduction may be necessary to avoid sedation, poor feeding, and other behavioral changes. The mother's dosage can be reduced, or bottle feeding can replace breast feeding partially or totally.

VIII. EFFECTS OF EPILEPSY ON PREGNANCY

The importance of adequate seizure control must be balanced between the potential teratogenic risks of antiepileptic drugs and the effects that seizures may have on the mother and fetus. Factors to be considered are the risk of traumatic injury during a seizure, occurrence of status epilepticus [50], and the possible deleterious effect to the fetus of a generalized tonic-clonic seizure. The risk of injury from a seizure is not well defined. Although anecdotally reported, seizures clearly place the patient at increased danger of physical injury and reduce the expected life span [51]. Even a brief complex partial or absence seizure could result in injury if it occurs while the patient is walking down stairs or crossing a street in traffic.

Because of excessive motor activity and circulatory changes, generalized tonic–clonic seizures may also affect the fetus. Specific effects on placental blood flow have not been shown. However, marked cardiovascular changes, particularly hypertension, and increases in cerebral blood flow have been documented to occur in both animals and humans [52]. Signs of fetal distress, such as decelerated heart rate, which may be persistent beyond the extent of the seizure, have been documented following a single convulsion [52]. However, serious adverse effects of maternal convulsions on the fetus have been limited to a few case reports [53]. Although these reports indicate some fetal risk, in most women, in the absence of trauma, a convulsion does not result in detectable injury to the fetus [51].

Status epilepticus in pregnancy is associated with a high mortality for both mother and infant [52]. The probability of seizures during labor and the first postpartum day is tenfold the average seizure risk during the rest of the pregnancy, and relates to factors such as stress of labor, low serum AED levels from missed doses [26,54], and sleep deprivation [26].

A. Perinatal Complications

Studies of pregnancy outcome in epileptic women have yielded conflicting results in terms of incidence of spontaneous abortions, perinatal problems, and obstetric complications. However, some general conclusions may be drawn. Although the difference may be small, most types of complication occur more frequently in women with epilepsy [55].

The incidence of spontaneous abortions is difficult to estimate. The majority of reports indicate that the rate is probably not increased in epileptic women over the general population [27,52,56,57]. Induced abortions, however, were found to be greater in epileptic women [56]. Contributing factors include fear of seizures, AED teratogenesis, and inheritance of epilepsy. Other medical and social problems also contribute to the higher rate of induced abortions seen in this group of women [52].

Obstetrical interventions such as induced labor and cesarean sections are also increased in women with epilepsy [56,58–62], as are special procedures such as amniocentesis [60]. This is attributable to concern over the impact that maternal epilepsy could have on labor and delivery [59], as well as the unfamiliarity of the obstetricians with epilepsy in mothers [54].

This concern is largely unwarranted. Early induction may result in unnecessary cesarean (C)-section due to prolonged labor and uterine exhaustion. Elective C-section is indicated for maternal epilepsy only in the most poorly controlled cases, which are infrequent [54]. Emergent C-section may be necessary after a grand mal seizure during labor if fetal distress occurs or the mother is unable to cooperate postictally [54].

A wide variety of pregnancy complications have been studied and found to be increased among epileptic women, with an estimated risk of 1.5 to 3 times over the general population [54]. These include vaginal bleeding [52,58,61], premature and prolonged labor, the latter explained theoretically by weakening of uterine contractions by antiepileptic drugs [54], preeclampsia or toxemia [58,63], abruptio placentae [52,58], and especially perinatal mortality (stillbirths), which have been found to be increased in every large retrospective study [52], unlike infant mortality, which is not increased in epileptic women [56]. The risk of perinatal mortality is estimated to be 1.2 to 3 times that in the general population [64].

B. Anticonvulsant-Induced Hemorrhagic Disorder

Anticonvulsant-induced hemorrhagic disorder (AIHD) of the newborn is a unique phenomenon that occurs in infants of epileptic mothers treated with phenytoin or phenobarbital [65,66]. There has been no published reports concerning a vitamin K–deficient clotting disorder with valproic acid or carbamazepine. The hemorrhage with AIHD occurs during the second to fifth day of life and often involves unusual sites of bleeding, such as the pleural or abdominal cavities [67]. This is to be distinguished from hemorrhagic disease of the newborn in which the bleeding is evident within the first 24 h of life. AIHD is due to a deficiency of vitamin K–dependent clotting factors (II, VII, IX, and X) and a prolonged prothrombin time. This has been felt to be produced by induction of fetal microsomal enzymes, resulting in an increase in oxidative degradation of vitamin K [67]. Women taking AEDs during pregnancy should receive vitamin K prior to delivery. This can be given 5 mg/day orally for the 2 weeks before delivery. If compliance is a concern, 10 mg of vitamin K should be given intramuscularly at 2 weeks and 1 week before expected delivery.

IX. TERATOGENESIS

A. Historical Perspective

The earliest mention of the possible teratogenic effect of an anticonvulsant was in 1884 by Beraud in a child whose mother was treated with bromide [68]. The next reported association was not until 1963 in a mother who had been treated with mephenytoin during her pregnancy [69]. The child was born with microcephaly, submucous cleft palate, IQ of 60, malrotation of the intestine, and speech defect. Following this, several infants exposed in utero to AEDs were reported to have congenital heart defects, oral facial clefts, and/or bone marrow aplasia [70–72]. In 1964, after reviewing 426 pregnancies in 246 mothers with epilepsy, Janz and Fuchs concluded that AEDs were without an increased risk of malformations [73]. The malformation rate was only 2.2%, which was not significantly above that of the general population. However, subsequently, an increased rate of malformations has typically been found in infants of mothers with epilepsy [74–79], although the etiology for this is still debated.

Anomalies are abnormalities of structure which, while varying from normal, do not constitute a threat to health. They represent variations within a spectrum of appearance and structure that deviate by varying degrees from the norm. These are also known as "teratogenic disruption syndromes" [80]. Patterns of anomalies in infants of mothers with epilepsy (IME) have been reported for the major AEDs and include the fetal hydantoin [81], phenobarbital [82], valproate [83], primidone [84], and carbamazepine [85] syndromes. The features of distal digital hypoplasia were reported in infants exposed to hydantoin and barbiturates in 1973 [86] (seven infants) and 1974 [87] (eight infants). The term *fetal hydantoin syndrome* was coined by Hanson and Smith in 1975 [81]. They reported on five IME exposed in utero to AEDs. The infants had multiple systemic

Table 2 Patterns of Anomalies in the Fetal Hydantoin Syndrome

Growth and performance
Motor or mental deficiency
Microcephaly
Pre/postnatal growth deficiency
Craniofacial
Short nose with low nasal bridge
Hypertension
Epicanthic folds
Low-set and/or abnormal ears
Wide mouth
Prominent lips
Cleft palate
Metopic sutural ridging
Wide fontanels
Limb
Hypoplasia of nails and distal phalanges
Fingerlike thumb
Abnormal palmar creases
Five or more digital arches
Other
Short or webbed neck ± low hairline
Coarse hair
Widely spaced, hypoplastic nipples
Rib, sternal, or spinal anomalies
Hernias
Undescended testes

abnormalities of the face, cranium, distal digital and nail hypoplasia, intrauterine growth retardation, and mental deficiencies (Table 2). Details of this report are important to review. Only one mother was treated with phenytoin in monotherapy and she was taking only 100 mg/day. The others were on multiple AEDs, including barbiturates, phensuximide, and mephenytoin. This report has had a long-term impact on the treatment of women with epilepsy. Because of this article, phenytoin has, in the past, been considered as more teratogenic than the other AEDs. Unfortunately, the conclusions made were not specifically supported by the cases reported. Several factors were not considered in this report and include polypharmacy, exposure to phenobarbital, race, nutrition, socioeconomic level, and prenatal care. Despite this, the authors described their cases as suffering from a fetal syndrome produced only by hydantoin. Hanson concluded that the syndrome consisted of three general characteristics: dysmorphic features, delayed development, and major malformations.

B. Dysmorphic Syndromes

The causal relationship of dysmorphic features by the AEDs and the existence of a specific AED syndrome was questioned in a study by Janz [88]. He studied infants of (1) mothers treated with AEDs, (2) mothers with epilepsy but not treated with AEDs, (3) fathers with epilepsy, and (4) controls. The infants were examined for presence of major malformations and dysmorphic features by a physician who was blinded to the mothers' medical background. Most of the features of the "hydantoin syndrome" were found in all four groups. Only distal digital and nail hypoplasia was specifically found in the IME treated with AEDs. Dizygotic twins exposed in utero to phenytoin have been reported to have different dysmorphic features [89], indicating a genetic etiology, not just a nonspecific adverse drug effect. Gaily et al. [90] extended the methodology employed by Janz. Infants were examined blinded to the mothers' medical history, but the mothers were also examined for the presence of dysmorphic features. An increased number of dysmorphic features were found in the IME, but these features were specifically more common when the mothers also had the same trait. They concluded that most features are inherited and not related to AED exposure, even with high phenytoin levels. Only distal digital and nail hypoplasia correlated with in uterine exposure to the AEDs.

C. Major Malformations

Major congenital malformations are defined as physical defects requiring medical or surgical intervention to avoid major functional disturbance. Trimethadione (TMO) was the first AED clearly demonstrated to have a teratogenic effect. In 1970, German et al. [91] described 14 pregnancies in which TMO was used in the first trimester. Only 2 of 14 children exposed in utero to TMO were normal. One had multiple hernias and diabetes, 8 had developmental defects, 3 were spontaneously aborted. Only 3 of the 14 survived infancy. Subsequent authors have reported other severe malformations from TMO, including craniofacial anomalies, delayed growth and psychomotor development, clefting, and congenital heart defect [92–94]. Distal digital and nail hypoplasia, which have typically been observed with the other AEDs, have not been found with TMO [80,91]. The occurrence of the fetal trimethadione syndrome, with a high morbidity and mortality, has been confirmed by others [92–94]. TMO and its chemically related compound paradione are now considered the most teratogenic of the AEDs and specifically contraindicated in pregnancy. Because of the high fetal mortality and malformation rate, intrauterine exposure to TMO is sufficient reason to terminate a pregnancy. These drugs were introduced in the 1940s for treatment of petit mal epilepsy [80], which can now be treated more safely and effectively with ethosuximide and valproic acid.

In a case-controlled study, Speidel and Meadow [95] concluded that the incidence of congenital malformations was increased two-fold in infants of mothers treated with AEDs. The increase was at least partially attributable to the drugs, and no single abnormality was specific for any AED [95]. In 1978, Annegers et al. [96] studied several groups, including mothers with active epilepsy who took no AEDs during pregnancy and mothers whose epilepsy had resolved or not yet developed at the time of their pregnancy [96]. In the study groups, elevated rates of certain types of malformations were found which included congenital heart disease, cleft lip or palate, and ureteral duplication. They concluded that despite the strong association of malformations with AED treatment, epilepsy per se could still be a significant factor in the genesis of malformations [96].

Numerous studies have focused on the relative importance of genetic and AED treatment. In the older literature the reported malformation rate has been approximately 2.5% in the general population, 4.0% in women with epilepsy untreated, and 6 to 8% in women with epilepsy taking AEDs during their pregnancy [74–78]. The Collaborative European Pregnancy study over the last decade found a 1.75% incidence of malformations in the general population [97]. This is lower than reported in older studies and probably represents overall better outcome from improved prenatal care. The 3.0 to 6.0% malformation rate in women with epilepsy treated with AEDs also represents a lower rate. However, the ratio between the two groups has remained about the same. The incidence of malformations in IME is two- to threefold increased over the general population [48,80,95,96,98,99]. Factors that have been found to further increase the malformation rate are maintaining high plasma AED levels during pregnancy [100] and polytherapy [101]. Malformation rate as high as 23% has been reported in women concurrently treated with four AEDs during their pregnancy [117].

The most commonly reported malformations in association with AEDs has been orofacial clefts (cleft lip and/or palate), compromising some 30% of these defects [80,102]. In a study analyzing the prevalence of clefting in siblings and children of 2072 epileptics using a national cleft register, the observed/expected ratio of clefting was increased only in the cases of maternal epilepsy and was highest in cases where anticonvulsants were given before and during pregnancy. The authors concluded that clefting is not a consequence of epilepsy per se but is attributable to anticonvulsant treatment [103], which is in agreement with most of the rest of the literature. This concept stands in contrast to the 1984 analysis of 315 families ascertained through a proband with clefting [102]. They concluded that environmental and genetic factors were more significant in producing clefting defects and that the role of anticonvulsant drugs had been overemphasized. The overall incidence of clefting has dropped in IME over the past four decades, suggesting that maternal health and other factors are also very important.

The next most common congenital malformation is heart defects, with a 1.5 to 2% prevalence [80,102]. The relative risk is threefold over the general population [104]. An increased incidence of neural tube defects (NTD) was first identified from the spina bifida registry in the Rhônes–Alps region of France. This finding was substantiated in the findings from the Collaborative European Pregnancy study [97]. They reported a 1.5% incidence with the use of valproate. This study also found a 0.5 to 1.0% incidence of neural tube defects with the use of carbamazepine. Rosa [105], in a study of Medicaid patients in Michigan, substantiated the finding that spina bifida is increased with intrauterine exposure to CBZ. He also reviewed the literature and concluded that the incidence of spina bifida was 1 out of 68 pregnancies with valproate, 1 out of 109 pregnancies with carbamazepine, and 1 out of 748 pregnancies with the other AEDs.

It is difficult to separate the effects of maternal seizures from those that the AEDs may have on pregnancy and perinatal outcomes. In monkeys [106] and mice [107], adverse fetal outcomes such as stillbirths and developmental delays did not relate to seizure occurrences but to high serum phenytoin levels. Maternal seizures have not correlated with complications of pregnancy in humans [54]. In the absence of direct injury to the mother or fetus, maternal seizures do not affect the incidence of perinatal complications or malformations [54,96,106].

A multifactorial inheritance has been suggested for most malformations, such as neural tube defects, congenital heart defects, and GI anomalies [97]. However, familial X-linked as well as autosomal dominant cleft palate have been described. The latter has a gene locus on the short arm of chromosome 6, which is the same location as juvenile myoclonic epilepsy (JME). Thus an association between cleft deficits and treatment with phenytoin or valproate (which have been used to treat the seizures in JME) may result from the occurrence of the two disorders on the same gene and not necessarily secondary to intrauterine drug exposure. Current concepts today for AED teratogenesis invoke a multiplicity of factors, including genetics transmission of the malformation, genetic susceptibility to AEDs, and environmental factors.

D. Growth Retardation

The incidence of intrauterine growth retardation, small birth weight, and small head circumference has been reported to be increased in women with epilepsy [60,108]. Hiilesmaa et al. were first to report that infants exposed intrautero to carbamazepine or phenobarbital had small head circumferences [109]. Other studies have also found that an association between exposure to CBZ or PB in monotherapy was more associated with smaller head and reduced birth weights than the other AEDs [110]. Gaily et al. [111] looked at 144 children of mothers with epilepsy and also examined the parents. Mean head circumference was

Table 3 Demographics of Infants of Mothers with Epilepsy and Controls Matched by Age, Race, and Parity

	Number of cases	Average (range) gestation (weeks)	Weight (g)	Average (range) head circumference (cm)
Epilepsy		39 (33–43)	3515	34.5 (32–39)
CBZ	19	40	3145	35.0
PHT	32	39	3367	35.5
PB	15	39	3214	34.5
VPA	9	39	3387	34.5
Control 1	57	39 (33–43)	3182	33.9 (28–37)
Control 2	59	39 (32–43)	3286	34.1 (27–37)

lowest in children of mothers treated with phenobarbital or carbamazepine. However, the head circumference of the parents in this subgroup was also smaller. When this factor was included in the analysis, no drug effect was evident. The phenobarbital-exposed group had the lowest mean value, and although genetics was the major determinant of head size, a mild drug effect could not be excluded. We have studied a group of women with epilepsy treated with CBZ, PHT, valproate (VPA), or PB in monotherapy. For each woman with epilepsy, two controls were identified from the same clinic and matched for age, race, and parity. No difference was found in length of gestation, head circumference, and birth weight between groups (Table 3). An increase in adverse pregnancy outcomes, including decreased head circumference, has also been found in offspring of epileptic women noted treated with AEDs [108,112]. When an appropriate control group is selected, many of the previously reported adverse outcomes are not found.

Gaily et al. [113] studied intellectual performance in children of epileptic mothers and found no increased risk of low intelligence attributable to fetal exposure to AED or maternal convulsions. In both the study and control groups, they found an association between high numbers of minor anomalies and lower IQ. Lower intelligence correlated with a high number of minor anomalies, but this association was also found in controls. They concluded that a genetic link explained the connection of epilepsy in the mother and low intelligence in the infant.

E. Perinatal Complications

Low birth weight (<2500 g) and prematurity [2,54,114–117,150], stillbirth [73,116–118], and neonatal and perinatal death [27,54,73,115,116,119,120,150]

Table 4 Proposed Mechanism for AED Teratogenesis

1. Folate deficiency
2. Genetic defect in epoxide hydrolase
3. Defect in free-radical scavenging enzyme activity (FRSEA)
4. Embryotoxic metabolites of the AEDs
5. Inhibition of protein synthesis
6. Alteration in lipid metabolism
7. Trace metal depletion
8. Alteration in intracellular pH

have been reported to be increased in women with epilepsy. Yerby et al. [60] analyzed the birth certificates from 1980 to 1981 in the state of Washington. They found a 2.5- to 3.7-fold increased risk of low Apgar scores and asphyxia among epileptic mothers. In our experience, women with epilepsy have twice the incidence of a complicated labor or a perinatal complication. The patient with epilepsy is more likely to be in a lower socioeconomic class [121]. This probably affects prenatal care and nutrition. However, low birth weights, Apgar scores, and increased incidence of asphyxia have not been found to be specifically explained by maternal race, parity, age, previous fetal loss, or socioeconomic status [60]. Women with epilepsy clearly constitute a high-risk group and should be monitored closely throughout their pregnancy.

X. MECHANISMS OF TERATOGENESIS

The first proposed mechanism of AED-induced teratogenesis was interference with folate utilization, proposed initially for phenytoin. However, over the last decade a body of evidence has accumulated supporting a number of additional hypotheses on the mechanisms of teratogenesis (Table 4).

A. Folate Deficiency

Studies on folate in mothers with epilepsy have had mixed conclusions. Dansky et al. [122] found significantly lower blood folate concentrations in women with epilepsy with abnormal pregnancy outcomes. However, Strauss et al. [123] found that folates were not lower during pregnancy in epileptic women who were not given folate supplement. Treatment of mice with folic acid alone reduced malformation rates in pups exposed to phenytoin [124] or valproate [125] in utero. Biale and Lewenthal [126] reported a 15% malformation rate in IME with no folate supplementation, while none of 33 folate-supplemented children had congenital abnormalities. Phenytoin interferes with folate absorption from the GI tract and conversion from dihydrofolate to tetrahydrofolate, which is the biologically active form. A relative folate deficiency has also been suggested to occur with the barbiturates, carbamazepine, and valproic acid [127]. Although low serum and plasma levels have not been found uniformly, folate still appears to play an important role. In a study of more than 22,000 women, the incidence of neural tube defects was reduced by 75% in women who received multivitamins and folate in the first 6 weeks of pregnancy [128]. Multivitamin and folate supplementation is presently accepted as standard therapy during pregnancy. Since several of the AEDs may impair the utilization of folate, supplementation should definitely be given to all women with epilepsy when pregnant. Considering that pregnancy is not always planned, the daily addition of a multivitamin and folate preparation to the patient's medical regimen is recommended in all epileptic women who are fertile when AED treatment is initiated.

B. Epoxides

A large number of drugs are metabolized to an epoxide intermediate. These reactions are catalyzed by the microsomal monoxygenase system [129,130]. In general, arene oxides are unstable epoxides formed by aromatic compounds. Various epoxides are electrophilic and may elicit carcinogenic, mutagenic, teratogenic, and hepatotoxic effects by covalent binding to critical cell macromolecules [131,132]. Epoxides are detoxified by (1) conjugation to dihydrodiols catalyzed by epoxide hydrolase in the cytoplasm, and (2) conjugation with glutathione in the microsomes (mediated by glutathione transferase). One of the epoxides of carbamazepine (CBZ-E) is, however, very stable. CBZ-E builds up in the plasma and levels can be measured. This epoxide has been investigated as a marker for teratogenic effect, but a definite relationship has not been demonstrated [133]. Arene oxides are obligatory intermediates in the metabolism of aromatic compounds to *trans*-dihydrodiols. Phenytoin also forms a *trans*-dihydrodiol metabolite in several species of animal [134]. The evidence that epoxide metabolites of phenytoin are teratogenic can be summarized as follows. Phenytoin has an epoxide metabolite that binds to tissues. Inhibition of epoxide hydrolase increased the rate of orofacial clefts in experimental animals and increased lymphocyte cytotoxicity. Buehler et al. [135] measured epoxide hydrolase activity in amniocytes and concluded that a deficiency in enzyme activity may be a marker for infants at increased risk to develop AED-induced malformations. Epoxide formation alone cannot completely explain the teratogenicity of the AEDs. Lymphocyte cytotoxicity related to epoxide metabolites correlates with major but not minor malformations [122]. Malformations have been described with in utero exposure to ethotoin, mephytoin, and valproate which are not metabolized through an arene oxide intermediate [136,137]. Trimethadione is clearly teratogenic but has no phenyl rings and thus cannot form an arene oxide metabolite. Therefore, alternative mechanisms must exist for the teratogenic effect of some AEDs.

C. Free Radical Intermediates of AEDs

Some drugs are metabolized or bioactivated by cooxidation. This occurs during the synthesis of prostaglandins catalyzed by prostaglandin synthetase (PGS). These metabolites serve as electron donors to peroxidases, resulting in an electron-deficient drug molecule which by definition is called a free radical. To complete their outer ring, free radicals add electrons by binding covalently to cell macromolecules, nucleic acids (DNA and RNA), proteins, cell membranes, and lipoproteins. This process thus may produce a cytotoxic effect.

Phenytoin is cooxidated, producing reactive free-radical intermediates [138]. Other AEDs with ring structures (e.g., carbamazepine and barbiturates) may participate in this same reaction. Substances that can reduce free-radical tissue levels include acetylsalicylic acid (irreversibly inhibits PGS), caffeic acid (antioxidant), and α-phenyl-*N*-*t*-butylnitrone (free-radical spin trapper). Pretreatment of pregnant mice with these compounds reduces the number of phenytoin-induced cleft lip/palates seen in their offspring [138]. Similar free-radical studies have not been done with other AEDs. Yerby et al. [139] reported on a child with a ventricular septal defect exposed in utero to carbamazepine and phenobarbital. He was found to have low levels of free-radical scavenging enzymes which had been inherited from his father. This may be one method in which genetic succeptability to environmental toxins could be explained. Tissue levels of free radicals can be reduced by treatment with vitamin C, vitamin E, zinc, and selenium. These are contained in most multivitamin preparations and is another reason that multivitamin supplementation is indicated in fertile women with epilepsy.

D. Other Mechanisms

Additional mechanisms have been proposed for teratogenesis. VPA has been found to be embryotoxic in rats [140–142]. The 4-en metabolite, which accumulates in embryonic tissue, has a similar potency as a teratogen. The 2-en and 4-en metabolites are produced by ω-oxidation. Conversion to these metabolites by ω-oxidation can be enhanced by coadministration of other medications that induce the hepatic P450 enzyme system. Valproamide, which has an amine group attached to the carboxy segment of VPA, and the 2-en metabolite do not have a teratogenic effect in animal. To prevent enhanced metabolism through the ω-pathway and possible increased teratogenesis, valproate should be used in low doses and in monotherapy.

Intracellular pH in the fetus affects several cellular functions, including rate or proliferation and intracellular communication [143]. Intracellular pH may be increased by teratogenic levels of VPA, acetazolamide, and dimethadione (metabolite of TMO) [144]. Interference with lipid metabolism (VPA) and protein synthesis (PB) have also been suggested as mechanisms of teratogenesis. All these effects appear to be a concentration-dependent phenomena, and low-dose therapy may reduce adverse effects. Phenytoin and valproate have also been suggested to sequester Zn and other trace metals, resulting in a relative deficiency [145]. These act as cofactors in enzymatic reactions, and a deficiency potentially affects fetal development. The multivitamin replacement therapy routinely prescribed during pregnancy should counter these effects and is another reason to give vitamin supplement to fertile women with epilepsy.

XI. TREATMENT PLAN DURING PREGNANCY

Both pregnancy complications and rates of malformation are increased in women with epilepsy and treated with AEDs. The contributors to birth defects must be multifactorial. Generalized convulsions pose clear risks for maternal injury and miscarriage [146–148]. For most women, anticonvulsant therapy needs to be continued during pregnancy and the outcome is improved with the use of AEDs in monotherapy [149,150]. Risks of adverse outcome can be reduced by careful prenatal care, good seizure control, and maintenance of high serum folate levels. Patients should start taking on a daily basis prenatal vitamins with 1 mg of folate prior to conception. Women taking VPA or CBZ should be informed of the additional risks of spina bifida. The unique nature of this defect permits detection in the prenatal period. A combination of real-time ultrasonography and amniocentesis for α-fetal protein concentration between 16 and 18 weeks gestation will detect over 90% of all cases of spina bifida. Additionally, women should be advised of the association of digital hypoplasia with PHT. Despite the very real risks, over 90% of women with epilepsy taking AED will deliver children free of congenital malformations.

Neural ectoderm begins as a flat sheet of cells and over the first 4 weeks of development folds up and forms a tube. By the end of the fourth week this process is complete. Development of the major organ systems continues into the second month and is determined largely by the end of the ninth week of pregnancy. Therefore, interventions aimed at reducing the incidence of major malformations must be initiated very early in pregnancy or, preferably, prior to conception. Following are general guidelines for the treatment of the woman with epilepsy before and during pregnancy.

1. *Counsel the patient.* The patient and her spouse must be advised of the two- to threefold increase in rate of malformation in women with epilepsy taking AEDs. It is important to outline that the increase in risk is only in part attributable to medications and that other factors, such as nutrition and maternal health, are also crucial. A careful genetic history should be obtained to determine if the parents are at increased risk genetically for malformations. Both sides of the coin should be presented: that an increase incidence of malformation

is present but steps can be taken to reduce this risk. More than 90% of infants born to women with epilepsy are normal.

2. *Continue AEDs*. Seizures pose a potential threat to the health and welfare of the mother and fetus. Since seizure frequency may increase, medications should not be discontinued routinely. Stopping AEDs should be considered only in those patients in which this would be reasonable to do so even if they were not pregnant.

3. *Simplify the drug regimen*. The patient should be treated with as few medications (preferably one) and with as low a dose as clinically advisable. No single AED is best for all pregnancies. The drug of choice is that AED which best controls the patient's seizures. Thus low-dose monotherapy can be used, which minimizes the risk of malformation.

4. *Monitor plasma AED levels*. Dosage of medication should be altered only as dictated by (a) changing seizure frequency or (b) increasing blood levels (unlikely to occur). AED dosage changes should be guided but not dictated by the plasma drug level.

5. *Ultrasound and* α-fetal protein monitoring. If valproic acid or carbamazepine is taken in the first trimester, a careful ultrasound examination should be done at 16 to 18 weeks of gestation. Draw serum α-fetal protein levels when the patient is first seen in pregnancy and again 4 weeks later. Look for an increase in the α-fetal protein level greater than expected during pregnancy. Ultrasound or α-fetal protein studies will detect the presence of spina bifida in most cases. If either study is abnormal, an amniocentesis can be done to measure α-fetal protein in amniotic fluid. However, routine amniocentesis in all women with epilepsy is not recommended, as the risk of the procedure is usually greater than the increase in sensitivity in the detection of neural tube defects.

6. *Prescribe supplemental vitamins, iron, and folate*. Much of the crucial fetal development often occurs before the woman is sure that she is pregnant. Thus supplementation should be initiated prior to conception. All women of childbearing potential prescribed AEDs should take a multivitamin and folate preparation on a daily basis.

7. *Good nutrition and adequate sleep is essential*. The patient must avoid use of other medications except as directed by a physician. Care must be taken to avoid medications that may affect the formation and degradation of epoxide metabolites (e.g., cimitidine and erythromycin). Consumption of alcohol should be avoided, as this has been associated with fetal anomalies. Alcohol may also stimulate hepatic pathways, altering the metabolism of the AEDs and thus altering the risk of a malformation. Adequate nutrition is essential for proper development of the fetus.

8. *Terminate pregnancies with exposure to TMO*. Fetal exposure to trimethadione early in pregnancy results in a very high incidence of major

malformations and fetal deaths. Elective termination of a pregnancy is recommended in this instance.

REFERENCES

1. Hauser WA, Kurland LT. The epidemiology of epilepsy in Rochester, Minnesota, 1935 through 1967. Epilepsia 1975; 16:1–66.
2. Svigos JM. Epilepsy and pregnancy. Aust New Zealand Obstet Gynaecol 1984; 24:182–85.
3. Rosciszewska D. The course of epilepsy at the age of puberty in girls. Neurol Neurochir Pol 1975; 9:597–602.
4. Holmes GL. Effects of menstruation and pregnancy on epilepsy. Semin Neurol 1988; 8(3):234–39.
5. Newmark ME, Penry JK. Catamenial epilepsy: a review. Epilepsia 1980; 21:281–300.
6. Logothetis J, Harner R, Morrell F, Torres F. The role of estrogens in catamenial exacerbation of epilepsy. Neurology (Minneapolis) 1959; 9:354–60.
7. Holmes GL, Donaldson JO. Effect of sexual hormones on the electroencephalogram and seizures. J Clin Neurophysiol 1987; 4(1):1–22.
8. Backstrom T, Landgren S, Zetterlund B, Blom S, Dubrovsky B, Bixo M, Sodergard R. Effects of ovarian steroid hormones on brain excitability and their relation to epilepsy seizure variation during the menstrual cycle. In: Porter RJ, Mattson RH, Ward AA Jr, Dam M, eds. Advances in epileptology. 15th Epilepsy international symposium. New York: Raven Press, 1984:269–77.
9. Backstrom T. Epileptic seizures in women related to plasma estrogen and progesterone during the menstrual cycle. Acta Neurol Scand 1976; 54:321–47.
10. Browne TR, Feldman RG. Epilepsy: diagnosis and management. Boston: Little, Brown and Company, 1983:333–39.
11. Laidlaw J. Catamenial epilepsy. Lancet 1956; 2:1235–37.
12. Ansell B, Clarke E. Epilepsy and menstruation. The role of water retention. Lancet 1956; 2:1232–35.
13. Holmes GL, Kloczko N, Weber DA, Zimmerman ZW. Anticonvulsant effects of hormones on seizures in animals. In: Porter RJ, Mattson RH, Ward AA Jr, Dam M, eds. Advances in epileptology. 15th Epilepsy international symposium. New York: Raven Press, 1984:265–68.
14. Carrington RE. In Wilson JR, Carrington ER, eds. Obstetrics and gynecology, 7th ed, St. Louis, MO: CV Mosby Company, 1983, 60–70.
15. Backstrom T, Jorpes P. Serum phenytoin, phenobarbital, carbamazepine, albumin, and plasma estradiol, progesterone concentrations during the menstrual cycle in women with epilepsy. Acta Neurol Scand 1979; 59:63–72.
16. Backstrom T, Zetterlund B, Blom S, Romano M. Effects of intravenous progesterone infusions on the epileptic discharge frequency in women with partial epilepsy. Acta Neurol Scand 1984; 69:240–48.
17. Locock C, in discussion, Sieveking EH. Analysis of 52 cases of epilepsy observed by the author. Lancet 1857; 1:528.

18. Shavit G, Lerman P, Korczyn AD, Kivity S, Bechar M, Gitter S. Phenytoin pharmacokinetics in catamenial epilepsy. Neurology (Cleveland) 1984; 34:959–61.
19. Mattson RH, Cramer JA, Siconolfi BC, Caldwell BV. Medroxyprogesterone therapy for catamenial epilepsy. In Porter RJ, Mattson RH, Ward AA Jr, Dam M, eds. Advances in epileptology 15th Epilepsy international symposium. New York: Raven Press, 1984:279–82.
20. Mattson H. Overview of the interrelationship among seizures, hormones, and pregnancy. Adv Epileptol 1984; 197–99.
21. Herzog AG. Clomiphene therapy in epileptic women with menstrual disorders. Neurology 1988; 38(3):132.
22. Schmidt D, Beck-Mannagett G, Janz D, Koch S. The effect of pregnancy on the course of epilepsy: a prospective study. In: Janz D, Bossi L, Dam M, Helge H, Richens A, Schmidt D, eds. Epilepsy, pregnancy, and the child. New York: Raven Press, 1982:39–49.
23. Gjerde IO, Strandjord RE, Ulstein M. The course of epilepsy during pregnancy: a study of 78 cases. Acta Neurol Scand 1988; 78:198–205.
24. Bardy AH. Incidence of seizures during pregnancy, labor and puerperium in epileptic women: a prospective study. Acta Neurol Scand 1987; 75(5):356–60.
25. Bardy AH. Seizure frequency in epileptic women during pregnancy and puerperium: results of the prospective Helsinki study. In: Janz D, Bossi L, Dam M, Helge H, Richens A, Schmidt D, eds. Epilepsy, pregnant, and the child. New York: Raven Press, 1982:27–31.
26. Canger R, Avanzini G, Battino D, Bossi L, Franceschetti S, Spina S. Modifications of seizure frequency in pregnancy patients with epilepsy: a prospective study. In: Janz D, Bossi L, Dam M, Helge H, Richens A, Schmidt D, eds. Epilepsy, pregnancy and the child. New York: Raven Press, 1982:33–38.
27. Knight AH, Rhind EG. Epilepsy and pregnancy: a study of 153 pregnancies in 59 patients. Epilepsia 1975; 16:99–110.
28. Remillard G, Dansky L, Andermann E, Andermann F. Seizure frequency during pregnancy and the puerperium. In: Janz D, Bossi L, Dam M, Helge H, Richens A, Schmidt D, eds. Epilepsy, pregnancy and the child. New York: Raven Press, 1982:15–26.
29. Schmidt D, Canger R, Cornaggia C, Avanzini G, Battino D, Cusi C, Beck-Mannagetta G, Koch S, Rating D, Janz D. Seizure frequency during pregnancy and puerperium. The role of noncompliance and sleep deprivation. In: Porter RJ, Mattson RH, Ward AA Jr, Dam M, eds. Advances in epileptology. 15th Epilepsy international symposium. New York: Raven Press, 1984:221–25.
30. Ramsay RE. Changes in hormone levels and anticonvulsant metabolism during pregnancy. Adv Epileptol 1984; 15:233–37.
31. Lefebvre G, Delagrave N, et al. Epilepsy and pregnancy. Apropos of 50 cases. J Gynecol, Obstet Biol Reprod 1989; 18(8):1031–36.
32. Bag S, Behari M, Ahuja GK, Karmarkar MG. Pregnancy and epilepsy. J Neurol 1989; 236(5):311–13.
33. Battino D, Binelli S, Bossi L, Canger R, Como ML, Croci D, Cusi C, DeGianbattista M, Pardi G, Avanzini G. Monitoring of antiepileptic drugs and hormones in pregnancy epileptic women. In: Porter RJ, Mattson RH, Ward AA Jr, Dam M, eds.

Advances in epileptology. 15th Epilepsy international symposium. New York: Raven Press, 1984:227–32.
34. Ramsay RE. Effect of hormones on seizure activity during pregnancy. J Clin Neurophysiol 1987; 4(1):23–25.
35. Nau H, Schmidt-Gollwitzer M, Kuhnz W, Koch S, Helge H, Rating D. Antiepileptic drug disposition, protein binding and estradiol/progesterone serum concentration ratios during pregnancy. In: Porter RJ, Mattson RH, Ward AA Jr, Dam M, eds. Advances in epileptology. 15th Epilepsy international symposium. New York: Raven Press, 1984:239–49.
36. Stock B, Dean M, Levy G. Serum protein binding of drugs during and after pregnancy in rats. J Pharmacol Exp Ther 1980; 212(2):264–68.
37. Leppik IE, Rask CA. Pharmacokinetics of antiepileptic drugs during pregnancy. Semin Neurol 1988; 8(3):240–46.
38. Bardy AH, Teramo K, Hiilesmaa VK. Apparent plasma clearances of phenytoin, phenobarbital, primidone, and carbamazepine during pregnancy: Results of the prospective Helsinki study. In: Janz D, Bossi L, Dam M, Helge H, Richens A, Schmidt D, eds. Epilepsy, pregnancy, and the child. New York: Raven Press, 1982:141–45.
39. Koerner M, Yerby M, Friel P, McCormick K. Valproic acid disposition and protein binding in pregnancy. Ther Drug Monit 1989; 11(3):228–30.
40. Lander CM, Livingstone I, Tyrer JH, Eadie MJ. The clearance of anticonvulsant drugs in pregnancy. Clin Exp Neurol 1981; 17:71–78.
41. Knott C, Williams CP, Reynolds F. Phenytoin pharmacokinetics during pregnancy and the puerperium. Br J Obstet Gynecol 1986; 93(10):1030–37.
42. Philbert A, Andersen J, Norgaard-Rasmussen S, Flachs H, Dam M. Disposition of phenytoin during pregnancy: a pharmacokinetic study. In: Porter RJ, Mattson RH, Ward AA Jr, Dam M, eds. Advances in epileptology. 15th Epilepsy international symposium. New York: Raven Press, 1984:251–57.
43. Bardy AH, Hiilesmaa VK, Teramo KA. Serum phenytoin during pregnancy, labor and puerperium. Acta Neurol Scand 1987; 75(6):374–75.
44. Yerby MS, Friel PN, Miller DQ. Carbamazepine protein binding and disposition in pregnancy. In: Wolf P, Dam M, Janz D, Dreifuss FE, eds. Advances in epileptology. 16th Epilepsy international symposium. New York: Raven Press, 1987:547–49.
45. Kaneko S, Otani K, Fujita S, Fukushima Y, Sato T, Ogawa Y. The pharmacokinetics of primidone during pregnancy. In: Porter RJ, Mattson RH, Ward AA Jr, Dam M, eds. Advances in epileptology. 15th Epilepsy international symposium. New York: Raven Press, 1984:259–63.
46. Tsuru N, Maeda T, Tsuruoka M. Three cases of delivery under sodium valproate: placental transfer, milk transfer and probable teratogenicity of sodium valproate. Jpn J Psychiatry Neurol 1988; 42(1):89–96.
47. Meyer FP, Quednow B, Potrafki A, Walther H. Pharmacokinetics of anticonvulsants in the perinatal period. Zentralbl Gynakol 1988; 110(19):1195–1205.
48. Yerby MS. Problems and management of the pregnant woman with epilepsy. Epilepsia 1987; 28(Suppl 3):S29–36.

49. Kuhnz W, Koch S, Helge H, Nau H. Primidone and phenobarbital during lactation period in epileptic women: total and free drug serum levels in the nursed infants and their effects on neonatal behavior. Dev Pharmacol Ther 1988; 11(3):147–54.
50. Ramsay RE, Strauss RG, Wilder BJ, Willmore J. Status epilepticus in pregnancy: effect of phenytoin malabsorption on seizure control. Neurology (NY) 1978; 28:85–89.
51. Hauser WA, Hesdorffer DC. Epilepsy: frequency, causes, and consequences. New York: Demos Publications, 1990:297–326.
52. Teramo K, Hiilesmaa VK. Pregnancy and fetal complications in epileptic pregnancies: review of the literature. In: Janz D, Bossi L, Dam M, Helge H, Richens A, Schmidt D, eds. Epilepsy, pregnancy, and the child. New York: Raven Press, 1982:53–59.
53. Minkoff H, Schaffer RM, Delke I, Grunebaum AN. Diagnosis of intracranial hemorrhage in utero after a maternal seizure. Obstet Gynecol 1985; 65(3 Suppl): 22S–24S.
54. Hiilesmaa, VK. Pregnancy and birth in women with epilepsy. Pregnancy, teratogenesis, and epilepsy, an international symposium, Santa Monica, CA, July 14, 1990:100–101.
55. Morris HH. Epilepsy and pregnancy. Cleve Clinic J Med 1989; 56(Suppl Pt 2):S195–201.
56. Anderman E, Dansky L, Kinch R. Complications of pregnancy, labour, and delivery in epileptic women. In: Janz D, Bossi L, Dam M, Helge H, Richens A, Schmidt D, eds. Epilepsy, pregnancy, and the child. New York: Raven Press, 1982:61–74.
57. Annegers JF, Baumgartner KB, Hauser WA, Kurland LT. Epilepsy, antiepileptic drugs, and the risk of spontaneous abortion. Epilepsia 1988; 29(4):451–58.
58. Egenaes J. Outcome of pregnancy in women with epilepsy—Norway 1967 to 1978: complications during pregnancy and delivery. In: Janz D, Bossi L, Dam M, Helge H, Richens A, Schmidt D, eds. Epilepsy, pregnancy, and the child. New York: Raven Press, 1982:81–85.
59. Battino D, Bossi L, Canger R, Como ML, DeGiambattista M, Oldrini A, Pardi G, Pifarotti G. Obstetrical monitoring of pregnancy in 59 patients with epilepsy. In: Janz D, Bossi L, Dam M, Helge H, Richens A, Schmidt D, eds. Epilepsy, pregnancy and the child. New York: Raven Press, 1982:99–101.
60. Yerby M, Koepsell T, Daling J. Pregnancy complications and outcomes in a cohort of women with epilepsy. Epilepsia 1985; 26(6):631–35.
61. Conley NJ, Olshansky E. Current controversies in pregnancy and epilepsy: a unique challenge to nursing. J Obstet Gynecol Neonat Nurs 1987; 16(5):321–28.
62. Davies SM. Epilepsy and pregnancy. Am Fam Physician 1986; 34(5):179–83.
63. Koch S, Gopfert-Geyer I, Jager-Roman E, Rating D, Steldinger R, Helge H. Obstetric complications in pregnancies of epileptic mothers and their obstetric histories. In: Janz D, Bossi L, Dam M, Helge H, Richens A, Schmidt D, eds. Epilepsy, pregnancy, and the child. New York: Raven Press, 1982:91–97.
64. McCormick KB. Pregnancy and epilepsy: nursing implications. J Neurosci Nurs 1987; 19(2):66–76.

65. Deblay MF, Vert P, Andre M, Marchal F. Transplacental vitamin K prevents haemorrhagic disease of infant of epileptic mother. Lancet, 1982; 1:1247.
66. Keith DA, Gallop PM. Phenytoin, hemorrhage, skeletal defects and vitamin K in the newborn. Med Hypotheses 1979; 5:1347–51.
67. Bossi, L. Neonatal period including drug disposition in newborns: review of the literature. In: Janz D, Bossi L, Dam M, Helge H, Richens A, Schmidt D, eds. Epilepsy, pregnancy, and the child. New York, Raven Press, 1982:327–41.
68. Beraud R. De L'épilepsie dans ses rapports avec la grossesse et l'accouchement-bromuration pendent la grossesse. Delahaye A, Lecrosnier E, libraires-editors, Paris, 1884.
69. Muller-Kuppers M. Embryopathy during pregnancy caused by taking anticonvulsants. Acta Paedopsychiatr 1963; 30:401–5.
70. Pantarotto MF. A case of bone marrow aplasia in a newborn attributable to anticonvulsant drugs used by the mother during pregnancy. Quad Clin Obstet Gynecol 1965; 67:343–8.
71. Centa A, Rasore-Quartino A. La sindrome malformativa "digitocardiaca" (Hott–Oram): forme genetiche e fenocopie. Probabile azione teratogrena dei farmaci antiepilettici. Pathologica 1965; 57:227–32.
72. Melchior IC, Svenswark O, Trolle D. Placental transfer of phenobarbitone in women and elimination in newborns. Lancet 1967; 2:860–61.
73. Janz D, Fuchs M. Are anti-epileptic drugs harmful when given during pregnancy? Ger Med Methods 1964; 9:20–22.
74. Meadow SR. Anticonvulsant drugs and congenital abnormalities. Lancet 1968; 2:1296.
75. Bodendorfer TW. Fetal effects of anticonvulsant drugs and seizure disorders. Drug Intell Clin Pharm 1978; 12:14–21.
76. Smithells RW. Environmental teratogens of man. Br Med Bull 1976; 32:27–33.
77. Janz D. The teratogenic risk of antiepileptic drugs. Epilepsia 1975; 16:159–69.
78. Lakos P, Czeizel E. A teratological evaluation of anticonvulsant drugs. Acta Paediatr Acad Sci Hung 1977; 18(2):145–53.
79. Fedrick J. Epilepsy and pregnancy: a report from the Oxford record linkage study. Br Med J 1973; 2:442–48.
80. Kelly TE. Teratogenicity of anticonvulsant drugs I: review of the literature. Am J Med Genet 1984; 19:413–34.
81. Hanson JW, Smith DW. The fetal hydantoin syndrome. J Pediatr 1975; 87:285–90.
82. Seip M. Growth retardation. Dysmorhic facies and minor malformations following massive exposure to phenobarbital in utero. Acta Paediatr Scand 1976; 65:617–21.
83. DiLiberti JH, Farndon PA, Dennis NR, Curry CJR. The fetal valproate syndrome. Am J Med Genet 1984; 19:473–81.
84. Myhre SA, Williams R. Teratogenic effects associated with maternal primidone therapy. J Pediat 1981; 99:160–62.
85. Jones KL, Lacro RV, Johnson KA, Adam SJ. Pattern of malformations in the children of women treated with carbamazepine during pregnancy. N Engl J Med 1989; 320(25):1661–66.
86. Loughnan PM, Gold H, Vance JC. Phenytoin teratogenicity in man. Lancet 1973; 1:70–72.

87. Barr M, Poznanski AK, Schmickel RD. Digital hypoplasia and anticonvulsants during gestation: a teratogenic syndrome? J Pediatr 1974; 84:254.
88. Janz D. Personal communication. Presentation to International symposium on epilepsy and pregnancy, Montreal, Canada, 1983.
89. Phelan MC, Pellock JM, Wance WE. Discordant expression of fetal hydantoin syndrome in heteropaternal dizygotic twins. N Engl J Med 1982; 307(2):99–101.
90. Gaily E, Kantola-Sorsa E, Granstrom ML. Intelligence of children of epileptic mothers. J Pediatr 1988; 113:677–84.
91. German J, Kowal A, Ehlers KH. Trimethadione and human teratogenesis. Teratology 1970; 3:349–62.
92. Zackai EH, Mellman WJ, Neiderer B, Hanson JW. The fetal trimethadione syndrome. Pediatr 1975; 87(2):280–84.
93. Brown NA, Shull G, Fabro S. Assessment of the teratogenic potential of trimethadione in the CD-1 mouse. Toxicol Appl Pharmacol 1979; 51:59–71.
94. Feldman GL, Weaver DD, Lovrien EW. The fetal trimethadione syndrome. Am J Dis Child 1977; 131:1389–92.
95. Speidel BD, Meadow SR. Maternal epilepsy and abnormalities of the fetus and newborn. Lancet 1972; 2:839–43.
96. Annegers JF, Hauser WA, Elveback LR, Anderson VE, Kurland LT. Congenital malformations and seizure disorders in the offspring of parents with epilepsy. Int J Epidemiol 1978; 7(3):241–47.
97. Delgado-Escueta A. Pregnancy, teratogenesis, and genetics in epilepsy. Neurology (Suppl) 1992.
98. Kelly TE, Edwards P, Rein M, Miller JQ, Dreifuss FE. Teratogenecity of anticonvulsant drugs II: a prospective study. Am J Med Genet 1984; 19:435–43.
99. French Chapter of ILAE. Teratogenic risk of antiepileptic drugs, with special reference to sodium valproate therapy. Adv Epileptol 1984; 15:299–307.
100. Dansky L, Andermann E, Anderman F, Sherwin AL, Kinch RA. Maternal epilepsy and congenital malformations: correlation with maternal plasma anticonvulsant levels during pregnancy. In: Janz D, Bossi L, Dam M, Helge H, Richens A, Schmidt D, eds. Epilepsy, pregnancy, and the child. New York: Raven Press, 1982:251–58.
101. Lindhout D. Teratogenicity of anticonvulsant drugs. Review and recent findings with implications for counseling and pharmacotherapy of epileptic women of child-bearing age. In: Moss AJ, ed. Pediatrics update, reviews for physicians, 1987 ed. New York: Elsevier, 1987:129–47.
102. Kelly TE, Rein M. Edwards P. Teratogenicity of anticonvulsant drugs IV: the association of clefting and epilepsy. Am J Med Genet 1984; 19:451–58.
103. Friis ML, Hom NV, Sindrup EH, Fogh-Andersen P, Hange M. Facial clefts in sibs and children of epileptic patients. Neurology 1986; 36(3):346–50.
104. Kallen B. Maternal epilepsy, antiepileptic drugs and birth defects. Pathologica 1986; 78:757–68.
105. Rosa FW. Teratogenesis in epilepsy: birth defects with maternal valproic acid exposures. In: Porter RJ, Mattson RH, Ward AA, Dam M, eds. Advances in Epileptology. 15th Epilepsy international symposium. New York: Raven Press, 1984:309–14.

106. Philips NK, Lockard JS. A gestational monkey model: phenytoin versus seizures and neonatal outcome. Porter RJ, Mattson RH, Ward AA In: Dam M, eds. Advances in epileptology. 15th Epilepsy international symposium. New York: Raven Press, 1984:325–30.
107. Finnell RH, Chernoff GF. Mouse fetal hydantoin syndrome: effects of maternal seizures. Epilepsia 1982; 23:423–29.
108. Mastroiacovo P, Bertollini R, Licata D. Fetal growth in the offspring of epileptic women: results of an Italian multicentric cohort study. Acta Neurol Scand 1988; 78(2):110–14.
109. Hiilesmaa VK, Teramo K, Ganstrom ML, Bardy AH. Fetal head growth retardation association with maternal antiepileptic drugs. Lancet 1981; ii:165–67.
110. Bertollini R, Kallen B, Mastroiacovo P, Robert E. Anticonvulsant drugs in monotherapy. Effect on the fetus. Eur J Epidemiol 1987; 3(2):164–72.
111. Gaily EK, Ganstrom ML, Hiilesmaa VK, Bardy AH. Head circumference in children of epileptic mothers: contributions of drug exposure and genetic background. Epilepsy Res 1990; 5(190):217–22.
112. Fabris C, Licata D, Stasiowska B, Tanzilli S, Bertollini R. Newborn infants from epileptic mothers: malformation and auxonologic risk. Pediatr Med Chir 1989; 11(1):27–31.
113. Gaily E, Kantola-Sorsa E, Ganstrom ML. Intelligence of children of epileptic mothers. J Pediatr 1988; 113(4):677–84.
114. Levy RH, Yerby MS. Effects of pregnancy on antiepileptic drug utilization. Epilepsia 1985; 26(Suppl 1):525–57.
115. Bjerkedal T, Bhahna L. The course and outcome of pregnancy in women with epilepsy. Acta Obstet Gynecol Scand 1973; 52:245–48.
116. Nelson KB, Ellenberg JH. Maternal seizure disorder, outcome of pregnancy, and neurological abnormalities in the children. Neurology 1982; 32(11):1247–54.
117. Nakane Y, Okuma T, Takahashi R, Sato Y, Wada T, Sato T, Fukushima Y, Kumashiro H, Ono T, Takahashi T, Aoki Y, Kazamatsuri H, Inami M, Komai S, Seino M, Miyakoshi M, Tanimura T, Hazama H, Kawahara R, Otsuki S, Hosokawa K, Inanaga K, Nakazawa Y, Yamamoto K. Multi-institutional study on the teratogenicity and fetal toxicity of antiepileptic drugs: a report of a collaborative study group in Japan. Epilepsia 1980; 21:663–80.
118. Nakane Y. Congenital malformation among infants of epileptic mothers treated during pregnancy: the report of a collaborative study group in Japan. Folia Psychiatr Neurol Jpn 1979; 33(3):363–69.
119. Higgins TA, Comedford JB. Epilepsy in pregnancy. J Irish Med Assoc 1974; 67:317–29.
120. Speidel BD, Meadow SR. Anticonvulsant drugs and congenital anomalies. Lancet 1968; 2:1296.
121. Hiilesmaa VK, Teramo K, Bardy AH. Social class, complications, and perinatal deaths in pregnancies of epileptic women: preliminary results of the prospective Helsinki study. In: Janz D, Bossi L, Dam M, Helge H, Richens A, Schmidt D, eds. Epilepsy, pregnancy, and the child. New York: Raven Press, 1982:87–90.
122. Dansky LV, Andermann E, Rosenblatt D, Sherwin AL, Andermann F. Anticonvulsants, folate levels, and pregnancy outcome: a prospective study. Ann Neurol 1987; 21:176–82.

123. Strauss R, Ramsay RE, Willmore LJ. Hematologic effects of phenytoin therapy during pregnancy. Obstet Gynecol 1978; 55:682–85.
124. Zhu M, Zhou S. Reduction of the teratogenic effects of phenytoin by folic acid and a mixture of folic acid, vitamins, and amino acids: a preliminary trial. Epilepsia 1989; 30(2):246–51.
125. Trotz M, Wegner Chr, Nau H. Valproic acid–induced neuroal tube defects: reduction by folinic acid in the mouse. Life Sci 1987; 41:103–10.
126. Biale Y, Lewenthal H. Effect of folic acid supplementation on congenital malformations due to anticonvulsive drugs. Eur J Obstet Gynecol Reprod Biol 1984; 18(4):211–16.
127. Calandre EP, Jorde F, Rodriguez E. Serum folate concentrations in epileptic patients treated with carbamazepine and valproate (abstr). Epilepsia 1991; 32:75.
128. Milunsky A, Jick H, Jick S, Bruell CL, MacLaughlin DS, Rothman KJ, Willett W. Multivitamin/folic acid supplementation in early pregnancy reduces the prevalence of neural tube defects. JAMA 1989; 262(20):2847–2852.
129. Jerina DM, Daly JW. Arene oxides: a new aspect of drug metabolism. Science 1974; 185:573.
130. Sims P, Grover PL. Epoxides in polycyclic aromatic hydrocarbon metabolism and carcinogenesis. Adv Cancer Res 1974; 20:165.
131. Nebert DW, Jensen NM. The Ah locus: genetic regulation of the metabolism of carcinogens, drugs, and other environmental chemicals by cytochrome p-450 mediated mono-oxygenases. CRC Crit Rev Biochem 1979; 6:401–7.
132. Shum S, Jensen NM, Nebert DW. The Ah locus: in utero toxicity and teratogenesis associated with genetic differences in metabolism. Teratology 1979; 20:365–76.
133. Lindhaut D, Höppener RJEA, Meinardi H. Teratogenicity of antiepileptic drugs combinations with special emphasis on epoxidation (of carbamazepine). Epilepsia 1984; 25:77–83.
134. Chang T, Savory A, Glazko AJ. A new metabolite of 5,5-diphenylhydantoin (Dilantin). Biochem Biophys Res Commun 1970; 38(3):444–49.
135. Buehler BA, et al. Prenatal prediction of risk of the fetal hydantoin syndrome. N Engl J Med 1990; 322(22):1567–72.
136. Finnell RH, DiLiberti JH. Hydantoin-induced teratogenesis: are arene oxide intermediates really responsible? Helv Paediatr Acta 1983; 38(2):171–77.
137. Wells PG, Kupfer A, Lawson JA, Harbison RD. Relation of in vivo drug metabolism to stereoselective fetal hydantoin toxicology in mouse: evaluation of mephenytoin and its metabolite, nirvanol. J Pharmacol Exp Ther 1982; 221:228–34.
138. Kubow S, Wells PG. In vitro bioactivation of phenytoin to a reactive free radical intermediate by prostaglandin synthetase, horseradish peroxidase, and thyroid peroxidase. Mol Pharmacol 1989; 35:504–11.
139. Yerby M, Pippenger CE, Johnstone D, MacFarlan WD, Canthon ML, Johnson E, Levy R, Kerr BM. Association of a deficiency of free radical scavenging enzymes with development of congenital malformations in infants exposed to antiepileptic drugs in utero (abstr). Epilepsia 1991; 32:71.
140. Rettie AE, Rettenmeir AW, Beyer BK, Baite TA, Juchau MR. Valproate hydroxylation by human fetal tissues and embriotoxicity of metabolites. Clin Pharmacol Ther 1986; 40:172–77.

141. Nau H, Scott WJ. Weak acids may act as teratogens by accumulating in the basic milieu of the early mammalian embryo. Nature 1986; 323:276–78.
142. Nau H, Löscher W. Pharmacologic evaluation of various metabolites and analogs of valproic acid: teratogenic potencies of mice. Fundam Appl Toxicol 1986; 6:669–76.
143. Aerts RJ, Durston AJ, Moolenaar WH. Cytoplasmic pH and the regulation of the dictyostelium cell cycle. Cell 1985; 43:653–57.
144. Collins MW, Scott W, Pitter E, Nau H, Wittfoht W. Correlation of teratogenic potency with alteration of intracellular pH by C-8 carboxylic acids. Teratology 1986; 33:45C.
145. Hurd RW, Wilder BJ, Perchalski RJ, McDowell RL. Phenytoin alters skin copper, zinc and calcium levels: implications for drug side effects (abstr). Epilepsia 1991; 32:76.
146. Higgins TA, Comerford JB. Epilepsy in pregnancy. J Irish Med Assoc 1974; 67:317–29.
147. Stumpf DA, Frost M. Seizures, anticonvulsants, and pregnancy. Am J Dis Child 1978; 132:746–48.
148. Burnett CWF. A survey of the relation between epilepsy and pregnancy. J Obstet Gynecol 1946; 53:539–56.
149. Klinger W. Anticonvulsive therapy and complications of pregnancy in epileptic patients. Psychiatrie Neurol Med Psychol 1989; 41(7):400–405.
150. Kallen B. A register study of maternal epilepsy and delivery outcome with special reference to drug use. Acta Neurol Scand 1986; 73(3):253–59.

17

Access to Community Support Services

NANCY SANTILLI
University of Virginia Health Sciences Center
Charlottesville, Virginia

NYRMA HERNANDEZ
Epilepsy Foundation of America
Landover, Maryland

I. INTRODUCTION

Families who have children with epilepsy are often in need of support systems to ensure their child does not suffer any unnecessry consequences as a direct result of the seizures or their secondary effects, regardless of the type and severity of seizures. Additionally, families need community support services to help cope with the impact of the disorder on their own lives. These services are needed immediately after diagnosis, during the difficult treatment process, and throughout the child's developmental years and family transitions. Seizures may be accompanied by other disabilities.

All families deal with similar medical and social concerns associated with epilepsy. Some families have additional special needs and demands placed on them because of the disorder's broad spectrum. Regardless of the disability, families present with uniquely different backgrounds, strengths, resources, needs, and ways of coping. Many will confront difficulties in living daily with epilepsy, but additionally, they may experience stress accessing and utilizing the medical and social support systems.

Ethnic and cultural values have a strong impact on the way families react to epilepsy. Studies suggest that fear, misunderstanding, and stigma about epilepsy are more prevalent among some ethnic and minority groups, making adjustment an even greater challenge for the family. These perceptions may influence the way that various ethnic groups label and recognize seizure symptoms and seek medical care. Such perceptions may also influence the groups' interactions with the medical system, compliance with treatment, and the use of traditional health practices. Extensive family support systems abound among these ethnic groups, offering the potential for excellent support [1].

Research findings in the area of social supports and resources demonstrate that when these are accessed and used effectively, they directly influence the family's well-being and health. Dunst et al. [2] report that

> the adequacy of different types and forms of support, especially aid and resources that match family identified needs, promotes parent and family well-being, decreases time demands placed upon a family, promotes positive caregiver interactive styles, enhances positive parental perception of child functioning, and influences a number of child-behavior characteristics, such as temperament and motivation.

The recognition that the best health care for a child is family-based and is responsive to the child's multiple needs requires that the family be viewed in the context of its formal and informal social support systems. Formal resources include professionals, agencies, and institutions. Informal resources include neighbors, the church, the circle of friends, extended family members, and other support networks of special meaning to the family. In epilepsy, the comprehensive nature and impact of the disorder often require that in addition to medical services, health care encompasses counseling; social services; support networks; education; advocacy; employment, legal, recreational, and financial assistance; and respite care.

It is often difficult for professionals to be aware of the range, quality, and relevance of resources and services needed by families of children with epilepsy. As a general principle, however, it is important to encourage and assist the family in seeking such services on their own. Families will know best what their needs are and if and when those needs are being met. Professionals can work with families to access the services they need and to help determine if their needs are met by such services. This places the family in the position of acting in an advocate role rather than in a dependent role. In this way the family can work to avoid problems by timely intervention through the use of suitable community resources.

It is important to note that access to services is often restricted to age, level of disability, and varying eligibility requirements. The broad spectrum of epilepsy presents special challenges to eligibility and to the access of services by both families and professionals. Access to special education and related services under the Education of the Handicapped Act will not be available to all children with epilepsy, but only to those whose condition is shown to severely affect their educational performance.

Eligibility criteria determine if someone can benefit and is entitled to a particular service. While eligibility for federal programs varies, they all share a common theme of assessing a person based on functional abilities rather than using a categorical approach to eligibility (i.e., having a specific diagnosis).

Additionally, in many instances, states have policies that affect eligibility for people with seizure disorders. The functional approach is generally favored by many in the disability community because it avoids labeling people. It also tends to target services for people with the most severe disabilities, as measured in functional terms.

The challenge of the functional approach is determining how persons within the broad spectrum of seizure disorders can meet the existing functional tests. The types of tests used by a state determine whether a person is functionally impaired and can affect the ease with which people with epilepsy can show that they qualify for services. Many states, for example, currently utilize tests specifically designed to measure the functional capacity of persons with mental retardation. This type of test will fail to assess accurately the extent to which persons with epilepsy, other than those who have mental retardation, are functionally impaired.

A problem exists where epilepsy may be recognized as a qualifying disability, but the applicant must still prove that the epilepsy is severe enough to be given priority for services. Often in these situations, assessments of severity are made by looking only at the frequency of seizures. For example, in the medical listings for social security, the severity of the epilepsy is determined almost solely on whether a person has seizures on a frequent basis. Other factors are not generally considered. Some state vocational rehabilitation programs will not serve a person who is not currently having seizures (those whose seizures are controlled on medications) because they are not viewed as disabled. However, those very same states, as well as other states, will not serve a person who is having active seizures because they are not viewed as being employable. The professional can play an important role in helping the person with epilepsy and the family understand the eligibility criteria, their application, and how the medical and social aspects of the seizure disorder relate to those requirements.

Informal support systems and resources are also valuable sources of support. In fact, one of the most effective ways in which families provide and receive support and develop coping skills is through parent and family networks. These networks are based on the philosophy that families of a child with a disability have something in common with other families in similar circumstances. Families who are living through the experience of raising a child with epilepsy gain a special understanding of the problems involved and of ways to cope with them. Families who are dealing with the initial diagnosis of epilepsy or a particular crisis, or parents who are struggling with acceptance, can be helped by other parents who share their insights and experiences.

An environment that provides empathy, eases frustration, alleviates fear, overcomes social isolation, and gives encouragement can be offered through parent and family networks. A two-way interaction of giving and receiving support

LLYFRGELL U.C.N.W. LI

and sharing information and expertise is fostered through parent-to-parent assistance, support meetings, and phone networks. Networks can also provide parents with an opportunity to gain additional confidence to seek and find the best solutions for their particular child and family and to advocate for better services for those with epilepsy [3].

It should be recognized, however, that whereas parent networks are immensely valuable for many parents, they are not necessarily the answer for all parents. Some parents choose not to join parent networks for reasons of personal privacy. Others may choose not to join initially—because they are not emotionally ready, or the timing is not right. These parents should nevertheless be provided with information about the network, in case they reconsider in the future. There are also parents who join the network but choose not to be involved in its advocacy activities.

These family networks can be found in the form of support groups, telephone networks, and parent-to-parent or child-to-child match. They can be specific to the particular medical condition or disability, or they may be organized across disabilities.

The Association for the Care of Chidren's Health (ACCH) has identified eight principles of family-centered, community-based, coordinated support networks:

1. Recognition that the family is the constant in the child's life, while the service systems and personnel within those sytems fluctuate
2. Facilitation of parent/professional collaboration at all levels of health care:
    a. Care of an individual child
    b. Program development, implementation, and evaluation
    c. Policy formulation
3. Sharing of unbiased and complete information with parents about their child's care, on an ongoing basis, in an appropriate and supportive manner.
4. Implementation of appropriate policies and programs that are comprehensive and provide emotional and financial support to meet the needs of families.
5. Recognition of family strengths and individuality and respect for different methods of coping.
6. Understanding and incorporating the developmental needs of infants, children, and adolescents and their families into health care delivery systems.
7. Encouragement and facilitation of parent-to-parent (and family-to-family) support.
8. Assurance that the design of health care delivery systems is flexible, accessible, and responsive to family needs [4].

In addition to those principles mentioned above: Other family members, such as brothers and sisters, grandparents, aunts and uncles, and caregivers outside the family, play an important role in the children's lives and should also be encouraged to be part of the epilepsy family network. Regardless of the degree of disability imposed by the seizure disorder, all families of chidren with epilepsy face common medical and social concerns, yet because of the broad spectrum of the disorder, some families may also have special needs and demands placed on them [3].

Efforts to promote collaboration and coordination of resources are essential to an effective community service network, not only to avoid duplication of efforts and expenses, but to support and complement the families' own resources and facilitate an optimum utilization of those resources which are available. Effective communication, coordination, and collaboration cannot be emphasized enough. It is at the core of access and utilization of resources and networking among professionals, agencies, and families. An attitude of partnership and a shared commitment to the best outcome for the child and the family should guide all collaborative efforts.

Usually, even in the smallest of communities, there are a number of public and/or private programs available to meet many basic family needs. Almost all communities have at least one identified resource to help its residents in locating the needed services. These information and referral services have comprehensive community information with staff that are skilled in assessing needs and matching them to available services. Voluntary organizations and disability groups can serve an excellent role in identifying these resources. For example, EFA's local affiliates in many states serve as the community focal point for identifying and helping families access needed resources and for helping families to identify those needs. Many epilepsy affiliates also provide a focus for ongoing needs assessments and for developing collaborative relationships among community agencies. Epilepsy clinics can also serve this role in some communities.

It is best when looking at resources to evaluate them from a national, state, and local level. Following is a listing of national organizations that may be a resource to professionals and to families with children with a seizure disorder.

II. NATIONAL CONTACTS

THE EPILEPSY FOUNDATION OF AMERICA, 4351 Garden City Drive, Landover, MD 20785; (301) 459-3700, 1-800-EFA-1000 (Toll Free Information Service) and 1-800-EFA-4050 (National Epilepsy Library)

The Epilepsy Foundation of America (EFA) provides numerous services throughout the country to people with epilepsy and their families. It has working relationships with various federal, state, and local government units. It has established professional ties with national and international organizations. It is the most readily available specific national resource for the family and the professional.

EFA has a national, state, and local structure. Its state and local organizations are independently operated but bound to the national organization by an affiliation agreement. Affiliates can provide information on community services in addition to their own programs. Some of the services provided by local organizations are (1) information and referral services, (2) school alert—an educational program to improve the school environment for the child with epilepsy, (3) epilepsy month—a program of intense public information and education, (4) speakers' bureau—an educational service to provide trained speakers to talk to groups and clubs about epilepsy, (5) professional education—a variety of programs for all professional and lay groups about epilepsy, (6) advocacy—activities to support both individuals and families and legislative and executive advocacy, (7) recreation, (8) self-help, (9) parent and family support services, (10) employment services, and (11) residential programs sponsored by some affiliates. Each affiliate may not offer all of the above but will offer a number of the services listed. This is determined by local need and ability to support such programs. The foundation offers the best ''one-stop shopping'' resource for the family and professional in need of services.

There are a number of unique programs offered at the national level that are of special interest to families. They include the following:

Research. The foundation supports a number of individual research projects annually and produces a quarterly newsletter for the scientific community. Many of these research projects focus on issues of particular concern for families.

Professional education and training. Professional education materials, audiovisual and print, are produced and distributed nationwide for use by physicians, nurses, and other professionals. Educational seminars are also sponsored. An international visiting professorship program is also operated to foster the exchange of knowledge among nations.

Membership. Membership in EFA is open to all. Benefits include subscription to ''Epilepsy USA,'' the EFA newspaper which covers such topics as research, legal issues, affiliate news, and new developments, to name a few. Members also participate in the American Association of Retired Persons (AARP Prescription Pharmacy Program) and benefit from special alerts, such as those related to medication recalls.

National epilepsy library. (1-800-EFA-4050). The National Epilepsy Library provides the latest in research and treatment information, as reflected in the professional literature, for the primary care physician and the neurological research and scientific community as well. It is also the most comprehensive resource of information on the psychosocial aspects of epilepsy.

Information and referral. This service is offered through a toll-free information line 1-800-EFA-1000, to assist callers in identifying current information on resources in their own area. It also provides the latest information about epilepsy. Besides having access to skilled information specialists in epilepsy, Spanish-speaking professionals and material are also available. EFA's National Toll-Free Service also maintains a nationwide database of community resources and provides information and referral services to families and the general public, particularly in communities without an EFA affiliate.

Family video library. This series consists of short, educational videotapes that address epilepsy-related issues of concern to families.

Parent and family networks. This network is a program sponsored both by EFA and its affiliates which helps put families in touch with one another so that families facing epilepsy problems for the first time can benefit from others who have been there.

Legal information services. EFA's Legal Advocacy Program provides free information for people with legal questions, their attorneys, outside agencies, and government officials.

Employment assistance and placement. This program offers job search assistance, training in job-seeking skills, employer education, and follow-along services to persons with seizure disorders.

Epilepsy family action services. Ths program strives to develop creative outreach approaches and services to young children and their families and also initiates and strengthens collaboration with relevant professionals and organizations and coordinates services to supporting families.

Videos, pamphlets, posters, and books. This catalog lists all EFA materials. To place an order, or for further information, call 1-301-577-0100.

ASSOCIATION FOR THE CARE OF CHILDREN'S HEALTH, 7910 Woodmont Avenue, Suite 300, Bethesda, MD 20814; (301) 654-6549

This organization works with the health care community to meet the multiple needs of children and their families through education, advocacy, and research programs. They have a large number of publications, including a bimonthly newsletter and a parent resource guide.

ASSOCIATION FOR RETARDED CITIZENS, 2501 Avenue J, Arlington, TX 76011; (817) 640-0204

This organization offers diverse services for children who have some form of mental retardation. It also provides information about all types of developmental delays. There are a number of local affiliates on both the state and community levels.

THE ASSOCIATION FOR CHILDREN AND ADULTS WITH LEARNING DISABILITIES, 4156 Library Road, Pittsburgh, PA 15234; (412) 341-1515

This is a grass-roots national organization with over 500 local offices meeting the needs of people with learning disabilities, including information, advocacy, school program development, legislative action, and publications.

COUNSEL FOR EXCEPTIONAL CHILDREN, 1920 Association Drive, Reston, VA 22091-1589; (703) 620-3660

This is a national organization with almost 1000 local chapters directed specifically toward the educational needs of children. They have a number of excellent publication products and computer searches available through them.

MAINSTREAM, 1030 15th Street NW, Suite 1010, Washington, DC 20005; (202) 898-0202

The organization's basic goal is to mainstream people with disabilities into society. It provides a job placement and development service, an information program, a newsletter with articles on disability related issues, and a disability awareness training program.

NATIONAL INFORMATION CENTER FOR HANDICAPPED CHILDREN AND YOUTH (NICHY), P.O. Box 1492, Washington, DC 20013; (703) 522-3333

This organization provides free information to parents of handicapped children. It answers specific questions and assists with information and referral and a wide variety of disabilities.

SIBLINGS FOR SIGNIFICANT CHANGE, 823 United Nations Plaza, Room 808, New York, NY 10017; (212) 420-0776

This is an organization dedicated to siblings of the disabled. It provides information services, access to legal-aid counseling programs, and community education.

III. STATE AND LOCAL CONTACTS

In each community there is usually at least one or two service agencies to help in identifying services available. EFA's national network of 86 affiliates across the country are the primary point of contact for people with epilepsy and their families in many communities. In addition, other sources may be available for accessing services, such as an *information and referral services agency*, or a local *United Way agency* can be of help. They are often listed under "Social Service" or with the Chamber of Commerce. These offices maintain current listings of all services available in a given geographic area by developing a resource directory of services available for the residents. Many offer formal and referral services and may serve as the main contact for the community.

Community services can be assessed by identifying categories of services that are available. For example, *the state department of health and human services* can encompass a number of divisions that provide services for children and their families. Agencies coming under this category could include maternal and child health services, developmental disability services, vocational rehabilitation, protection and advocacy services, and mental health and mental retardation services.

A number of health services available in each state can be obtained by contacting a local health department. They can inform the family of the services available in their community or direct them to services that are available more regionally. They include such services but are not limited to dental care, family planning, health clinics that include children's specialty service, home health services, immunizations for childhood disease and overseas travel, Medicaid screening, public health nursing, child development evaluation, obstetrical and pediatric care, WIC vouchers, and nutritional counseling.

State developmental disabilities agencies have been designed for the purpose of providing funding for direct services to people with developmental disabilities. Most of the programs are administered by private, nonprofit agencies and provide such services as diagnosis, evaluation, recreation, group homes, information and referral, advocacy and protection, and social services. Programs are provided either directly by the state office or through grant funding for development of new programs within the state. The agency usually works very closely with local groups and has a good working knowledge of the services provided around the partcular state.

The *state vocational rehabilitation agency* provides counseling, education, training, and medical evaluation along with other services needed to prepare people for work.

The *state protection and advocacy offices* (PAOs) are set up for persons who have developmental disabilities. The services offered through these vary according to state. The main purpose of PAO is to advocate on behalf of individuals in areas of education, health, residential, vocational and social services involving activities of daily living. Legal services are also provided. These offices were established to protect the rights of those with developmental disabilities.

The state agency responsible for *mental health and mental retardation*, in many states, oversees and supports a comprehensive array of outpatient and inpatient mental health services as well as a full complement of services for those with mental retardation. These can include, but are not limited to, case management services, residential services, medication clinics, preadmission screening, client advocacy, and social recreational programs. They usually work very closely with community services boards to ensure that services are provided within the local community when possible.

The *state department of education* has the sole responsibility of providing educational services to all children in a given state. These services can begin as early as at birth and extend until 21 years of age for those qualifying for special education. Early intervention programs may not always be listed with the department of education and may exist under community service boards, in institutions of higher learning, or through voluntary nonprofit organizations. As states sign on to the new education law, P.L. 94–457, each state will decide who will be responsible for these early intervention programs. In some states this will fall under the state department of education, whereas in others it will exist under other state agencies, such as mental health and mental retardation and developmental disabilities.

Families who have a child with epilepsy face quite a challenge. During different stages of development both the child's and the family's needs will change considerably. To support a family in its efforts to provide the child with the best opportunities for a normal life, it is helpful to develop a checklist of concerns that frequently emerge and need attention. There are nine areas to which health care providers often refer families for services: health care, education, counseling and supportive resources, financial aid, legal assistance, employment, epilepsy education, and family services. Each of these areas will be dealt with separately in order to streamline the professional's response to the consumer's concerns.

A. Health Care

The majority of individuals with seizures receive their primary care from pediatricians and/or family practitioners. They do not benefit from ongoing comprehensive multidisciplinary care offered by many of the epilepsy centers. Thus it is imperative that whoever is the primary care provider for the treatment of epilepsy in children be cognizant of the fact that even the child with well-controlled seizures often has secondary complications related to the epilepsy and its treatment. Thus from time to time they may benefit from an annual evaluation at a comprehensive epilepsy center, especially during a period of significant change in their medical condition and/or functioning abilities. To identify some of the national and regional services available, it is probably best to contact either the Epilepsy Foundation of America (which has been discussed previously) or the National Association for Comprehensive Epilepsy Programs. The Epilepsy

Foundation of America maintains a national database which is continually updated and expanded with information on hospitals, clinics, and individual neurologists who have indicated that they are treating people with epilepsy. Staff at the foundation are prepared to provide three or more names with service descriptions as provided by the physician or facility. The National Association of Comprehensive Epilepsy Programs has defined the various levels of care available to individuals with seizures. They have outlined the times in treatment when referral to the next level of care should be made. They maintain a list of comprehensive epilepsy programs and have developed the criteria in establishing what constitutes a comprehensive center.

The family can contact their local health department to learn more about specialty programs that might be available to children with seizure disorders and/or developmental disabilities in addition to the services provided for routine health maintenance for their child. Since children have medical needs that extend beyond their seizure disorder it is necessary to be aware of the other health maintenance programs available in the community. These include identifying pediatricians and family practitioners who have extended their services to include developmental evaluations for their clients. In addition, families need to be aware of dental practices that will care for children who have seizure disorders. By contacting the local dental association, those dentists specializing in pediatric care and willing to accept patients with developmental disabilities are frequently identified. Often, the local pediatrician and/or family practitioner can help identify dental services in the community that are willing to care for these children.

B. Education

Since epilepsy and its treatment can affect a child's education development in several ways, numerous questions often arise regarding determining the appropriateness of the services provided and/or referral to needed services. Under federal and state laws, schools must provide appropriate education and special services to any children whose disability impinges on their ability to benefit from regular classroom instruction. Parents often approach doctors regarding difficulties children may be experiencing in school. The following resources can be suggested to families:

1. Local Director of Special Education or State Office of Special Education

Each school district can identify that person in their area. A family can request that their child be evaluated for the services provided. In each locality there is usually a parent advisory committee to the special education program, and it can be most helpful for parents to contact the chairperson or individual committee members in order to have the parents' perspective of how to work through the system. A number of lay organizations have handbooks on how the educational process for special services operates and potential rights and responsibilities. It is to the family's advantage to obtain copies of those books to assist them in understanding their position. Public Law No. 94–457 requires that communities provide the services for children starting at 2 years of age up through 21 years of age.

2. Parent-Infant Development Programs

These are home-based early intervention programs designed to prevent or reduce developmental delays in chilren aged birth through 2 years of age. These delays may be a result of congenital, acquired, medical, or environmental conditions. The focus of instruction is family centered to meet the needs of the individual family. Trained outreach workers work on a one-to-one basis with the parent and child at home. Developmental screening is available. In some areas where these services are offered, through such lay organizations as the Association for Retarded Citizens, center-based programs are available. In either case these groups will usually work closely with day care providers to develop a comprehensive plan that can be followed through by all care providers.

3. Head Start Programs

These are early intervention programs designed to give children at risk a head start in their educational programs. Enrollment is usually limited to 3- and 4-year-olds and is based on financial status.

4.Day Care/Preschool Services

A large number of these programs have developed throughout the country. They are both home and institution based, with private and public support. Each center has its own philosophies and rules regarding enrolling children with developmental disabilities. It is often necessary for the health care provider to work closely with this group of child care workers and educators so that parents can have access to these services while allowing the child to be mainstreamed appropriately.

C. Counseling Resources

The family and often a child with epilepsy are in need at some point of counseling to assist them in making the adjustment to living with a seizure disorder. Since counseling services can vary significantly, it is important to be sensitive to individual family needs when suggesting services. It is important that the resources have some general understanding of epilepsy and its special consequences. Services can be provided by a variety of professionals and community settings. A number are listed below.

1. *Social workers*. These professionals can often be found in many settings. They are located in private practice, community and university hospitals, health departments, and through local social service departments. A number of large

employer groups do offer some employee counseling services through their human resource departments. These professionals are very helpful in identifying and referring families to other community service programs as needed.

2. *Psychologists*. These persons can often provide counseling, therapy, and psychological/educational testing. If the latter is needed, it is best to identify a neuropsychologist who may be able to do a more comprehensive evaluation and thus develop a more effective treatment and habilitation plan.

3. *Psychiatrists*. These specialists may be employed for children and families with complex and/or overwhelming problems. They are often helpful with children who have a dual diagnosis of behavior and/or mental health problems in addition to their seizure disorder.

4. *School counselors*. These persons are frequently available in each school district and can act as a liaison between the home, school, and medical community. They can assist the child, their family, and the teacher in supporting the child in the school environment for optimum learning.

5. *Clergy*. This group may be considered as a counseling resource and can be explored with individual families based on their religious preference and the services available through their religious community. A number of religious communities are now offering support programs to persons with handicaps and their families.

6. *Mental health clinics*. These clinics are usually operated as part of the community service programs and are staffed by various disciplines. Services are usually available on a sliding-scale basis.

7. *Family service agencies*. These agencies provide individual and family counseling through special programs in which they meet the diverse needs of our present-day families.

8. *Support networks*. Over the years numerous types of support networks have been developed to meet the varying needs of a community. Support networks usually fall into the following categories.

a. *Self-help groups*. These are primarily run by and for those with a personal involvement. Professionals may participate in an advisory or training capacity, but the leadership is vested in the group.

b. *Parent and family networks*. These networks offer a large array of services for the diverse needs of families. They are based on the philosphy that families have something in common with other families in similar circumstances. These networks provide an opportunity for families to share experiences and feelings. There are a variety of parent and family networks approaches or models. The Epilepsy Foundation of America promotes and assists with the development of three basic models: (1) parent/family partners based on one-to-one interactions, (2) parent/family support groups, and (3) parent telephone networks [3].

Support groups and networks usually meet on either a weekly or a monthly basis. These meetings are usually announced regularly in the local newspaper in the community service section.

9. *Counseling groups*. These are professionally run groups which deal with a variety of audiences, goals, and purposes. They may be organized specifically for teenagers, siblings, parents of a newly diagnosed child, families with severely disabled children, young adults, and married couples.

10. *Social or recreational groups*. The primary focus is to provide an opportunity for families and children to get out and meet others. They may also include an educational and socialization experience, such as specialized camps. They may be sponsored through local parks and recreation departments, religious organizations, or nonprofit advocacy groups, such as EFA affiliates across the country.

Other necessary resources to support families may include:

In-home health care services
Respite care programs
Transportation assistance
Financial assistance
Toy lending libraries

Families and professionals need full access to information if they are to work as partners in a coordinated network approach to community resources. In addition to the information on national, state, and local services and regarding the various professional resources, there are a few other mechanisms to learning about and accessing and utilizing appropriate resources. Newsletters, for example, are effective ways to keeping informed. They are especially useful in widely dispersed areas, isolated from major medical centers and from other resources. Family resource libraries can also be organized locally by nonprofit groups, parent networks, or epilepsy clinics. These are a good way to ensure that families and professionals have ready access to information. EFA's National Epilepsy Library can be an effective source of staying abreast of the latest developments in epilepsy.

Public information and education and working with the media are other successful vehicles for keeping families, professionals, and the communities informed of services and new developments. EFA affiliates typically carry on public information campaigns, particularly during November, which is Epilepsy Month.

In summary, family-based, coordinated care for children with seizure disorders depends on an informed, coordinated system of informal and formal support. The critical factor lies in the recognition that the best health care for a child with seizures is family-based, that it be viewed comprehensively within the context of both natural and informal support systems, and that it incorporates both medical and social resources.

One recent development of great significance to access to services and resources for people with disabilities is passage of the Americans with Disabilities Act of 1990 (ADA). The act prohibits discrimination against qualified people with disabilities in employment, public services, transportation, public accommodations, and telecommunications services. The law gives civil rights protections to people with disabilities simliar to those provided to persons who are discriminated against because of their race, sex, national origin, or religion.

Except for the employment section of the act, the law applies equally to children with disabilities, with excellent collateral benefits for their families. State and other federal laws that provide equal or greater protections for the rights of children and adults with disabilities are not invalidated or limited by the Americans with Disabilities Act. Further, the ADA does not require a person with a disability to accept an accommodation, aid, service, benefit, or opportunity that the person does not choose to accept.

The passage of the Americans with Disabilities Act represents another major step against discrimination and in favor of integration into society of children and adults with disabilites and their families. The Epilepsy Foundation of America played a major national leadership role in the enactment of this legislation and will continue to work hard to ensure that the intent and the vast protections of the law are realized.

REFERENCES

1. Association for the Care of Children's Health. Guidelines and recommended practices for the individualized family-services plan. 1989.
2. Dunst, Trivette, Deal. Enabling and empowering families: principles and guidelines. Cambridge, MA: 1988.
3. Epilepsy Foundation of America. Epilepsy parent and family networks. Landover, MD: EFA, 1989.
4. Epilepsy Foundation of America. Annual report. Landover, MD: EFA, 1990.
5. Hauser WA, Hesdorffer DC. Epilepsy: frequency, causes and consequences. New York: Demos Publications, 1990.
6. Shelton, Jeppson, Johnson. Family-centered care for children with special health care needs. Washington, DC: Association for the Care of Children's Health, 1989.

18

Legal Issues Facing Children with Epilepsy

DAVID FIELD OLIVER
Smith, Gill, Fisher & Butts
Kansas City, Missouri

I. INTRODUCTION

Young people with epilepsy can face difficulty in getting a driver's license, obtaining employment, and getting insurance. In each case they may be faced with written applications that ask if they have a seizure disorder. They will worry that if they answer "yes," they will not be able to drive, get a job, or get insurance. If they answer "no," they will worry about what happens if they have a seizure while driving or on the job, and if their insurance claim may be denied if they have a seizure and the insurance company discovers that they falsely answered a question about seizures on their application. The physician should be sensitive to these concerns and take the initiative in discussing these issues with the patient.

These can be real problems. But they are problems that can be solved. People with epilepsy have been discriminated against in obtaining driving privileges, employment, and insurance—and continue to be. Stereotypes and ignorance abound regarding epilepsy. The modern trend, however, reflected in many state and federal laws, is to protect people with epilepsy from discrimination. People can get a driver's license if their seizures are controlled; their employment rights are protected by laws; and insurance protection is available. This chapter cannot be a legal treatise but will provide a practical approach to the physician on the legal issues regarding driving, employment, and insurance.

If a young patient is diagnosed as having a seizure disorder, a conference with the patient and family should be held where these issues are discussed openly and honestly. The family may be confused and uncertain as to what to do and may, in fact, not know what to ask or do. If this is the first experience they have had with epilepsy, they may have stereotypical views of what their child can and cannot do. They should be encouraged to discuss these issues with their child and seek assistance from others, if necessary. The physician obviously cannot provide legal advice but can provide general advice and support and indicate how they can get legal advice.

The Epilepsy Foundation of America is an excellent source of information in these areas. It publishes booklets on the legal rights of persons with epilepsy. It can be reached by calling (301) 459–3700 or by writing the Epilepsy Foundation of America, Legal Advocacy Department, 4351 Garden City Drive, Landover, MD 20785. Staff members deal with these problems on a daily basis and are always willing to help persons with epilepsy and their families. And if the physician has a question, this is a good resource for him or her. Most communities have local affiliates of the Epilepsy Foundation of America. They can also be excellent sources of information for the young patient or family. Phone numbers and addresses can be found in the phone book or can be obtained from the Epilepsy Foundation of America.

If a young patient experiences a real problem in getting a driver's license or feels that he or she has been discriminated against in employment or insurance merely because of the fact that he or she has epilepsy, he or she should be encouraged to seek legal advice. Again, the Epilepsy Foundation of America can help or a private attorney can be consulted. Most states have not-for-profit legal services corporations that provide free or low-cost legal assistance if the patient or family cannot provide a private attorney.

Federal law requires each state to have "protection and advocacy agency" for persons with developmental disabilities. Epilepsy may qualify as a developmental disability in some circumstances. The state "protection and advocacy agency" can answer many questions the young patient or family may have about their rights under federal and state laws. The governor's office will provide the phone number and address for the agency.

II. DRIVING

Every state has certain eligibility rules for obtaining a driver's license if a driver has a seizure disorder. The physician should encourage the young patient and his or her family to find out what these eligibility rules are. A call to the department of motor vehicles is a good place to start, or a driver's education instructor at school would be a good person to discuss this with. A frank discussion should be held with the patient and family and the physician should be direct with his or her opinions whether or not the patient should drive. As a general rule, if the seizures can be controlled by medication for whatever period the particular state requires, the patient should be told that he or she can apply for a driver's license.

All states require that a resident be a certain age and have passed a driver's examination before getting a driver's license. The examination usually includes a written exam, a vision exam, and an actual performance showing driving skills. The written exam and driving skills performance usually are not required to renew a license.

States also generally require that a driver not have any disability that would prevent proper operation of a motor vehicle. Epilespy can be such a disability. In the past, many states prevented anyone with epilepsy from getting a driver's license, believing the mere fact that the person had epilepsy would prevent the person from operating a motor vehicle properly. However, most states now allow persons whose seizure disorders are controlled by medication to obtain a driver's license if certain requirements are met. The requirements vary by state and range from requiring that a driver be seizure free for a specified period of time to requiring a person with a seizure disorder to submit a medical report to a medical advisory board to determine his or her ability to drive. In those cases the physician will be asked to submit a written report on his or her evaluation of the patient's ability to operate a motor vehicle. Some states require yearly reports on the driver's condition.

III. EMPLOYMENT

Almost all states have laws that prohibit employment discrimination on the basis of handicap. The definition of what a handicap is varies state by state, but epilepsy can be considered a handicap under these laws. Federal law also protects the rights of certain handicapped individuals, including the right not to be discriminated against in any area of employment. The laws can be complicated and confusing, and if a real problem of discrimination against the young patient because of epilepsy has occurred, the physician should advise the patient to seek legal assistance.

An employment problem usually arises when the young patient is applying for a job and is asked to fill out a written employment application. Very often there will be general questions such as "Do you have a handicap?" or "Have you had any nervous disorders?" This presents the young patient with a difficult choice. If he or she puts "epilepsy" on the application, the person may think that he or she will be turned down for the job. If the person does not put down the epilepsy, is hired, and then has a seizure on the job, he or she may worry about being fired. The natural tendency may be to try to hide the epilepsy or think it is none of the employer's business. The family may encourage the person to hide the condition, as well. The physician should encourage the patient and family to be open and honest. Most employers will respond positively.

In general, the physician can tell the young patient and family that a job applicant does not have to answer questions unrelated to his or her ability to perform the particular job. General questions about past and present medical conditions should not be asked by the employer and do not have to be answered. A practical solution to the problem would be a letter from the physician to a prospective employer providing a brief history of the seizure disorder and an explanation of how the seizures are controlled by medication. Young patients should be encouraged not to hide the fact that they have epilepsy, but to deal with it honestly and openly. Most employers will respond positively, and if they do not and the patient feels that he or she is being discriminated against, assistance can be obtained from the Epilepsy Foundation of American, one of its local affiliates, or a lawyer, to make certain that the employer is acting within the law.

IV. INSURANCE

The rising cost of health insurance is a concern to everyone and may be of particular concern to the family of a young patient who has been diagnosed with a seizure disorder. If a parent has a group health insurance through an employer, or private health insurance, the young patient may be covered under dependent coverage if the policy states that they are covered. Group health insurance plans differ, but such coverage will provide some assistance to the family.

If the family does not have group health insurance, or if the young patient does not have coverage on his or her own, there may be difficulties in obtaining such coverage because of exclusions for preexisting conditions. The family should be encouraged to consult with the employee benefits department of the parent's employer or talk with an insurance agent they have used in the past to see if coverage can be arranged.

Some states have enacted laws that establish shared-risk health insurance plans. Such laws are similar to assigned-risk auto insurance plans, in which people who cannot otherwise obtain insurance coverage can be assigned to a specific insurance program that has been created by state law. Premiums may be higher than regular insurance, but coverage is available. The family should check with the Epilepsy Foundation of America or the state insurance commissioner to find out if their state has such health insurance plans.

The main problem is that the insurance industry has treated people with epilepsy as all the same and has made assumptions that all persons with epilepsy present the same insurance risk. The insurance industry does not always recognize that there a number of forms of seizure disorders and that most can be controlled by medication.

Similar problems exist in obtaining life insurance. Most states make it illegal for life insurance companies to refuse to accept life insurance applications from those who are physically disabled. Most life insurance applications ask if the applicant has epilepsy. The application should be answered truthfully, or the company could deny coverage of a claim if it turned out that death was caused by epilepsy (even if that is a remote possibility) and the applicant said that he or she did not have epilepsy. Premiums for such coverage may be higher, but the increased cost must be based on some statistical evidence that physical disability (in this case epilepsy) results in an increase in risk to the insurance company.

Index

About the Editors

Jerome V. Murphy is Chief, Section of Neurology, Children's Mercy Hospital, Kansas City, Missouri, Professor, University of Missouri, School of Medicine at Kansas City, and Clinical Professor, Departments of Neurology and Pediatrics, University of Kansas, School of Medicine, Kansas City. The author or coauthor of over 100 professional papers and presentations, he is a member of the Child Neurology Society, the Society for Pediatric Research, the American Academy of Neurology, and the American Epilepsy Society, among other organizations. Dr. Murphy received the M.D. degree (1962) from Johns Hopkins University, Baltimore, Maryland.

Fereydoun Dehkharghani is Director, Clinical Neurophysiology Laboratory, Children's Mercy Hospital, Kansas City, Missouri, and Associate Professor of Pediatrics, University of Missouri, School of Medicine at Kansas City. A member of the Child Neurology Society and the American Academy of Neurology, Dr. Dehkharghani is the author of several professional papers on neonatal neurology. He received the M.D. degree (1965) from Meshad University, Iran.